NECROPOLIS

NECROPOLIS

Disease, Power,
and Capitalism in the
Cotton Kingdom

KATHRYN OLIVARIUS

The Belknap Press of
Harvard University Press
Cambridge, Massachusetts
London, England
2022

Library of Congress Cataloging-in-Publication Data

Names: Olivarius, Kathryn Meyer McAllister, 1989– author.
Title: Necropolis : disease, power, and capitalism in the Cotton Kingdom /
Kathryn Olivarius.
Description: Cambridge, Massachusetts : The Belknap Press
of Harvard University Press, 2022. | Includes index.
Identifiers: LCCN 2021044327 | ISBN 9780674241053 (cloth)
Subjects: LCSH: Race discrimination—Louisiana—New Orleans—History—
19th century. | Yellow fever—Louisiana—New Orleans—History—19th century. |
Immunity—Social aspects—History—19th century. | Slaves—Louisiana—
New Orleans—History—19th century. | Social stratification—Louisiana—
New Orleans—History—19th century. | New Orleans (La.)—
Race relations—History—19th century.
Classification: LCC E185.93.L6 O45 2022 | DDC 305.8009763/3—dc23/eng/20211018
LC record available at https://lccn.loc.gov/2021044327

To my family and especially to Joe

Contents

Author's Note

I started writing *Necropolis* almost a decade before Covid-19 arrived in the United States in 2020. If there are aspects to this story that feel contemporary, it is because they are. Two centuries ago, humans took advantage of epidemics in ways that caused misery, enriched the few, and increased inequality. Today, we have sadly seen many similar patterns unfold. I wish this story and its themes felt more like anachronism.

If the outcome of a person's experience with yellow fever is known, I note it in the text. For example, Benjamin Henry Latrobe (d. YF 1820) means Latrobe died from yellow fever in 1820; J. D. B. De Bow (a. YF 1847) means De Bow fell sick with yellow fever in 1847 but survived and became "acclimated."

NECROPOLIS

INTRODUCTION

A Rising Necropolis

One January morning in 1825, a white, seventeen-year-old boy from Newton, New Jersey, woke up with a case of "Mississippi fever"—an insatiable urge to head west and south.[1] Indifferent to warnings about the South's sultry climate and enraptured by promises of exorbitant slave- and plantation-based wealth, he packed up his belongings, hugged his mother goodbye, and made his way to New Orleans. But every other boy seemed to have the same idea. Hundreds of them, fresh off boats from Dundee or Boston, jostled for work on the levee, papering the city's many cotton offices with inquiries. Promising to start right away and work year-round, this stranger was snapped up by Wadsworth & Vandergriff, one of Louisiana's premier dry goods firms, at a wage of $1.50 a day. He was good at clerking, able to differentiate between "prime" and "fair to middling" cotton by the feel of the fiber. He grew wise to the tricks of upcountry planters and could haggle up prices with the Barings Bank agents sending shiploads of goods to Europe. One balmy night in May, the stranger walked back to his boardinghouse ($3.80 per week) near Jackson Square, admiring the Creole women, listening to the raucous cheers of men playing *vingt-et-un,* and gazing up at the spire of St. Louis Cathedral at twilight. The reputation of New Orleans back up North—as a place where people lived fast and died young—must have been exaggerated, he thought. The stranger sat on the levee and watched flatboats descend the Mississippi River. He was sure his future was bright—and that of New Orleans too.[2]

The stranger could not pinpoint precisely when things began to change. He noticed the first pang of unease in late June, when every dwelling seemed to have a *chambre garnie* or "to let" placard in the window. He noticed it again on July 1, when all the city's normally deafening church bells went quiet in unison. It was disquieting that everyone in his congregation renewed their baptismal vows and embraced at the end of the service as if for the last time. Smaller things bothered him, too: his neighbor's preoccupation with estates and wills; the sudden profusion of black armbands; ragged children begging door-to-door; coffin-toting slaves. One morning, three of his fellow lodgers decided to leave town. They asked the stranger to safeguard their possessions, promising they would be back soon. They clasped his hand and hurried off to the docks, fighting their way through the scrum onto the first departing boat. That night the remaining tenants made fun of the "truants" for their cowardice. The stranger agreed that their departure seemed hasty, even an overreaction. But he quietly wondered what they knew that he did not. And by late July it was like a candle had been extinguished: New Orleans, the great emporium of western commerce, had become a ghost town.[3]

Suddenly the stranger's whole life was eclipsed by yellow fever, a "demon king" that descended upon the city every second or third summer and sparked terror across the tropical Atlantic. At Maspero's, the coffee shop, businessmen discussed the latest death tolls.[4] The stranger caught terrifying snippets—"Three new cases last night"—"It was real yellow fever now, no mistake"—"A very complicated form"—"Quite an aggravated type"—"Worse than '17"—"I'm safe—I've had it." The stranger joined in the gossip. Creoles and old-timers who had been "acclimated" to the virus years before told the boy to be careful, as yellow fever proved fatal to many. In fact, they conceded with eyes downcast, about half of all people who got the fever died. At first the stranger welcomed their counsel, noting down their precise medicinal regimens. But soon he grew weary, even overwhelmed, by the relentless onslaught of contradictory advice on how best to weather the epidemic. Eat only fruit or only meat? Take exercise or stay indoors? Use a French doctor or a Black nurse? It was just too much, too hard to process, too numbing. Besides, in a place where everyone was a self-styled yellow fever expert, it seemed increasingly clear that no one *really* was.[5]

The stranger lay awake at night listening to distant cannon fire, rockets discharged by the city guard to dispel the disease-causing miasmas emanating from the nearby swamps. Every hour or so, he leaped out of bed and peered into the mirror, searching for any sign of yellowing skin or bloodshot eyes. Nothing, yet. He sprinkled some chlorate of lime on the floor before returning to bed, pulling the mosquito netting tight around his mattress. In the morning he scurried to work through deserted streets. Most of the stores he passed were empty or staffed by just a clerk or two, the factors and merchants having traveled north or to their country plantations for the season. At the office he picked up a newspaper—quite thin these days—but put it down before reaching the obituaries. He tried to do some work but was distracted. He took up pen and paper to write a letter home but found he had no energy, having "worked his spirits down to zero." All he could manage were a few limp lines to a friend up north: "I am well and Harty [sic] as I ever was in my life."[6]

The stranger mentioned to his boss, a New Yorker with ten years' tenure in Louisiana, that he was considering leaving town, just for a few weeks. Or maybe he would ride out to Lake Pontchartrain for the day? Some fresh air would be good, he said. A chance to clear his head. His boss was sympathetic, recalling his own brush with yellow fever back in 1817, the last big one. He told the stranger to follow his conscience; he should go if he needed to. But he also reminded the stranger that his job was not guaranteed. It was nothing personal. But there were plenty of fully acclimated, brave, bilingual men who would gladly fill his shoes. The stranger, feeling both disposable and defiant, decided to stay put.[7]

A few days into August, the stranger felt anxious and hot around the collar. He told his co-clerk that he just needed a minute to lie down, that the spell would pass. But soon he was gripped by an intense headache, muscle pain, nausea, and chills. He could not see straight, so he lay down on the floor. It was like a "civil war" was raging in his stomach. Was this it? Should he have left town? Had keeping his job been worth risking his life? With his skull now feeling as if "filled with molten lead," the stranger conceded it was too late for regrets. And anyway, this was a disease that other sorts of people died of. He was young and healthy. He was determined to survive and become an "acclimated citizen."[8]

The concerned coworker carried the ailing stranger back to his boarding-house and called for a doctor, rooting around in the stranger's belongings for the pouch of money he had squirreled away with $50 (about a month's wages) inside for just such a medical emergency. By the afternoon, the patient was delirious and boiling hot. A Black nurse was called for—at $3 a day—to deliver blankets one moment, ice the next. Then the doctor arrived and, after receiving his initial payment of $10, found the patient "restless—talkative—ill-natured."[9] The innkeeper, suspicious of the commotion, came to the door and was horrified to see a man so obviously sick in her house. She threatened to evict the stranger before he infected others. The doctor dismissed her concerns, insisting that yellow fever was not contagious. But he sent the coworker off to inquire at Davidson's Infirmary, a private establishment with a good yellow fever record. A fruitless exercise as their wards were already full, as were the wards of the Circus Street Infirmary, Touro Infirmary, and St. Philips Street Hospital. It was no matter, as the stranger probably could not afford them anyway. The doctor implored the innkeeper to let the stranger stay, warning that without her kindness he would end up in the Charity Hospital, an institution so poorly funded and understaffed that it was common to "see the living babe sucking death from the yellow breast of its dead mother."[10] The innkeeper relented, pocketing a $3 bribe on her way out.

It was evening now and the stranger was not improving. The doctor directed the nurse to restrain the patient as he applied mustard powder to his abdomen, blistered his hands and feet with a red-hot iron, and poured ice water over his head. Next the stranger was force-fed purgatives. His fever was so high at this point—104°F—that the doctor decided to bleed him. One pint, then two, then three. The stranger lost consciousness. When he revived, the doctor bled him again. The nurse protested. This approach was reckless, she insisted. The doctor loudly chastised her, making sure those loitering outside the door heard him. But he quietly changed course, opting now for leeches. Before leaving for the night, the doctor instructed the nurse to swaddle the stranger in thick woolen blankets. Around midnight the boy was suddenly agitated and wide awake. He struggled to push off his heavy covers, to get up from his sweat-soaked mattress and run into the street. This spurt of energy was taken as a promising sign by his coworker. Perhaps he had turned a corner? No, replied the nurse, who had noticed the stranger's yellowing eyes and skin. This was jaundice, a sign of organ failure.[11]

By morning the stranger was exhausted. He knew he was probably dying. But thinking of his mother far away, he struggled through the "Pain & nervousness" to keep his eyes open. The stranger's boss arrived with the doctor around 10 a.m. and found the boy awake but distressed. The boss apologized that business had prevented him from coming sooner. The stranger grabbed his hand and whispered "that he was sick and very poor." He did not want to end up in Potter's Field, the swamp repository for New Orleans indigents where bodies tended to "reappear," floating up from water-logged graves. Please, would the boss ensure that he received a proper Protestant burial in an aboveground tomb?[12] "Don't give up hope yet, boy!" the boss insisted. He had seen many survive more serious cases than this—"it is the fear, not the fever, that kills," he said. The stranger laughed nervously at this. Then he began to cry. It was blood, not tears, oozing from his eyes, leaking from his ears and nose, even from his gums. Those in the room begged the doctor to intervene. But the doctor shook his head, indicating that further intervention was pointless. The only hope now was prayer.

At this point the stranger's tale would progress in one of two predictable ways. One version sees the stranger improve. The sleep-deprived nurse tends to him during his groggy convalescence, feeding him beef tea and lemonade. The burns on his palms scab over and a rosy hue returns to his cheeks. He can eventually take a few steps unaided. Within a week, the doctor says he is out of danger, shakes his hand, and declares him "acclimated," safe from all future attacks of yellow fever. Soon the doctor will send his itemized bill.

In the other version, the stranger's condition continues to deteriorate. He starts to regurgitate black vomit: thick, congealed blood, the consistency and color of coffee grounds. It covers his body and bed, staining the mattress. The stranger curses, hiccups, and belches. He shrieks, convulses, and groans. Then he goes quiet, lapsing into a coma, his once-muscular frame reduced to an unearthly skeleton. He dies with eyes bulging and his mouth frozen wide as if he is silently screaming. The "sad, sullen, and perturbed" corpse, banana-yellow and frozen by rigor mortis, remains in the room until a coffin ($15), hearse ($6), and cemetery plot ($70–$100) can be procured. The stranger's few personal effects—perhaps some clothing or a silver watch—are pawned to cover the $60 he still owes to the doctor and nurse. The boss, in keeping with local custom, ponies up for the funeral and burial. It would not be a lavish affair; the boy had few mourners anyway.[13]

The stranger's body is pushed into its vault in Girod Cemetery by two enslaved men, workers fortified by whiskey and cigars to dull the endless horror of their task. An old woman passing by kisses the stranger's coffin, a proxy for the blessings of his mother far away. She sings some words from the book of Luke—*weep not for the dead but for the living*—as she walks to the next graveside. Later the boss would write to the stranger's mother in New Jersey: "While the tears Tremble down my cheeks . . . it Becomes my painfull duty with much regret to Announce to you the death of your Son, who Departed this Life . . . of the Yellow Fever."[14] He will insist on the stranger's bravery and serenity in the face of death and will ask her to reimburse him for the funeral. Enclosing a lock of the stranger's hair with his account, the boss will hand the envelope to his new clerk to mail, this one a fresh teenager from Dublin.[15]

Every city had its archetypes. Old New York had its Five-Points goons, its slick Bowery Boys, its Wall Street tycoons. Nineteenth-century Boston had its hucksters, its brahmins, its brawling Irishmen. And New Orleans had princes of cotton, Creole capitalists, quadroons, and rowdy boatmen. Many of the Crescent City's characters, however, were marked and made by yellow fever. Everyone knew the "Acclimated Man" by sight. He was the confident fellow—a yellow fever survivor—who strutted about town during epidemics with a "tremendously bold swagger," convinced of his own invincibility. They also knew the "Anti-Panic Man," who suppressed information about yellow fever to keep attracting men of capital, talent, or wealth to the Gulf Coast, luring some to their deaths. Most pitied and familiar of all the New Orleans archetypes was the "Unacclimated Stranger," a foreigner whose fear of yellow fever was eclipsed by the seductive dream of slave-based Southern riches.[16] His journey down the Mississippi—the "father of rivers"— often carried him to his grave in the "Necropolis" of the United States.[17]

Whenever the conversation at dinner dulled, or when the counting house quieted at night, or when enslaved men piled sugarcane onto carts under the baking Louisiana sun, or when mothers wanted their children to behave, this story—of the unacclimated stranger and his terrible death—was sure to be recited. The best raconteurs practiced their delivery, adding dramatic tension through each worsening symptom: pausing deliberately to give listeners hope, inventing a cast of supporting characters—a jilted lover or a long-lost friend—to heighten the drama. In some versions the stranger might have a beautiful, pregnant wife, or he might undergo a deathbed conversion. And though the stranger of city lore was normally rendered as white, free, and male—the nexus of identities most associated with potential and power in antebellum New Orleans—there were many real-life variations on the theme. There was Solomon Northup, a Black violinist kidnapped from upstate New York to Louisiana, and later the author of *Twelve Years a Slave,* who was forced to pick cotton through his spiking fever. When he collapsed, not even a whip could rouse him. There was Ellen McDonald,

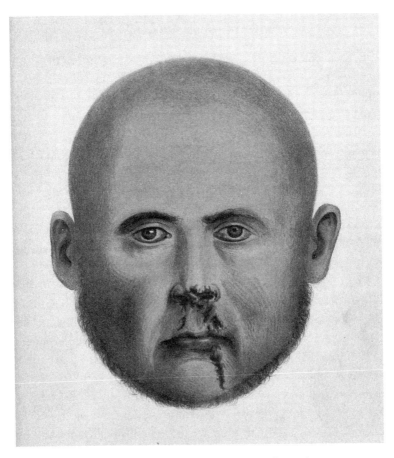

"Features, complexion, and hæmorrhagic appearance of a Madeira immigrant in advanced stage of yellow fever," Daniel Blair, *Some Account of the Last Yellow Fever Epidemic of British Guiana* (London, 1850), plate IV.

an Irishwoman who, in a fit of fever-induced delirium, slit her own throat and died. There was "Black Mary," an enslaved woman who sickened with yellow fever in 1853, the illness taxing her body to such an extent that she was forced into premature labor. And there was Maria, a poor Spanish woman, who died in a small, dark room only a few hours after her husband Pedro died, as "a scarlet foam oozed slowly from her mouth."[18] Some yellow fever sufferers got better. But in thousands of versions of this tale—the stories of those unlucky people who died of yellow fever in the nineteenth-century Deep South—the story crescendoed to the same tragic climax: black vomit and death.

Immunocapitalism

This book is not a history of yellow fever, nor is it a history of Southern public health.[19] It is the story of why so many unacclimated strangers died in nineteenth-century New Orleans and how their collective deaths exacerbated inequality in an already violent and unequal slave society. Past epidemics and pandemics, from the Plague of Justinian to the Black Death to the Spanish Flu of 1918, have sometimes been described as "great levelers": moments of vast suffering and mass death that flattened social and economic asymmetries, increased the bargaining power of surviving workers, renewed people's sense of common humanity, and reaffirmed their subservience to an omnipotent God.[20] Fast-killing fevers could potentially shape empires and "equalize" societies, too. J. R. McNeill has shown that "lowly mosquitoes and mindless viruses" determined the outcomes of multiple imperial struggles in the eighteenth-century Atlantic. And Vincent Brown has argued that once conquered, highly unequal eighteenth-century Caribbean slave societies could be leveled by mass mortality; the unrelenting attrition of fevers—malarial, bilious, and yellow—finally undermined the privileges accorded to whiteness, equalizing all people in the face of death.[21]

Graveyard equality might have been a consolation to some. But for those living in antebellum New Orleans—the hub of America's flourishing slave, cotton, and sugar kingdoms and the nation's deadliest city *by far*—the constant possibility of painful death made for more inequality, not less. Here, disease did not attack and destroy existing class and racial structures; it was part of their very foundation. As many historians have shown, New Orleans was an outlier among American cities, characterized by its Caribbean-esque tripartite social structure of whites, *gens de couleur libres,* and Black slaves. But as yellow fever epidemics increased in frequency and ferocity in the six decades before the Civil War, the city also became stratified between those whites who possessed immunity to the disease (the "acclimated"), those who remained vulnerable to the virus (the "unacclimated"), and those (Black slaves and most free people of color) whose immunity status would only socially and economically benefit others.

These labels *mattered.* They mattered because which side of the immunity divide a person landed on measurably impacted their lives and prospects. Here, a white person was virtually *required* to survive yellow fever, to enter the elite. And once acclimated, the city's Creole and American merchants, planters, and enslavers embraced epidemic yellow fever as a blessing, not a curse, finding that it could "solve" any number of political, financial, and social problems that would have otherwise burdened the kind of hegemony and profits they sought. Betraying their hardened attitudes to human life—evidenced in their indifference to the suffering of enslaved people—local elites embraced yellow fever risk, mobilized disease for discriminatory ends, and used their own alleged immunity as proof that they deserved success, consolidating their power atop the cotton market, the most lucrative sector of antebellum America's export economy. Taking advantage of the diseased reality around them, New Orleans elites differed from leaders of other major American port cities in spearheading policies that systematically heightened inequality, enriched themselves, enhanced white supremacy and wealth, undercut the majority, and etched epidemiological discrimination into law.

White elites claimed that the apparent logic of yellow fever on the lower Mississippi seemed to demand, and therefore to justify, the existence of highly asymmetrical social and labor relationships. They even claimed that marginal groups—the poor, *gens de couleur libres,* the enslaved, and recent immigrants—were biologically different from them and inferior. Elites capitalized on mortal risk and equated immunity (obtained only by surviving yellow fever) with creditworthiness, reliability, and political potency, and so linked each person's potential worth to a sometimes imprecisely understood or wrongly claimed acclimation status. Instead of trying to curb the disease, powerful and immune people in the Cotton Kingdom prospered by monetizing the ensuing chaos and personal horror that disease caused.[22]

In this system of class rule, which I call *immunocapitalism,* disease was endowed with spiritual purpose.[23] It provided ideological legitimation for vast inequality. Elites insisted that newcomers had to brave yellow fever alone. Unacclimated "strangers" were considered outsiders—undeserving, untested, effeminate, and illegitimate. They could not get certain jobs, live in certain neighborhoods, vote, or socialize with the acclimated. Some elites even argued that yellow fever was a social panacea because it efficiently weeded out lesser men. One physician writing under the pen name Cenci described the commonly held nativist view: *"A good, scorching yellow fever is the best thing in the world for New Orleans! That is a sort of crucible, a fiery furnace, separating the pure metal from its alloy!"*[24] If yellow fever was incurable, and acclimation was the difference between stigma and privilege, it was no wonder that people actively sought sickness as a pathway to prosperity, agreeing with the words of Dr. Edward Hall Barton, president of

New Orleans's 1841 board of health: "The VALUE OF ACCLIMATION IS WORTH THE RISK!"[25]

White elites' claim that Black people had "perfect" and natural immunity to yellow fever became the backbone of an increasingly elaborate—if strained—justification for widespread and permanent racial slavery. Only inherently immune Black people, the logic went, could safely cultivate epidemiologically fraught spaces immediately around New Orleans, for white people lacked the constitution to work in a subtropical climate, collapsing under the "torrid" sun and unable to breathe in the "deleterious gases" lingering in the atmosphere.[26] Black slavery, proslavery theorists said, was therefore classified as positively natural, even *humanitarian,* for it protected the health of whites, insulating them from labor and spaces that would kill them. In this view, slavery was not only essential for personal and national prosperity but positively beneficial and divinely ordained. White elites thus used yellow fever to justify the expendability of certain white laboring lives and the exploitation of enslaved Black ones, reinscribing an already obvious message: in New Orleans, certain people were decidedly less equal than others.[27]

Yellow fever influenced the pace and schedule of the cotton and slave markets based in New Orleans. It was a major professional consideration for clerks and bookkeepers and an unfortunate reality for business owners and partners. The virus embedded itself into all interpersonal relationships and formed a key aspect of a person's identity, prescribing many of their choices and actions.[28] Yellow fever also mediated the relationship between state and citizen, setting the conditions for citizenship itself and delineating the size and responsibilities of government. It produced politicians who were apathetic about the welfare of their poor, free Black, and recently immigrated constituents, and who left those people to beg for help from private charities and the Roman Catholic Church.

That many people died in pursuit of immunity did not matter. There were always shiploads of people arriving to replace the dead, some willing and enthusiastic, others desperate or enslaved. Elites in New Orleans insisted that disease, like hurricanes or floods, was a problem with no solution. Profoundly uninterested in public health, politicians maintained that most tax revenue spent on quarantines, hospitals, garbage removal, and sanitation was wasted. Never mind that quarantine had often worked to suppress yellow fever in New York or Genoa or Charleston, or that Philadelphia suffered less serious outbreaks of yellow fever after it constructed a waterworks following the epidemic of 1793. As cities and municipalities across the Atlantic world exerted increasing influence over their public's health, New Orleans doubled down on inaction, maintaining with righteous fatalism that the state bore no responsibility for the health of its inhabitants. Instead, it was the individual's personal duty to get acclimated. New Orleans's approach had terrible knock-on effects for the health of cities upriver. But deaths in Natchez or Vicksburg did not move those who would have been able to change New Orleans. The commercial-civic elites were perversely incentivized to do nothing. The region's sclerotic health system, undergirded by ideologies of disease denialism and tax aversion, well suited a lopsided slave society that at its core ignored the human cost of amassing wealth.[29]

Yellow fever also played a key role in shaping the South's aggrieved sectional identity in the years leading up to the Civil War. Defenses of slavery and defenses of the diseased status quo began to align around each other and cross-fertilize, culminating in a vision of sectional distinctiveness and grievance that underpinned secession. Yellow fever was thus not background noise to the more resonant stories of the nineteenth century—westward expansion, the explosion of racial slavery, commodities, and civil war—but a crucial plot point in each.

The question of health—who has it and who does not and why—always contains political elements. But this kind of health—the immunity people acquired to a disease that killed half of all it infected—was mobilized by elites to further divide and exploit the population. Yellow fever was, simply, no great leveler in antebellum New Orleans. Quite the opposite. Within this system of immunocapitalism, it became economically, socially, and politically profitable for a set of powerful, white, opportunistic actors to operate in such a profoundly unhealthy space.

"A Place of Immense Business"

On December 20, 1803, France ceded official control of Louisiana to the United States. Overnight the territory of the United States doubled, and New Orleans became the nation's ninth-largest city and an immensely valuable strategic possession. Since the early eighteenth century, control over New Orleans had been synonymous with control of the Mississippi River, the world's fourth-largest river system, whose fertile valley drains an area stretching 1,250 miles across North America's heartland, from the Rockies to Appalachia and from the Great Lakes to the Gulf of Mexico. During the eighteenth century, every empire in the Atlantic world coveted the bounty pouring out of the Mississippi Valley—pelts, grain, timber, and food. Louisiana fed and provisioned the Caribbean, enabling those tropical islands to focus on producing lucrative commodities like sugar and coffee. Given existing trade routes, it made sense for a goods depot to be located somewhere close to the Gulf of Mexico, low down on the Mississippi River. But there were few good physical locations for such a place. The site chosen in 1718 for *La Nouvelle-Orléans* was the best of a bad lot. It sat on a large, swampy river bend about thirty leagues from the Gulf of Mexico. And though the fort immediately faced a fifteen-foot levee—the natural dirt and silt barrier at the river's edge—most of the town sat at a precarious one foot above sea level.[30]

New Orleans's main ecological limitation—overwhelming amounts of water from the sea, river, sky, and ground—was obvious, prompting more than one disgruntled traveler to suggest it was the most "disagreeable place on the face of the whole globe," more bilgewater than backwater.[31] As Frenchmen fought bloody battles against the Natchez and Choctaw Indians, dispossessing them of swampland they hoped to drain and turn into profitable plantations, they also battled Louisiana's stifling heat and humidity. Spaniards, who took control of the city in 1763 as part of the settlement of the French and Indian War, grumbled that hurricanes periodically destroyed large swaths of town as well as surrounding plantations. Colonists hated that tobacco rotted in the ground before it matured. They hated the mosquitoes, too. They complained that their floorboards rotted out every few years and that a pair of leather boots left outside would be covered in mildew by morning. The soil was so soft and waterlogged, most planters did not bother to shoe their horses. Visitors routinely noted that even when the river was held back by levees, water seeped through and made the roads so muddy that they became impassable after just a light shower. Rainwater flowed *away* from the river and collected in stagnant, garbage-laden pools. People traversed the *Vieux Carré* on wooden risers, hoping not to fall into the morass. When levees broke, the deluge washed out sewage ditches, creating a smell so fetid people could not breathe. Officials in Paris and Madrid bemoaned that New Orleans was so filthy that no sane person would go there. The colony's last Spanish governor warned in 1795 that if some drainage was not undertaken in New Orleans, it would be "necessary to abandon the town in less than three or four years."[32]

By the nineteenth century, however, imperial powers were willing to put up with almost any environmental risk at New Orleans for two reasons: cotton and sugar, sources of immense wealth. Frustrated by the continued weakness of tobacco crops and responding to the market gap left by Saint-Domingue's revolution—in which the world's most profitable sugar colony exploded in a fierce and sustained slave revolt—Creole planter Étienne de Boré and his enslaved striker (the production overseer) successfully granulated sugar for the first time in late 1795, on his plantation just outside the city. De Boré's success set off a chain reaction: by 1797, fifty sugar mills had been built along the lower Mississippi, collectively churning out about half a million pounds of "white gold" each year. By 1802 Louisiana boasted seventy-five sugar plantations, producing more than six million pounds of sugar per year. Then came cotton. In 1795 Eli Whitney's recently patented cotton gin appeared in the Natchez region of Mississippi, about eighty miles upriver from New Orleans. The gin revolutionized the process of cotton cultivation, increasing productivity by a factor of fifty, making cotton, a once marginal regional crop, a viable commodity for even the cash-short planter.[33]

These two crops—aided by new technologies, rich alluvial soil, and the labor of enslaved Africans—promised transformative wealth for white American and Creole individuals and glory for nations with footholds in the Mississippi Valley. Initial dispatches from the southernmost reaches of Louisiana, written on the brink of this commodity revolution, brimmed with optimism. W. C. C. Claiborne, the first American governor of Orleans Territory, pronounced Louisiana a "desirable country" where the value of the 1801 cotton crop was worth "upwards of eight hundred thousand dollars." At 22 percent of all Louisiana exports, New Orleans cotton exports were still small by comparison to Charleston, South Carolina, which exported some twenty million pounds of cotton in 1801. But Claiborne projected that, with markets so "immediate and lucrative," cotton production would soar and make New Orleans the American *El Dorado.* Soon Claiborne marveled to President Thomas Jefferson that "the facility with which the sugar Planters amass wealth is almost incredible." It was not "uncommon," said Claiborne, for a white man with "20 working hands" to make upward of $10,000 a year, though he knew of "several planters whose field Negroes do not exceed forty" who made more than $20,000.[34] On the eve of the Louisiana Purchase, this vision of New Orleans as a "place of immense business" had taken hold across the Atlantic world, capturing the imaginations of profit-seekers who spoke of "fortunes acquired there as if by magic," just as earlier generations of dreamers had spoken about the goldfields of Mexico. One traveler to New Orleans prophesied early in the nineteenth century that "in the course of fifty years" New Orleans "will probably be, in a mercantile point of view, second to none in the world."[35]

French prefect Pierre Clément de Laussat, the man responsible for orchestrating the transfer of Louisiana to the United States, observed that thousands of people from points north and east were "swarming" into Louisiana like the "holy tribes invaded the land of Canaan."[36] People concentrated most densely in and immediately around New Orleans, by this point a polyglot city where trilingual free people of color, Indigenous fur traders, and flatboat men with a Kentucky twang could be heard haggling over prices on the levee. Increasingly, immigrants were not just Americans; they were Black and white French-speaking refugees escaping revolutionary Saint-Domingue (9,000 refugees from the colony landed in 1809) and immigrants from Bremen, Sligo, and Bordeaux escaping famine and political turbulence in Europe. By 1840 the city's population had swelled to 102,000 and on the eve of the Civil War to more than 168,000, including about 15,000 enslaved people and 10,000 *gens de couleur libres*—the largest concentration of free Black people in the Deep South. In all, more than 550,000 whites freely immigrated to the United States through New Orleans between 1803 and 1860, making it the country's second most popular port of entry after New York City.[37] Many of these people simply passed through on their journeys to Texas or California, but enough stayed to provide a consistent immigration-fueled white working class. New Orleans also became the nation's largest slave market during the antebellum period. Every inch of the city—from the slave marts of Esplanade, to the grand lobby of the St. Charles Hotel, to the street corners of Marigny—was a potential site of human sale. Tens of thousands of people, forced to build Thomas Jefferson's "empire for liberty," were thus sold each year in the city before they were moved across the region to cultivate commodities, day in and day out.[38]

Sugar had fueled the early growth of American New Orleans, but by the 1820s slave-grown cotton had eclipsed everything and sucked everyone into its orbit. And by the mid-1830s, New Orleans had become the leading export city of the United States, processing hundreds of thousands of bales of cotton from the growing Cotton Kingdom, which now stretched across upcountry Alabama and Mississippi, the blackland prairie of Arkansas, and rich lands of east Texas. Cotton—$25 million worth—passed through New

Orleans in 1841; fifteen years later, cotton exports exceeded $92 million. On the eve of the Civil War, approximately 3,500 vessels were steaming and sailing in and out of New Orleans each year, carrying an annual cargo worth $220 million. Soon it seemed as if the entire region was involved in a permanently expanding cycle of exploitation and profit. As traveler Joseph Holt Ingraham aptly described it, "To sell cotton in order to buy negroes— to make more cotton to buy more negroes, 'ad infinitum,' is the aim and direct tendency of all the operations of the thorough-going cotton planter; his whole soul is wrapped up in the pursuit."[39]

The market that developed in and around New Orleans—extractive, export-driven, violent, and dependent on slave labor—made some whites and a small handful of *gens de couleur libres* incredibly wealthy. A planter could make "eighty or a hundred thousand dollars per year" just from slave-grown cotton. Such an income allowed Louisiana's planters to "live in magnificent style" and winter in town "in gayety and fashion." Certainly, many whites were highly leveraged and intimately comfortable with risk. "Not one in fifteen, I am assured, is free of debt," wrote British visitor James Stirling in 1857. Ignoring the vast suffering of enslaved Black people (as well as the extreme poverty of starving Irish immigrants), Lillian Foster, a rich New Yorker who visited the city in the 1840s and 1850s, insisted there was no other place in the United States where a person could "kill time more agreeably" than New Orleans.[40]

King Cotton and Yellow Jack

That was unless yellow fever did not kill them first. Most New Orleanians quickly learned that the epithets given to their city abroad—the "burial place of America," its "widow-making capital," the "theatre of Pestilence," a "great charnel house," and the "head-quarters of Death"—were not abstractions. From 1796 onward, cases of yellow fever appeared every summer. Every second or third summer, the mosquito-borne virus became epidemic, killing about 8 percent of the city's burgeoning population and leaving countless more widowed, orphaned, and bereaved. Deaths didn't stop until November, following the first mosquito-killing frosts. During particularly bad fever seasons, as many as 20 or even 30 percent of "immunologically naïve" people—mostly Irish and German "strangers"—could die. In 1853, the year of the worst epidemic in the city, about 12,000 people perished over the course of three months, constituting around one-tenth of the city's

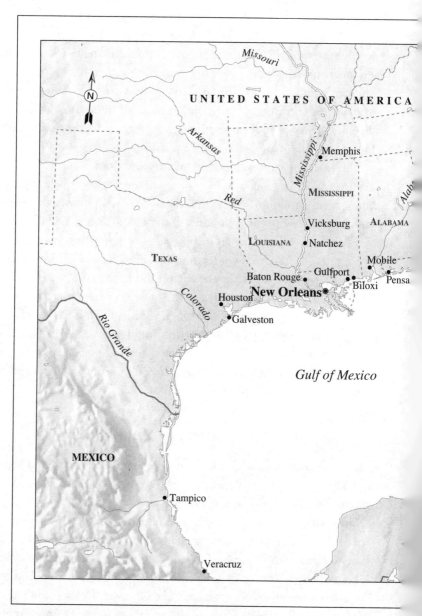

The "Yellow Fever South," ca. 1850.

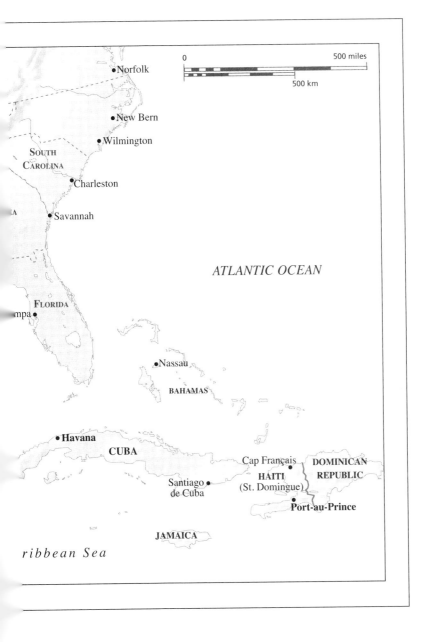

0   500 miles

500 km

•Norfolk

•New Bern

•Wilmington

SOUTH
CAROLINA

•Charleston

•Savannah

ATLANTIC OCEAN

FLORIDA

mpa•

•Nassau

BAHAMAS

•Havana

CUBA

Cap Français

DOMINICAN
REPUBLIC

HAITI
(St. Domingue)

Santiago •
de Cuba

•Port-au-Prince

JAMAICA

ribbean Sea

population and one-fifth of the Irish-born inhabitants. In mortality terms, the 1853 epidemic remains one of the worst natural disasters in American history.[41]

By relocating to what we might call the "Yellow Fever South"—a 4,000-square-mile patch on the lower Mississippi River that by the 1840s life insurers had carved out as the riskiest region in the nation—migrants effectively cut their life expectancy by twenty years.[42] The Yellow Fever South was centered in New Orleans, a city with regular Caribbean communication, and extended to the places over which New Orleans exerted considerable economic and therefore *epidemiological* influence. This immediately encompassed the subtropical area within ten miles of the Mississippi River, below the 32nd north parallel—the densest sugar-growing region in the United States. But it also included all urban areas proximate to New Orleans on the Mississippi River and the Gulf: Natchez, Vicksburg, Baton Rouge, Mobile, and Biloxi, the way stations of the larger Cotton Kingdom. These cities were so dependent on New Orleans and carried on such continuous trade with it that if an epidemic erupted in the Crescent City, it was only a matter of time until urban centers across a much larger region were scourged, and their hinterlands too, blurring the urban / rural divide. Surrounded by this terrifying, omnipresent, and seemingly unstoppable virus, people mordantly spoke of being subject to two tyrants: King Cotton and Yellow Jack.[43]

Yellow fever was petrifying because it was so mysterious. Even the most experienced doctors were flummoxed by this virus, calling it the "queerest disease in the world," like a "character actor on the stage, who comes out in different costumes and with different gestures and voices, but is the same man under it all."[44] There was no cure, no inoculation, no conclusive evidence of disease transmission, no consensus as to whether it was "miasmatic" or "contagious," and no satisfactory explanation for why it killed some and spared others. Physicians did not even agree as to whether yellow fever was a discrete illness; many considered it the dire endpoint on a fever spectrum. Symptomatically akin to malaria, yellow fever was also incredibly easy to misdiagnose. It was only at the very end of the nineteenth century that yellow fever's vector, the female *Aedes aegypti* mosquito, was discovered by Cuban researchers, and only in the 1930s was an effective vaccine developed.[45]

Whatever its presentation, yellow fever killed so horribly that "courageous, enduring women" and "strong fathers and husbands . . . who would face the grape-shot battery in battle . . . fled dismayed" from its approach. Victims experienced a sudden onset of intense headaches, muscle pains, jaundice, nausea, and chills. Within days, delirium set in. Victims seeped blood through their external orifices, wept tears of blood, and vomited up coagulated blood. As the liver and other organs shut down, the patient turned yellow, lapsed into a coma, then died. This process was so painful that even the pious screamed profanities as the end neared.[46] Remembering his time in New Orleans, Unitarian minister Theodore Clapp wrote that there was no death "more shocking and repulsive to the beholder . . . Scarcely a night passes now, in which my dreams are not haunted . . . by the distorted faces, the shrieks, the convulsions, the groans, the struggles, and the horrors which I witnessed thirty-five years ago."[47]

A Rigged Lottery

Today we know a great deal about how yellow fever kills. It does so by weaponizing our own immune systems against us. Yellow fever is an acute viral infection transmitted to humans through the bite of a female aedine mosquito, most commonly of the species *Aedes aegypti.* When the infected mosquito bites, it regurgitates a tiny amount of the virus into our bloodstream. The virus then circulates around the body and replicates in the dendritic cells of the skin, nose, lungs, stomach, and intestines. When the virus enters the lymph nodes and liver, it has effectively breached the castle; it infects hepatocytes—the cells responsible for protein and cholesterol synthesis and storage, detoxification, and the secretion of bile. As hepatocytes degrade, their nuclei fragment and the cells shrink. To combat the damage, the body's normal response is to release cytokines, pro-inflammatory molecules that orchestrate the immune response by mobilizing white blood cells and directing them to the site of infection. This reaction combats the infection effectively for some, who will get better. But sometimes an excessive release of these pro-inflammatory molecules—a "cytokine storm"—causes our immune systems to go into overdrive and attack the body's own tissues rather than the virus. This is the toxic phase of the illness, and it is serious. Hyper-inflammation can cause multisystem organ failure, shock, and death. Sometimes this whole microscopic pageant unfolds over many weeks; other times, in just a few days.

No concept in this description—from the mosquito vector to the cytokine storm—was understood two centuries ago. But people in the past did understand that a person could not be reinfected with yellow fever; unlike cholera or plague, surviving yellow fever conferred lifetime immunity. Deep Southerners did not understand much about immunity—euphemizing it as "acclimation," "creolization," or "seasoning." But they did crudely grasp that surviving the disease was the key to long-term survival. Josiah Nott, a proslavery Alabama doctor who claimed to have cared for more yellow fever patients than any other man in the United States, captured the contemporary understanding, writing in 1847 that though people disagreed on definitions, acclimation was "the single point" on which the "value of all our conclusions" turn.[48]

Immunity was (and is) an objective biological reality. But it was (and is) invisible, presenting no lasting outward signs. Yellow fever survivors were not left with scars, rashes, or pockmarks. Sometimes it was even hard to tell if a person had been sick from yellow fever at all, because not everyone experienced its signature symptom of black vomit. Many people who suffered through serious bouts of "intermittent" or "breakbone" fever (malaria and dengue) mistook their illness for yellow fever, thereafter maintaining a false belief in their own security. Plenty of people became infected with yellow fever but remained asymptomatic. Without diagnostic blood testing or vaccination, immunity was impossible to verify. This all-important, life-saving protection—*yellow fever* immunity—remained subjective and performative, a matter of faith as much as fact.[49]

Though Deep Southerners did not have a stable concept of acclimation, they were well practiced at cloaking uncertainty in certain terms. And in a slave society where snap judgments were routinely wrapped in the language of scientific objectivity—and where a person's race, origin, slave status, wealth, and ancestry were all fundamentally guesses—New Orleanians became socialized to recognize immunity cues in others and developed methods for quickly predicting who was likely to be acclimated. If a man was Creole (born in Louisiana), had passed through multiple epidemic summers, or had lived in the tropics for many years, society generally afforded him the benefit of the doubt. He could *pass* as immune. If he was a newcomer, poor, foreign-born, or a drunk, he was assumed to be "unacclimated" until proven otherwise. As the Irish immigrant and former Georgia congressman Richard Henry Wilde aptly described it shortly before he died from yellow fever in 1847, "no one is regarded an *Inhabitant* or any thing but a mere Squatter, who has not passed a summer."[50]

Acclimation was the process of surviving yellow fever. It became *immunocapital* if it was recognized by others. When so acknowledged, white New Orleanians conceived of immunity literally as capital, their definitions mapping closely to those theorized by French sociologist Pierre Bourdieu. Immunity was immaterial, intangible, and immovable (it could not be transferred as material capital could). But it was merit-based (each person earned it) and encoded with pecuniary value no different from other forms of tangible capital, like machines or enslaved people. A white man with immunocapital found himself economically reborn; he made more money in better jobs, was promoted more readily, and had access to new lines of credit and insurance. His social standing also improved. With the acclimation "credential," he could mingle and marry within elite circles and was provided access to lucrative commercial and civic networks. Immune white individuals also possessed cultural capital. In declaring themselves acclimated, they made a claim about their innate worth and legitimacy—that they were good risks, people of character and grit permanently invested in this society and, in turn, worthy of investment.[51]

Surviving yellow fever had little to do with nineteenth-century medicine, personal choices, morality, or character. But the white immune elite had an uncanny knack for attributing their relative epidemiological luck to God's approval—of their lifestyle and the system of racial slavery that made it possible. In their carefully curated ideology, the immune elite stood atop the New Orleans pyramid, not because they were lucky, but because they were white in a majority Black city, and because they had made the moral *choice* to survive yellow fever. Here, white survivors were lauded as climatic heroes; acclimation was locally referred to as a "passport" to riches, a "rebirth," or the "baptism of citizenship."[52] The acclimated boasted of their acquired immunity as if it were the winning ticket in a lottery without losers.

Judge Richard Claiborne captured the dangers and seduction of immunocapitalism best. "New Orleans," he wrote in the 1810s, "may be compared to a Plate of Honey. Thousands of insects come & satiate themselves with the sweet food, and die—but where one dies, a thousand visit the delicious repast. So it is with men—where their interests lie, they'll come to the place, tho' death stare them in the face."[53] The cold facts of disease risk mattered little; the *myth* of immunological reward wielded far more power. Newly acclimated migrants—equipped with survivor's pride—also proved willing to buy into and sustain immunocapital and the hierarchy it created. *They* had survived yellow fever; others would have to survive as well. The system was harsh, yes. But as one traveler aptly described it, "New Orleans is a surprising evidence of what men will endure, when cheered by the hopes of an ever-flowing tide of all mighty dollars and cents."[54]

New Orleans's immunity lottery was rigged. The potentially massive re-wards of acclimation could be accessed by whites only. Enslavers argued that Black people were naturally resistant to this virus—or, in the words of proslavery theorist Samuel Cartwright, that all people of African descent were "perfect non-conductors of yellow fever."[55] Such public pronounce-ments cut a stark contrast with enslavers' private concerns. Planters' letters were filled with worries about what would happen to their capital—embodied in the people they enslaved—when epidemics descended. Some would only purchase Creole or "guaranteed acclimated" people. And some, knowing that fraudulent claims of acclimation were a dime a dozen in the slave market, spent large sums on doctors to usher their slaves through the acclimating process "safely." Moreover, these pronouncements contradicted what enslaved people experienced firsthand. Many Black people from the Upper South, ripped from families and friends and marched south to New Orleans, knew their skin color did not confer total protection against yellow fever. And many remembered that yellow fever was one of the most fear-some aspects of their forced relocation to the Deep South through the do-mestic slave trade or "Second Middle Passage." One formerly enslaved woman recalled, years after she made it through a bad epidemic, "You have never seen the like . . . The folks died in piles" with coffins piled "as high as a house."[56] Within immunocapitalism, it did not matter that Black people were clearly vulnerable to yellow fever. Rather, the devastation it visited on enslaved Black people was ignored or turned into a "heads-I-win, tails-you-lose" proposition where whites accrued all the benefits resulting from Black survival. Immunity increased the monetary value of slaves *to their owners* and strengthened a set of racialized assumptions about the Black body that bolstered racial slavery.

Alleged Black immunity accrued as a benefit to white enslavers, but New Orleans society conferred no such gains on free people of color. Many *gens de couleur libres* could boast of long family lineages in Louisiana. Like all Creoles and all people of African descent, they were assumed to have im-munity to yellow fever, something whites could only earn by dangerous trial. They were nevertheless deprived of the social and economic privileges immunity conferred on whites. This racist society was interested in constraining the freedoms and opportunities of free Blacks, not expanding them. From 1808 onward, free people of color were legally required to show deference to whites, they could not hold political office, and they could not vote. Oppression became especially acute by the 1850s when onerous limits were put on their rights and freedom of movement. By this time this group made up a small (and shrinking) proportion of the city's booming population, just 8.3 percent, and to be free and Black was increasingly classified as a "diseased" condition—a societal sickness. Many *libres* emigrated from New Orleans to escape the increasing racism. And though presumed-immune free people of color continued to dominate in certain industries (especially undertaking), and some grew wealthy through sugar and slavery, economic opportunities were now out of reach for most.[57] Thus, most people of African descent—whether free or enslaved—could possess immunity but not immunocapital.

New Orleans did not have to be this way. There were alternative possibilities the elite rejected—other ways of managing public health, of imagining self-making within a capitalist society, of thinking about disease and race, and of managing disease and poverty. But immunocapitalism did not seek to be thoughtful, because it was so furiously lucrative for the few and because it literally destroyed competition. The result was a system shockingly shortsighted and shallow-rooted. It would collapse if people stopped immigrating to New Orleans in large numbers, if the Yellow Fever South lost its enslaved labor force, or if New Orleans's dominance within the nation's cotton export economy eroded. All three processes did unfold after the Civil War, catching the elite off guard. In part this was because yellow fever narrowed people's imaginations, with many coming to accept that New Orleans—a city with triple the national mortality average—could be no other way than the way it was. Of course, that was untrue. Immunocapitalism was time-limited, arising in nineteenth-century New Orleans only because capitalists improvised economic and social systems in a particular ecological and political framework that allowed them with great success to establish their own prosperity on the backs of others.

All forms of capitalism—war, necro-, racial, slave-racial, industrial—arise not because of the irresistible logic of the market but because powerful actors mobilize the materials at their disposal to consolidate their dominance. This could be as true of disease as it was of laws, demographics, and

politics. From New Orleans's first undisputed yellow fever epidemic in 1796 until its last in 1905, the ruling class mobilized disease risk to their advantage. In this manner, immunocapitalism is reminiscent of what Naomi Klein called "disaster capitalism": when governments or regimes take advantage of major disasters—"shocks"—to enact policies and build systems the population would not normally accept. In the case of New Orleans, however, the "shocks" were not individual wars or invasions (as in Klein's modern narrative) but instead repeated epidemics that together formed a century-long war of epidemiological attrition. Brutality, simply, was accepted as a transaction cost of doing business in New Orleans. The results were wealth for the few, and misery for the many.[58]

Our Journey

Our story begins, in Chapter 1, right after the Louisiana Purchase. In the summer of 1804, almost every American agent in Louisiana—tasked with the military, administrative, and legal Americanization of the Southwest—was stricken by the "stranger's disease," throwing the entire imperial project into disarray. American politicians lamented that yellow fever branded them as usurping strangers among the Creoles—the native-born, French- and Spanish-speaking inhabitants who dominated the lucrative sugar industry and embraced a more complicated racial classification system. If the United States was going to successfully absorb Louisiana, an urgent solution was needed to the practical and political impediments thrown up by yellow fever. The solution found had two parts. First was mass acclimation. It became the patriotic duty of every white American to get sick and survive, so as to raise white Americans' political and economic position to equality with the region's *anciennes*. The second was to embrace domestic slavery. Anglo-Americans, building on a centuries-old argument developed in the Caribbean, claimed that *all* people of African descent were naturally immune to yellow fever. This, they said, justified the spread and entrenchment of Black slavery on a much larger scale across Louisiana, especially around New Orleans.[59]

We then move from the 1820s to the 1850s, focusing on different themes. Chapter 2 explores what it was like to live in the necropolis of the United States and how people experienced the *danse macabre* differently according to race, free-status, gender, ethnicity, religion, and wealth. What comfort could medicine or institutions offer? Responding to a serious plague with no confirmed cause and no cure, in a climate of state-sponsored disinformation about the progress of the disease, New Orleanians developed systems to cope with mass mortality. As epidemics set in by July and people either fled the city or sickened, the market's attention refocused on the region's third industry after commodities and slavery: health. Crops might fail, but sickness was more or less guaranteed, making doctoring the steadiest and one of the most lucrative professions in the Deep South. Yellow fever was so lucrative, in fact, that it became a physician's springboard to slave and land ownership, and thus political power. Scared, desperate, and delirious people proved willing to spend just about anything—a whole year's salary or more—on medical care. They also spent large sums on lawyers, lodging, and elaborate funeral arrangements. Poor and enslaved people, especially women, had few good options when they fell sick. Black women in particular spent each autumn caring for the sick and convalescent. Consequently, many Black people developed their own systems for thinking about illness and mourning that went against those prescribed by whites.

Because "all old residents know . . . that no person can be looked upon as a permanent citizen of New Orleans until he has undergone the acclimating process," Chapter 3 concerns disease risk and acclimation: how these terms were understood, leveraged, capitalized, and encoded with specific racial and social meanings.[60] In job interviews, white people carefully curated the details of their sickness and convalescence, citing grotesque symptoms and medicinal regimens to get a foot in the door. For whites, immunity translated into economic capital, with all desirable jobs going to those who claimed to be acclimated. Successful acclimations factored into the genesis stories of almost all of New Orleans's political and economic elite. Men claimed that their triumph over disease was a product of providential selection, manliness, morality, sobriety, and honor, making death a mark of damnation rather than luck. Simultaneously, proslavery theorists and physicians like Josiah Nott, Samuel Cartwright, and Philip Tidyman crafted an increasingly elaborate argument by the 1830s: God had made all Black people naturally immune to yellow fever so that slavery was their natural and deserved state. In public, most enslavers uncritically echoed this idea. In private, enslavers routinely lamented how vulnerable the people they owned were to yellow fever, that *their* disease risk was astronomical. No enterprising enslaver, therefore, would purchase a person without an express guarantee of acclimation. And many were willing to pay 25 or even 50 percent more for this security.

Why did politicians in America's deadliest city spend virtually nothing on public health? Chapter 4 explores how New Orleans sharply diverged from national trends in this regard. Ineffectual boards of health came and went, depending on the politics of the day; quarantines were attempted sporadically and without vigor; the Charity Hospital was a notorious death-trap. As Dr. E. H. Barton put it after the devastating 1853 epidemic, "New Orleans is one of the dirtiest, and . . . consequently the sickliest city in the Union, and scarcely anything has been done to remedy it."[61] What Barton failed to acknowledge was that this neglect was by design. Government officials saw their sole responsibility as protecting the market. They refused to spend tax money to protect lives—especially of the poor and newly arrived—by sanitizing and draining immigrant neighborhoods. The commercial-civic elite argued that health was personally established through acclimation, not publicly upheld. Despite evidence that public health measures had value against yellow fever in other cities, New Orleans leaders righteously insisted those examples were irrelevant. Instead, their best solution to yellow fever was not public health, but paradoxically, more yellow fever. In this view, water pumps and quarantines only delayed the inevitable sorting of human wheat from chaff. While some protested this system, most newcomers came to accept it. As unacclimated noncitizens as yet unable to vote, their practical choices were to embrace the filthiness of the urban condition and gain immunity, or flee, or die.

Chapter 5 concerns the ideology of disease denialism and its close intellectual relationship with Southern nationalism and proslavery thought. Following the 1853 epidemic, when more than 12,000 people died, critics claimed unchecked yellow fever was damaging New Orleans's civic credit. "We have lost the confidence of capitalists abroad," said one doctor, "our property has lessened in value at home; and all of our natural advantages have proved too weak to successfully combat with yellow fever."[62] But elites in the Yellow Fever South measured "public health" by economic prosperity, not mortality—and they needed a steady flow of immigration, both Black and white. Health "boosters" conducted a propaganda campaign aimed at downplaying the dangers of disease and countering the region's deadly reputation. This campaign was filled with lies and often slipped into bold claims for the health of the larger slave system. Denying the cruelties of slavery and the reality of disease were both part of the same intellectual venture: to project a sunnier and more meritocratic vision of the Cotton Kingdom as national tensions and sectionalism were rising.

Chapter 6 analyzes the progress of yellow fever—and the slow collapse of the system of immunocapitalism—during the Civil War and Reconstruction. Confederates hoped Union forces would be crippled by Yellow Jack. But under General Benjamin Butler's occupation of New Orleans—complete with a quarantine and strict sanitation measures—the city experienced its first significant decline in mortality in over six decades. The virus had not stopped the enemy; instead the enemy had stalled the virus. But such public health wisdom was conveniently forgotten after the war when yellow fever returned. Only now the old canards about yellow fever did not seem to hold up, or to fit the new legal and economic order of emancipation. Reflecting on the glory days of the Old South, apologists ridiculously argued that Blackness itself had not been the key to yellow fever resistance—*enslavement* had been. Slavery, in this view, had been a blessing to Black people, who were incapable of calibrating disease risk properly, and now—independent of white authority—would die on an unprecedented scale or even become "extinct." This was, of course, both ludicrous and unfounded. But it became an argument against extending freedpeople full citizenship, with its white proponents once again using false science about yellow fever to subjugate Black people politically and economically. The rigidity of immunocapitalism waned as New Orleans's importance within the national cotton export economy declined. This was especially pronounced after the region-wide epidemic of 1878, when white immigration slowed and Black people, fleeing violence and coercive labor, left the region in large numbers for the North and West.

1

Patriotic Fever

In mid-September 1804, syndic Juan de Castañedo reported to New Orleans's city council some troubling intelligence he had received: a group of armed Black men had been meeting in the home of Widow LeSassier on Rue L'Hôpital, just inside the city gate. Given the agitation of that summer—a short sea voyage away, the slaves of Saint-Domingue had successfully thrown off their white masters and declared the independent nation of Haiti—Castañedo grew concerned for the public's safety. He asked two friends, the Creole planters Claude Tremé and François Hulin, to join his inspection of LeSassier's residence. There they discovered a group of Black men "with no white to watch them." Searching the rooms and attic of the house, they uncovered a stockpile of thirteen guns, a sword, and one bayonet—hard evidence, thought Castañedo, that something nefarious was afoot. Alarmed, the city council investigated further. It determined that the guns actually belonged to Captain Robert Davis, a white American, who had purchased them to protect his ships against pirates. In an apologetic letter, Davis insisted that the unsupervised slaves were Creoles from the Bahamas, not the revolutionary crucibles of Saint-Domingue or Jamaica, and thus should not inspire fear. But Davis vowed to keep his weapons in a safer place in the future, as even "if his negroes [had] no evil intentions, there [were] many others disposed differently."[1]

City councilors seemed satisfied by Davis's explanation, but the majority of New Orleans's white residents—paranoids disposed to treat even the smallest of slave "infractions" with suspicion—were not. Many townspeople interpreted the discovery as the latest episode in a vast conspiracy stretching far beyond the walls of the French Quarter. All summer there had been reports of Black revolutionaries from Saint-Domingue pouring onto the levee, infecting "the slaves of this country" with their colorblind ideas of *liberté, égalité, fraternité*. For those looking for it, evidence of the Haitian contagion was everywhere. In late June the city council ordered the arrest of a Black man named Marseille, who was said to be without a "rightful master." When questioned (and perhaps tortured) by the mayor, Marseille confessed to having served "in the insurgent armies in San Domingo." Then in July two white men named Delery and Boulingy killed one unarmed slave and injured another, claiming their use of lethal force was justified because the men were running away. As Article 8 of the Public Orders of 1795 immunized whites against prosecution for killing escaping enslaved people, the murderers "could be assured that this affair would have no serious results for them." Suspiciously, however, no white man had come forward seeking financial restitution for property destruction—the death of this enslaved man. And by late summer, many whites complained that the epidemic of running away could no longer be ignored; emboldened slaves did "not hesitate to collor [*sic*] the white people and have even dared to raise and strike them with their sacrilegious hands."[2]

On sugar plantations surrounding New Orleans, whites complained about a new work-shirking attitude among the enslaved who "wander[ed] about at night without passports" and were said to be "in a shameful state of Idleness . . . stealing, drinking and rioting." Still others, demonstrating a "great Savageness of Character," had been overheard speaking "of eating human flesh" and boasting of their participation in "the horrors of St. Domingo." And in early August, New Orleans mayor Étienne de Boré, an extremely wealthy sugar planter, warned that a colored man named Dutaque, suspected of "having taken a very active part" in the revolution in Saint-Domingue, was aboard an inbound ship, his purposes for coming to Louisiana unknown. White fears spiraled. By September it was said that 6,000 enslaved Blacks and *gens de couleur libres* in and around New Orleans would imminently unite, rise up, plunder the city's arsenal, kill the white men, rape the white women, and burn the city to the ground.[3]

For America's fledgling territorial government, based in New Orleans, such unrest could not have come at a worse time. The United States had just taken formal possession of Louisiana and had only tenuous control over the space and its people. New Orleans sat more than 1,000 miles away from

Washington, D.C. There was no regular standing army there, and Spaniards in West Florida were threatening to attack, perhaps with their Houma Indian allies. Louisiana's court system—shifting from civil law to a civil-common law hybrid—was in chaos. The *anciennes* had shown little enthusiasm, and sometimes even downright disdain, for these new Americans claiming authority. When the city's various ethnic and racial factions were not fighting each other, they happily attacked W. C. Claiborne, the twenty-eight-year-old monolingual Virginian recently installed as acting governor of Orleans Territory, a man universally derided as incompetent. In fact, 250 influential Creoles were in the process of drafting a "Remonstrance" to the US Congress, a litany of complaints against Claiborne personally and American policy more generally.[4]

Worse still, New Orleans was in the grip of a violent yellow fever epidemic, the fourth in a decade. The summer's first victim—a well-connected Kentucky businessman named John A. Seitz—died on Louisiana's first Independence Day.[5] Townspeople were tempted to read political meaning into who the disease killed: yellow fever ravaged "strangers" from Northern states and Europe but it spared the Creoles, those Black and white people born in Louisiana. In mid-September, Claiborne told President Thomas Jefferson that New Orleans was the "Seat of Disease," estimating that yellow fever was killing seven or eight people per day, with new cases "hourly occurring." By early October, Claiborne had reassessed: one-third of all recently immigrated Americans and almost every newly arrived European had died. As the health situation deteriorated, a mass exodus ensued. Wealthy merchants and aldermen escaped to their country plantations to drink away the gloom. Those without funds or freedom were forced to remain.[6] Aware that the city's white population was rapidly diminishing—through death or distance—thirty panicking whites gathered in the parlor of Michel Fortier, a powerful Creole merchant and alderman appointed to the city's transition government. They drafted a petition to Claiborne, emphasizing that yellow fever had made New Orleans especially vulnerable to slave insurrection. Without "active Surveillance" over enslaved and free Blacks, accompanied by "Severe Justice" for the duration of the epidemic, Louisiana would surely fall "prey to the same Events which have laid waste" to the "Proud and rich Colony of San Domingo."[7]

Claiborne surely felt ill-equipped to handle this multifront emergency. But he was also savvy enough to know that if by some chance he handled this crisis well, it could boost his reputation and that of the United States.

He therefore made two decisions. First, he "put a public Musket in the hands of every White man in the City" to stop any revolting slaves and guarantee the "Lives & property of the Inhabitants!"[8] Second, he vowed to remain in town for the duration of the epidemic, against medical advice, just as his colonial-era predecessors had always done. Claiborne holed up with his young family in the Government Lot, a disgusting mansion known as the "most unhealthy" in town. Here, the brother of the last French governor, Baron de Carondelet, had died from yellow fever in 1796; so did Louisiana's last Spanish governor, Manuel Gayoso de Lemos, who fell victim to the scourge three years later.[9] The stench of putrefying waste and garbage emanating off the adjacent levee was overwhelming. The mosquitoes flitting about his chambers were maddening. Soon Claiborne was chilly and nauseous. Alternating between high fevers and bouts of delirium, he took to his bed, dictating orders to his private secretary—who also was feverish—to increase night patrols and arm the militia with powder and ball from the city's arsenal.[10]

Claiborne got lucky that summer in some respects. He survived his brush with yellow fever, and the slave rebellion never materialized. Even so, the epidemic took a staggering toll on him personally and professionally. On September 27, the same day Jefferson made Claiborne's temporary governorship permanent, yellow fever killed his first wife, Eliza, and their three-year-old daughter Cornelia (his brother-in-law also died in 1804; Claiborne's second wife, Clarisse, would die from yellow fever five years later). It also killed one-third to one-half of the new territorial government's officials, including the up-and-coming Joseph Briggs, Claiborne's private secretary, whose death left about a dozen administrative projects unfinished. Claiborne's two deputy clerks lay convalescent for months. His two chief liaisons to the city's merchant community—John Gelston of New York and Benjamin West of Philadelphia—perished, as did many hundreds of other ambitious white American men seeking a foothold in the cotton and sugar industries.[11] Worse still, yellow fever killed more than a hundred soldiers posted at the barracks just outside town. As Claiborne lamented to Jefferson, "Lower Louisiana is a beautiful Country, and rewards abundantly the Labour of man;—But the Climate is a wretched one, and destructive to human Life."[12]

Globally, 1804 was a bad yellow fever year. Historians estimate that this epidemic killed perhaps 125,000 people across southern Europe, West Africa, and the tropical Americas—part of a larger Caribbean-wide epidemic sparked by the Napoleonic Wars. Exactly how much of that Atlantic toll was exacted in New Orleans we will never know. In the chaos of regime change—as the vast 827,000-square-mile territory of Louisiana transferred from French to American rule—collecting accurate vital statistics in New Orleans was no one's priority. Many yellow fever deaths went unrecorded. Bodies were hastily buried in the overwhelmed Catholic and Protestant cemeteries. The city ordered enslaved workmen to toss the corpses of indigents into the Mississippi, to float down to the Gulf of Mexico along with the trash. Proportionally, 1804 had to have been one of the most convulsive years in New Orleans history. About a third of the city's population of 8,000 fled and between 1,000 and 1,500 people died—most of them newly arrived white Americans. America's imperial dreams had given way to an epidemiological nightmare.[13]

Give Me Liberty or Give Me Death!

News of the Louisiana Purchase had electrified the United States in 1803. But whether distracted by the complexity of incorporating Louisiana or blinded by the promise of Caribbean-style wealth, few Americans back east did due diligence on the disease question. Cotton might thrive there, but did people? The answer had long been a resounding no. Pathogens introduced by Hernando de Soto's expedition in 1540 and by later European explorers had decimated native peoples in the Lower Mississippi Valley, reducing a population that had stood as high as a million people to just 70,000 by 1700. As colonization and war accelerated in the eighteenth century, and as La Nouvelle-Orléans's population increased, the proliferation of diseases intensified. Mysterious fevers killed thousands of French voyageurs, Acadian farmers, Spanish soldiers, and African slaves. So many people died so fast, in fact, that Lower Louisiana became the deadliest major settlement on mainland North America, deadlier even than Jamestown, Virginia, in its sickliest years. Caught in a vast epidemiological web invisibly stretching across the tropical and subtropical regions of the Atlantic world, long-term residents of New Orleans came to accept fevers as a fact of life—like floods or fires.[14] James Pitot, a businessman and future mayor, expressed the people's resignation to their swampy environment in 1802, writing, "The roads have deep holes; the bridges are not maintained; and every time the Mississippi rises substantially, it causes crevasses that obstruct the roads and ruin the planters, leaving putrid remains of fish, snakes, and animals."

The ebb and flow of the river, the heat, and the stench, Pitot lamented, caused "periodic fevers that decimate the foreigner and bring desolation to the families of the colonists." There was simply nothing to be done about it.[15]

The first generation of white Anglo-Americans to head to New Orleans in 1803, however, discounted tales of the city's excessive fevers as exaggeration. Admitting that colonization was always a dangerous venture, especially in the torrid zone, they still preferred the myth that New Orleans was "in health a Montpelier"—a place of potential riches where "disease was scarcely known . . . where old age was the chief waste-gate of human life." When Claiborne arrived in New Orleans in early 1804, he relayed a version of this utopian fiction to Jefferson, writing that "the climate of lower Louisiana is unhealthy, but it is by no means so unfriendly to human life as has been represented."[16] But Claiborne, like seemingly everyone, was caught off guard by the sickly reality. Yellow fever nearly killed him in 1804. Then four more devastating epidemics struck in quick succession—in 1805, 1807, 1809, and 1811. By the time Louisiana applied for statehood in 1812, yellow fever, a disease once most associated with the Caribbean and occasional outbreaks in Philadelphia or Charleston, had become nearly synonymous with New Orleans—"as inseparably connected," said British traveler Thomas Hamilton, "as ham and chicken."[17]

Mass yellow fever death caused cascading structural problems for American government in Louisiana. It delegitimized American rule and embarrassed the United States' authority at the precise moment it sought to project confidence to the local Creole population and the wider world. The virus killed so many newly transplanted government officials that it slowed the wheels of the administration, disrupted commerce, and massively delayed land and legal reform. Yellow fever impeded the creation of a basic administrative state with a functioning court system, systematized land ownership, and a tax and tariff system able to handle the deluge of goods flowing through New Orleans. Arguably, it stalled Louisiana's application for US statehood. Most of all, the disease, which appeared to leave the Creoles unscathed, cast new Americans as unwelcome and unworthy invaders, unable to survive—let alone succeed—in subtropical New Orleans.[18]

The United States could not solve the yellow fever problem. No one could at that time. But America could not afford to lose its battle with disease. That would mean the loss of New Orleans and all the bounty flowing through it. Thus, by 1810, Anglo-Americans had devised ways to live with yellow fever—and generate power from it. The first "solution" to the yellow fever problem was acceptance: Americans had to embrace their diseased environment, just as Creoles across the Greater Caribbean had done for centuries, and then *actively* pursue immunity. This strategy was individually very risky—about half of all people who contracted yellow fever died. But faced with a disease no one understood and no one could cure, some took a conscious risk to remain, others just stayed put, and the cumulative result was acclimation *en masse,* which effectively naturalized surviving white Americans to Louisiana and raised their political position to equality with that of long-established residents.

America's second ostensible "solution" to yellow fever was to promote widespread racial slavery in the Deep South, supplied through the domestic slave trade after African slave trading was federally banned in 1808. Racialized perceptions of yellow fever immunity proved central in the logic underwriting the Lower Mississippi Valley's new regime of exploitative commodity production, with Black slavery being classed as essential to white liberty *and* the white public's health. Deploying the long-standing myth that all Black people possessed natural resistance to yellow fever—whether that person came from Senegambia or Maryland—white Louisianans claimed slavery was an economic and epidemiological necessity there more than anywhere else in the United States. While whites dropped dead, Black slaves could labor "safely" in the most dangerous, diseased, and environmentally exposed jobs. Without racial slavery, white Louisianans warned, the budding Cotton Kingdom would become a "waste land" with no value. But with it, the land could produce bounty even as epidemics raged. In embracing domestic rather than African slavery, Louisiana's planters tied themselves economically to the eastern United States—where most enslaved people came from. The subsequent Americanization of Louisiana's slaving industry would allow the United States to jettison the complex racial hierarchies of *casta* that had defined Louisiana's French and Spanish eras, subjugate the large and cosmopolitan free Black population, and potentially stem the Haitian threat.[19]

By the end of Louisiana's territorial period, sickly New Orleans had developed the preconditions for immunocapitalism. It had a deadly virus that conferred immunity on survivors, increasing control over the nation's cotton and sugar export industries; a small but powerful ruling class constituted of apparently immune (as well as apparently "white" people); and an abundance of people—free and forced—who would replace the dead following each epidemic. As New Orleans's elites embraced disease as a mode of class dominance, they made the Deep South, the center of Jefferson's utopian "empire for liberty," into its opposite: the beating heart of American slavery.

The Atlantic's Smallest Killer

No one outside of Africa knew yellow fever existed before the early seventeenth century, but the disease quickly demonstrated its ability to wipe out islands, armies, even empires. The yellow fever virus—a tiny parcel of RNA strands encased in a protein shell—has existed in its present form for about 3,000 years.[20] Most of the time, the virus sits dormant in the bloodstreams of monkeys living in jungle canopies. But sometimes a mosquito will take a blood meal from an infected primate, fly a short distance, then bite a human. If that infected person travels into a densely populated area—a town, city, barrack, or plantation—the disease can spread quickly and violently. Epidemic yellow fever in a nonendemic zone requires a trifecta of conditions to emerge: a hot and humid climate; a large, densely packed human population of nonimmunes; and a robust vector population. Such conditions could be met occasionally in northern latitudes like Canada or even Ireland, places where yellow fever did make rare seasonal visitations. More frequently, yellow fever struck cities in the subtropics like Buenos Aires, Charleston, and New Orleans—places hot enough in the summer months to sustain the mosquito's feeding and breeding activity, and where ships from warmer climates constantly reinforced the vector population. Most often, yellow fever struck the coastal lowlands of the Greater Caribbean, especially the port cities of equatorial West Africa, South America, and the West Indies, where mosquitoes lived and bred year-round.

Not just any mosquito could carry the disease. Yellow fever is primarily transmitted by the female *Aedes aegypti,* which is also the vector of other flaviviruses like dengue, Zika, and chikungunya. This is a mosquito of particular tastes. Native to Africa, this species—like all mosquitoes—cannot breed until the female takes a blood meal. But she will not eat unless she is warm enough, optimally between 63°F and 88°F. And unlike the swamp-loving, malaria-carrying *Anopheles,* she will lay eggs only in unpolluted water. She has a unique preference for manmade containers—the wooden cisterns, cement wells, and clay-lined pots typical of sugar plantations. But she can breed in any crevice holding even a small amount of rainwater. She is by nature a homebody, remaining within a twenty-meter radius for her entire two- to four-week life. Most of all, she is a picky eater. Though she can take a blood meal from a horse, cow, or pig, her feeding focus is humans. After two or three blood meals, she seeks out a suitable spot to lay her eggs—something she will do each week of her life. And as she ages, she grows more dangerous, for the longer she lives, the more likely she is to have bitten an infected person and harbor the virus.[21]

A. aegypti probably came to the Americas in the era of the transatlantic slave trade, stowing away with the densely packed enslaved captives and goods crammed below deck. During the sea voyage, mosquitoes sat on the walls of slave ships, occasionally fed on captives' blood, and laid their blackish larvae in one of the dozens of freshwater casks each ship carried. Second- or third-generation bugs disembarked in the Americas sixty days later.[22] The first Africans—and A. aegypti mosquitoes—to land in the Greater Caribbean, however, found themselves in ecologically unstable worlds, host to a motley assemblage of indigenous and invasive species jostling for a niche. After the "Great Dying"—the century following 1492 saw an unfathomable 80 to 95 percent of the Caribbean's Amerindians killed, either by invading Europeans or more often by the pathogens they carried—native peoples had all but disappeared from large parts of the Americas. Initially, few Europeans or enslaved Africans came to replace the dead. Cuba, the largest island in the Greater Antilles, had no more than 7,500 inhabitants in 1620. As late as 1640, the Caribbean's total population probably stood below 200,000 people, many of them indentured servants. Almost all wanted to return to Europe as soon as possible.

The sugar revolution of the mid-seventeenth century changed everything. Sugarcane is not native to the Caribbean, but European colonists found the grass grew well there due to sustained heat and fertile soil. Cultivating cane—transforming tall green stalks into sweet crystals—is backbreaking labor on a time crunch. Once cut, cane must be pressed and boiled within a day or else the juice ferments and is ruined. Sugar thus required lots of fuel and an abundant, coordinated labor force, working around the clock during the harvest—cutting, hauling, pressing, stoking, and stirring on an endless loop. With so much work to be done and so much money to be made, the sugar plantation complex ascended. Barbados, the first island to seriously adopt cane cultivation, saw its population soar from 1,400 in 1629 to 40,000 by 1642, an upsurge mirrored in Jamaica, the French colony of Saint-Domingue, the Spanish colony of Cuba, as well as most smaller islands. Enslaved Africans did nearly all the work. By 1750, Africans constituted three-quarters of the Caribbean's total population, and up to 90 percent on some islands.[23]

Sugar plantations proved voracious consumers of wood and people, and efficient producers of riches. As the plantation complex intensified and spread across the Caribbean, a dangerous ecological cycle emerged. Sugar meant more enslaved Africans; enslaved Africans meant more slave ships; and slave ships meant more *A. aegypti*. These bugs thrived in the tropics. Deforestation across vast acreages led to the eradication (or near eradication) of their bat and bird predators. With no direct competition, the *A. aegypti* had ample time to find people to feed on and comfortable places to breed. Sweaty, panting, nonimmune food sources were present in abundance—trench-digging soldiers and cane-cutting slaves. Caribbean port cities and sugar plantations contained millions of clean-water breeding places, especially the hundreds of clay pots (or concave pot fragments) that collected water during the rainy season. By the mid-seventeenth century, colonists frequently commented on the clouds of mosquitoes that hovered low to the ground or flitted around their cabins. The Caribbean had unwittingly put itself on the precipice of a disease disaster.[24]

Yellow fever's first recorded epidemic struck North America between 1647 and 1651, following a strong El Niño. No one recognized this disease. It killed over 6,000 people in Barbados alone, 14 percent of the island's population. British writer Richard Ligon landed at Bridgetown shortly after this epidemic and dubbed it a "plague," its horrors evoking biblical pestilence. Three thousand miles away, the Yucatecan Maya documented mass death from *xe kik* in 1648 in the Tizimin Codex, noting that year "Come is the quetzal; Come is the blue bird; Come are the yellow deaths; Come is blood vomit." As yellow fever cut its destructive path, it took on a panoply of monikers: *mal de Siam,* the peste, Barbados distemper, *petit fleur, Climat-feber,* Haemagestic pestilence, putrid bilious fever, Bulam fever. The Caribs of Guadeloupe knew it as *iepoulicáatina;* French-speaking Creoles called it *coup de barre.* But most Caribbean dwellers came to know it as *vómito negro,* so-called for its signature symptom.[25]

Yellow fever proved so deadly and destructive that it killed off entire remaining Indigenous communities and upended settlement schemes. Of the 2,500 Scots who sailed to the isthmus at Darien (Panama) in 1698–1699, 80 percent died from yellow fever. The battered survivors abandoned the colony. In 1764–1765, as many as 11,000 Europeans died in Kourou

(Guyana), which suffered a death rate somewhere between 85 and 90 percent. This was, according to J. R. McNeill, "the single most abysmal failure" in the history of European colonization. Yellow fever could even threaten well-established cities and empires. Geographer John Pinkerton noted that the native people of Mexico suffered from an "epidemical distemper" locally called *matlazahuatl*—though this was the same disease people in Veracruz called black vomit. Pinkerton claimed that this scourge swept away more than one-third of the population of *Ciudad de México* in 1736 and 1737. Though he doubtlessly overestimated, he also noted that the same ailment "almost depopulated" the Kingdom of Mexico three decades later.[26] Facing death at such a scale, it was hard not to be fatalistic.

Indigenous peoples and settler colonialists could not fathom this mysterious ailment's wreaking havoc one year but disappearing the next. It was as if the virus intended to lull people into a false sense of security—to trick them into letting their guard down. Despite the occasional disappearances of the disease, European soldiers and sailors (especially impressed young men making their first forays into the tropics) lived in perpetual terror of "Yellow Jack." They had good reason to be scared. As the Caribbean became richer, it became a theater for large-scale warfare, with European nations seeking to hold on to immensely lucrative, slavery-powered colonies and seize others. Yellow fever abounded. In 1690, during the Nine Years War, British captain Lawrence Wright managed to recapture St. Kitts from the French but lost half his men to yellow fever in the process. Two years later, Commodore Ralph Wrenn's losses from yellow fever were so heavy (half his men died, and eventually he himself died) that some of his ships just sank, lacking adequate crew to navigate away from reefs and shoals. A year later Rear-Admiral Sir Francis Wheler lost two-thirds of his men to yellow fever and malaria in Barbados, some 3,100 of 4,500 men. During the War of Jenkins' Ear in 1741–1742, probably 21,000 of the 29,000 British soldiers and sailors participating in Admiral Edward Vernon's Cartagena campaign died, almost all from yellow fever—just 1,000 died in battle. In 1762 the British seized the rich prize of Havana, along with a treasury of over £3 million in specie, tobacco, and sugar. But the victory came at a heavy cost. Seven thousand soldiers were stricken by yellow fever during the siege. In Cuba, yellow fever killed fourteen times as many British attackers as did Spanish guns. Given the catastrophic death rate, it is no surprise that European soldiers tried to avoid Caribbean duty and officers resigned commissions before those regiments shipped out.[27]

Colonial subjects could see their metropolitan overlords change rapidly. The same could not be said for their core modes of governance. None of these plantation societies governed through consent. Nor did sugar islands particularly value expertise or good administration—that would require higher taxes and Europeans committing to living on the islands long-term. As a rule, Caribbean slave societies, in which white planters monopolized all power, were glorified police states in which white wealth was built on Black terror. The choreography of power was nearly the same everywhere: imperial officials drew up *Codes Noirs* to enshrine enslavers' power over life and death; colonial assemblies established militias and slave patrols to weed out maroons and runaways; slave revolts were met with furious brutality.[28] As Daniel Defoe wrote in 1722, the key to dealing with Africans was to ensure they were "rul'd with a Rod of Iron, beaten with *Scorpions,*" or else they would "rise and murder all their Masters which their Numbers consider'd, would not be hard for them to do, if they had Arms and Ammunition sustainable to the Rage and Cruelty of their Nature." Most islands had meager state apparatus outside of that required to subjugate Africans or ship the products they cultivated back to Europe.[29] Edward Long, who published a three-volume *History of Jamaica* in 1774, lamented the lack of infrastructure; the hospitals, schools, and even government buildings of the British West Indies were decrepit or nonexistent. Welfare did not exist beyond the Church. Disease and violence were endemic. Wharfingers—ulcerous sailors abandoned by their ships when they no longer had value—begged on every beach from Grenada to Havana. Lucky ones might enter a poorhouse or special sailor's hospital. But many, unable to return home from island societies that did not care whether they lived or died, simply crawled into empty sugar casks to die.[30]

Racial Immunity

European physicians were key players in the transatlantic slave trade and mainstays of imperial navies. They had seen a lot of yellow fever by the eighteenth century. As eyewitnesses to the suffering—and probably survivors themselves—their testimony about symptoms, etiology, and effective treatments was given weight. There was little diagnostic or prophylactic consensus, but doctors noted certain consistencies: children tended to experience milder cases of yellow fever than adults; European newcomers were incredibly vulnerable; and yellow fever did not strike the same person twice. Physicians were also likely the germ of one hugely consequential and sticky idea about yellow fever—that it discriminated racially, killing white people in droves while sparing all or almost all Black people. This race-based theory of immunity probably arose, not because of European doctors' abject racism *per se,* but because it made sense of morbidity and mortality patterns that contemporary science could not otherwise explain and did so in a language of racial difference in which white imperialists were already fluent.[31]

It will be useful to break down this cyclical logic step by step. Everywhere yellow fever struck, death registers seemed to provide incontrovertible proof that the tropics were dangerous for everyone but were a veritable "charnel house" for whites. Following the 1699 epidemic in the majority-Black city of Charleston, for example, sextons estimated that yellow fever killed about 300 people, but that only one of them was nonwhite.[32] This striking racial disparity was probably not chiefly the result of erroneous data collection or bad methodology, but instead a reflection of New World demographics. Eighteenth-century physicians were most likely to encounter two groups in the Americas: first-generation "saltwater" slaves who had probably been exposed to yellow fever as children, in the cramped coastal slaving depots along the African coast, or during the Middle Passage across the Atlantic; and white Europeans—settler colonists, sailors, and farmers—with no previous exposure to tropical disease. This meant that many Black people arrived in the Americas after a grueling transatlantic journey already immune to yellow fever (and very often resistant to malaria), a protection virtually no white European shared.[33] The violence endemic to the sugar plantation-complex, combined with overwork, suicide, disease, and malnutrition, ensured that most of these newly arrived enslaved Africans would not live long in the Americas. Within a year of landing, up to one-quarter of all "New Negroes" died; the "lucky" ones could expect to live just five or six years. Enslavers simply bought new Africans to replace the dead. This, in turn, meant that established eighteenth-century Atlantic societies were predominantly African, not Creole. Physicians then extrapolated outward from their observations of Africans' seeming resistance to yellow fever to mean that *all* Black people—of any origin or parentage—were innately, even providentially, more resistant to yellow fever than all whites.[34] This belief then created a structural problem for understanding Black immunity in the past, and for historians seeking to understand it now: If Black people, by definition, could not die from yellow fever, sextons were not likely to attribute their deaths to it in mortality records. Then the same death registers counting no Black deaths from yellow fever were held up as proof that Black immunity existed. The cycle was self-perpetuating—and immensely useful to whites.

Such racialized thinking metastasized across the Atlantic world, and far beyond medical circles. Following Charleston's 1748 epidemic, Dr. John Lining of South Carolina, a slaveholder, avowed, "There is something very singular in the constitution of the Negroes, which renders them not liable to this fever . . . I never knew one instance of this fever amongst them." Writing years later, Thomas Trotter, a British naval doctor, agreed, stating that "African negroes" seemed entirely immune to "contagious fever." Even Robert Southey, the English poet laureate and author of *Goldilocks and the Three Bears,* chimed in, writing in 1804 that "diseases, like vegetables, choose their own soil; as some plants like clay, others sand, other chalk, so the yellow fever will not take root in a negro."[35]

In the United States, the theory of Black yellow fever immunity was explicitly put to the test in Philadelphia during the summer of 1793. That summer, the city was gripped by a devastating epidemic in which 5,000 people—one-tenth of its population—died and a further 17,000 fled to the countryside. With a city in chaos and not enough doctors and nurses to tend to the sick, America's premier physician Benjamin Rush asked the Black community to step in, assuming them immune or at least very resistant to the scourge. Rush published a pseudonymous article citing Lining's ideas, then approached his friend Richard Allen, founder of the African Methodist Episcopal Church, telling him that yellow fever "infects white people of all ranks, but passes by persons of your color." Philadelphia's Black population answered the call. But over 400 Black people died from yellow fever that summer. Then, adding serious insult to injury, Philadelphia mayor Matthew Clarkson accused Black survivors of profiteering off the epidemic by extorting money and goods from sick white people.[36]

Reflecting on the carnage of that summer, Rush later disavowed the idea of total Black immunity, with various qualifications. He and other doctors (many of whom moved south in the nineteenth century) should have listened to clergymen Absalom Jones and Richard Allen, who debunked white claims of Black immunity in their 1794 account of the epidemic, insisting that Black people had died from yellow fever in the same proportion as other racial groups. "Happy would it have been for you [white people], and much more so for us, if this observation had been verified by our experience," they wrote. Allen and Jones also rebutted the claims of extortion, noting the labor of Sarah Bass, "a poor black widow [who] gave all the assistance she could, in several families, for which she did not receive any thing," and Sampson, "a poor black man" who went house to house to help the distressed without fee or reward, only to be "smote with the disorder." The pamphleteers added a curt rejoinder: "We do not recollect such acts of humanity from the poor white people."[37] Philadelphia provided clear evidence that Black people could and did die from yellow fever. But the *theory* of Black immunity stubbornly persisted. François Marie Perrin du Lac, a French émigré and former administrator from Saint-Domingue, noted that Americans he met with on his travels in Louisiana in 1801 widely believed that when yellow fever struck, "negroes . . . seem[ed] privileged from the effects of the contagion."[38]

Louisianacide

Yellow fever's most consequential ravages took place on the French colony of Saint-Domingue, the western third of the island of Hispaniola. During the eighteenth century, Saint-Domingue was considered the "jewel" of the Antilles, the envy of nations. Half a million enslaved people, working in brutal conditions across 8,000 plantations, produced 40 percent of the world's sugar and 60 percent of its coffee. But on the night of August 21, 1791, the slaves exploded in revolt. A band outside Cap Français hacked an overseer to pieces, then went from plantation to plantation burning cane fields, razing boiling houses, and bludgeoning masters to death. Within a week, the insurgents had destroyed over 200 sugar plantations on what had recently been some of the most profitable agricultural land on the planet. By September the slave army numbered 80,000; by December the entire colony was convulsing. Despite planter attempts to quash the rebellion, the unrest dragged on for years, with refugees escaping to all corners of the Atlantic world—especially to Charleston, Cuba, and New Orleans. In 1794, Toussaint Louverture, the former slave and self-styled "First of the Blacks," abolished slavery across Saint-Domingue, permanently dismantling the cycle of profit and death that had made the *grand blancs*—the wealthy whites—of Saint-Domingue and the French metropole so wealthy.[39]

Napoleon Bonaparte, France's republican-turned-monarch, wanted Saint-Domingue back. He saw the resurrection of the sugar industry, and thus the reinstatement of slavery, as the easiest way to remedy France's war-induced financial problems. In 1801 Napoleon sent the largest invasion fleet that ever crossed the Atlantic—some 65,000 men, including Polish, Swiss, Italian, and German mercenaries—to Saint-Domingue under the leadership of his brother-in-law, Charles Leclerc. Their mission was to crush the slave army, subdue any resistance by deception or force, and eventually return all surviving Africans to bondage. In February 1802 Leclerc landed in Le Cap, which had once been a city larger than Philadelphia and with more jewelers than London. He found it a smoldering ruin. French forces flew into a genocidal rage against the former slaves. Toussaint was captured and spirited away to a chilly prison in the Jura Mountains on the French-Swiss border, where he died. But the slave army continued, and in the summer of 1802 the revolutionaries counterattacked, aided and abetted by the tiniest warrior, the mosquito. Over a period of nine months, yellow fever killed 35,000 to 45,000 French soldiers. Adding these deaths to those lost on the battlefield brought the total death toll of the French army in Saint-Domingue to about 55,000 (the deadliest Napoleonic campaign except for the disastrous 1812 invasion of Russia). Of the 840 Swiss mercenaries in Leclerc's army, only 11 returned to Europe—a death rate so miserable that Swiss mercenaries never again agreed to serve in the West Indies. Leclerc himself perished from yellow fever, his skin turning bright yellow as blood poured out of every bodily orifice. Following this and many military setbacks, France permanently abandoned its mission to retake Saint-Domingue.[40]

Saint-Domingue's loss rippled throughout the French empire and threw its geopolitical strategy into disarray. Of what worth was a supply colony like Louisiana, 7,000 miles from Europe, without Saint-Domingue to supply? France began an imperial fire sale, offering not just New Orleans but all of Louisiana to the United States for a mere $15 million. Bonaparte lamented his "Louisianacide" but conceded it was his best worst option: the sale would bring France much-needed cash and keep Louisiana out of enemy British hands.[41] The young United States could not believe its luck. It had long considered the occupying power of New Orleans a "natural and habitual enemy" and would probably have gone to war to claim it at a later date. But now, as Alexander Hamilton put it, because of "the deadly climate of St. Domingue" and "the courage and obstinate resistance made by its black inhabitants," Louisiana had transferred to American hands.[42]

Hamilton knew the power of yellow fever. He had seen it as a child in Nevis, and like many framers of the Constitution he had survived it, after contracting a serious case in Philadelphia during that fateful summer of

1793.[43] By the end of the eighteenth century, most urban Americans were familiar with the disease. Yellow fever probably arrived in Britain's mainland colonies by the 1650s; the first recorded epidemics hit New York in the summer of 1668 and Boston in 1691. Two years later a boat from the Antilles carrying infected people sparked an outbreak in Charleston. Ports across the Atlantic seaboard experienced several small epidemics throughout the eighteenth century and were hit with some big ones at century's end. Yellow fever killed 5,000 people in Philadelphia in 1793, 5,000 more in 1798 in both Boston and New York, and 1,000 in Baltimore in 1800. Charleston, Savannah, and Norfolk saw multiple epidemics in the 1810s, each triggered when a Caribbean sloop docked in port with sick people on board.[44]

Given New Orleans's regular maritime contact with the West Indies, it was only a matter of time until yellow fever struck the Gulf Coast, too. It is impossible to prove that these outbreaks before 1796 were *yellow* fever, though the immunity Creoles displayed during later epidemics strongly suggests they were. Fevers of various descriptions visited Biloxi, New Orleans, and Mobile in 1702, 1704, and 1707. Following a royal decree in 1737 that provided a ten-year exemption from customs duties for all products exchanged between Louisiana and the West Indies, sea traffic between Martinique, Guadeloupe, Saint-Domingue, and New Orleans increased. This meant more people—and more *A. aegypti* mosquitoes—in Louisiana. In 1739 Henri de Louboey, one of King Louis XV's lieutenants in Louisiana, wrote a letter to Paris, reporting on trade, crops, and the Chickasaw campaign. He also noted that "*La Contagion*" was spreading rapidly among New Orleans's 2,000 inhabitants, killing people of all ages and sexes. An experienced colonial official, Louboey had probably seen yellow fever before. He had no doubt that this "mal de Siam" was yellow fever, and that it had been imported to New Orleans on a ship from Saint-Domingue. This disease would return to New Orleans in 1766, the year Antonio de Ulloa arrived with troops from Cuba to take possession of Louisiana for Spain.[45] During the 1790s with revolution and war convulsing the Atlantic, yellow fever fell like a hammer across the Greater Caribbean. As nonimmunes poured into New Orleans, the city had small outbreaks, likely of yellow fever, in 1791 and 1793. And by 1796, New Orleans had unknowingly secured all three of the elements necessary for a much more serious yellow fever episode: a hot climate, a healthy vector population of mosquitoes, and a large, cramped, and susceptible human population. All it would take was the arrival of a few infected mosquitoes or a recently infected person to spark a disease disaster.

New Orleans's first indisputable yellow fever epidemic struck in mid-July 1796, an epidemic so deadly and unprecedented that New Orleanians still spoke of it decades later. Perhaps 1,000 Spanish soldiers garrisoned just outside the city sickened or perished. At least 638 civilians also died, including "all of the laborers" building the Carondelet Canal connecting the city to Lake Pontchartrain, the brackish estuary three miles from town. By late August about fifteen to twenty people were dying each day, leaving the city's 7,500 inhabitants, as Spanish intendant Juan Ventura Morales described it, "terrified" and "in a state of consternation."[46] The rich chewed on astringent tree bark like *quinquinia* and had their servants soak themselves head-to-toe in vinegar. But bodies piled up faster than they could be buried. By the epidemic's end in November, 6 percent of New Orleans's population had died, or roughly 10 percent of all whites and more than a quarter of the "strangers." No reliable record of Black deaths, whether free or enslaved, exists for 1796. This does not mean Black people did not die from yellow fever, just that these deaths were not recorded—a statistical deficiency reproduced in later epidemics. Three years later, in 1799, another epidemic of "this cruel malady" killed almost 8 percent of New Orleans's population—once again mostly "strangers," but also Manuel Gayoso, the last Spanish governor of Louisiana. When yet another epidemic broke out in 1800, New Orleanians feared yellow fever was not a passing novelty. Perhaps this deadly trend would continue—even worsen—into the nineteenth century.[47]

Territorialism in Territorial Government

The United States inherited New Orleans in 1803 within this new disease context. But exactly *whom* had the United States inherited and how would they be governed? A hastily compiled 1803 census counted 8,050 city residents—making New Orleans the ninth-largest city in the United States—inclusive of 3,248 whites, 1,335 free people of color, 2,773 slaves, and 700 "undomiciled" people.[48] Within these groups there was wide ethnic, linguistic, and cultural diversity. The majority of New Orleans residents were Black, and most were Creole (categories that overlapped). Strictly speaking, a Creole was any person of any race born in Louisiana—but the term was used more loosely to refer to French- and Spanish-speaking people, mostly Catholics, and those who claimed French and Spanish ancestry. Thus "Creole" encompassed white people from other parts of the French Caribbean and Cuba and *gens de couleur libres,* most of whom had at least one white ancestor, spoke French, often owned slaves and property, and might have been educated abroad. At the time of the Purchase, only 13.5 percent of Orleans Territory's population was described as "American," a shorthand for white, recently arrived, English-speaking Protestants. Two-thirds of New Orleans's enslaved population had been born in Louisiana, the Caribbean, or the United States, and variably spoke English, Spanish, French, or Creole—sometimes all of them. About 1,000 people in New Orleans were African-born and spoke a wide array of African languages.[49]

Could America handle a sudden influx of new, un-naturalized people concentrated on a distant subtropical frontier? What about the white Creoles, many of whom held alien beliefs typical of French aristocrats and Caribbean grandees? And what about the city's majority Black population—many of whom were free and some of whom were incredibly wealthy? Against opposition from New England Federalists, a nervous, Republican-dominated Congress determined that Louisiana's territorial status would be extended indefinitely, until the "Mass of the Inhabitants"—shorthand for white and Francophone Creoles—disabused themselves of their European prejudices and embraced American law and custom. After a probationary period, which Jefferson branded an "apprenticeship to liberty," Louisianans could be "admitted to the rights, advantages, and immunities of citizens of the United States."[50]

But apprenticeships take years and the United States was in a hurry. The Purchase agreement, after all, was just a flimsy piece of paper, a promise from Bonaparte made an ocean away. Transition would be an immensely tricky task. The United States had to win over the powerful Creoles and transform them—on a compressed timeline—from territorial subjects into American citizens. To dilute the power of these *anciennes,* the federal government had to encourage the mass immigration of American-born easterners and get them enmeshed in the cotton and sugar industries. All laws, property claims, and tax schedules had to migrate to an American standard, and Louisiana's cotton and sugar economies had to be tied indelibly to eastern markets. Outside New Orleans, powerful Indian nations factored heavily in America's geopolitical imagination. The federal government calculated that it had to extinguish the title or violently seize the lands of the Creek, Choctaw, and Chickasaw—people who, in the federal government's estimation, held too much valuable real estate and failed to use it productively. Trickiest of all, America needed to regulate slavery in a place where *casta*—Spain's multilevel system of racial classification—had predominated for ninety years, where the majority of the inhabitants were Black, and where the influence of Saint-Domingue was significant.[51]

Aware that the "greatest enmity exist[ed] between the Creoles & English & Americans" and wanting to get a sense of the broad shape of power within the city, Governor Claiborne had an aide compile a confidential dossier on 119 of New Orleans's richest and most powerful men. The description of sitting mayor Étienne de Boré as a "man of mean extraction, without abilities either natural or acquir'd" was one of the more generous. James Pitot (a. YF ca. 1796), a future New Orleans mayor, was characterized as a man of "vanity . . . pedantry & arrogance" who thought of France as the "first of nations & himself the first Frenchmen."[52] Many were derided as gamblers, alcoholics, and men of "Creole morals." It was said of the well-connected planter Breton Orgenois that he could only pass "for an Oracle where Apollo has few Temples." It was said of Jean Baptiste Poeyfarré, "If Ten thousand words & phrases [were] cut out of as many Books [and] should be all jumbled together without any Order," that would give an idea of his intellect. Claiborne wrote to Secretary of State James Madison, "The attainments of some of the first people consist of little else than a few exterior accomplishments. Frivolous diversions seem to be among their primary pleasures: and the display of wealth and the parade of power constitute their highest objects of admiration." In turn, many Creoles balked at the presumption that they—the *anciennes*—had to undergo some vague and condescending "apprenticeship to liberty" in their own homeland. As they were not a conquered but a *purchased* people, was it not the *Mericain coquins* (rogue Americans) who had to prove their worth to them?[53]

Who would hold political power in New Orleans—the *anciennes* or new Americans? Excluding Creoles by fiat from the territorial government presented both political and logistical problems for the United States. Importing people of skill, patriotic zeal, and republican sympathies from the East for official jobs took time—at least three months, longer if the job required Senate approval. To be effective, whoever held power would have to be seen as credible and impressive by the Creole majority. Claiborne sought to thread the needle. He pressed Jefferson to appoint Dr. John Watkins (d. YF 1812) as territorial secretary, the second most powerful job in the territory. Watkins was American, a first cousin of Kentucky's Henry

Clay. He had lived in Upper Louisiana since 1797 and in New Orleans since July 1803. Not only was Watkins trilingual, but he also had "great influence among the People," having recently married into the Creole Trudeau family. Well-qualified, well-spoken, and well-liked, Watkins was also staunchly pro-American, writing in 1805 that "the American population must be increased, it must be made to overballance [sic] that of every other description of persons."[54]

Jefferson, who had never been to Louisiana, chose a different course. All of Louisiana's territorial government offices—governor, secretary, as well as three Superior Court judgeships—would be filled by American citizens to whom he owed political favors. Because New Orleans would also house a branch of the federal district court, Jefferson used his discretion within the Justice Department to give those slots to allies. He also leaned on the Treasury Department to install his friends at New Orleans's Customs House. As an olive branch, Jefferson conceded that a handful of less powerful though still locally meaningful municipal officers in New Orleans—like the mayor, city councilors, and court recorders—could remain (for a time) the provenance of Creoles.

Jefferson's preference for appointing older and already established outsiders was probably a reaction to the uproar caused when Claiborne—a man Creoles derided as too young and spineless for such a position—was appointed governor. Though Claiborne had represented Tennessee in Congress in 1797, succeeding Andrew Jackson at the age of just twenty-three (and two years under the constitutionally mandated age of twenty-five), he was a virtual unknown in the eastern political world. After the election of 1800, Claiborne was appointed governor and superintendent of Indian affairs in the Mississippi Territory, where his two major political achievements seem to have been eliminating a gang of outlaws and implementing a smallpox inoculation program. These were no small feats. But Jefferson probably settled on Claiborne for the territorial governorship because he was already close by. Jefferson privately called Claiborne a "secondary character" and for months continued to beg the Marquis de Lafayette and James Monroe, men of gravitas, to take the job. Both refused.[55]

Claiborne was aware he did not have Jefferson's full confidence. And as a young, monolingual "stranger in the Country," he was prepared for some local hostility. But he scarcely imagined how bad it would be. He reeled from having to defuse tensions among ethnic groups he did not understand. Official interpreters deliberately misconstrued his remarks; he was the punchline of jokes; French newspapers mocked his social awkwardness and blamed him personally for everything from the haphazard migration of land titles to the lack of Creole political representation to the weather. Hand-bills openly preaching insurrection against Claiborne, akin to those "used in France during the Revolutionary War," appeared on street corners.[56] Claiborne's was not the proud face of American power Jefferson had desired. But by the summer of 1804, with the epidemic killing people left and right, an alleged slave revolt looming, and a Creole insurrection taking shape, Jefferson decided he had no choice but to permanently install Claiborne as governor. This did not go over well. One *Louisiana Gazette* editorial written by "Fidelis" satirized Elizabeth Claiborne's death, suggesting that Claiborne was glad his wife had died so that he could make an advantageous marriage in the Creole community. Claiborne's brother-in-law challenged Fidelis to a duel and died from a bullet to his heart.[57]

In 1804 Jefferson made territorial appointments at a dizzying pace. For territorial secretary, he cast aside Watkins, whom he had never met, for James Brown of Kentucky (a. YF 1804), a close acquaintance. He installed another family friend, Hore Browse Trist of Virginia (d. YF 1804) as customs collector, appointed Republican allies Mahlone Dickerson from Pennsylvania as the district attorney (declined) and Dominic A. Hall from South Carolina (a. YF childhood) as US district court judge. Ephraim Kirby of Connecticut (d. YF 1804) and John Prevost of New York (a. YF 1804) received appointments to the Superior Court. All of these candidates were not only members of Jefferson's Democratic-Republican party, but also loyal to him personally and ideologically. Jefferson hoped that their eminence would assuage the Creoles and their skills would get American Louisiana rolling.

Slavery's Capital

The people who really got American Louisiana rolling, however, were the more than 51,000 enslaved Black people sold in New Orleans between 1803 and 1820. These people—described as "bright young men" and "first-rate cotton pickers" by avaricious traders—arrived in New Orleans traumatized, homesick, and exhausted, having just endured the Middle Passage across the Atlantic or the "Second Middle Passage" from the upper to lower South. They were sometimes sold in family units, but more often individually. Then most would be marched out of town toward a frontier where a veritable army of forced laborers dominated the landscape. In the first decades of the nineteenth century, enslaved people often arrived at plantations to find nothing but some surveyors' markers. All the land had to be cleared, all the structures built. Food was scarce. And they were forced, under threat of severe violence, to do the backbreaking labor of clearing thick, old-growth forest to "whittle a plantation right out of the woods." "All I had to do," recalled a former slave named Henry Clay, was to "cut down trees and grub sprouts all day every day." As soon as a patch was cleared, enslaved people began trenching the earth to get a first crop in the ground, working through sickness and understanding that failure could be as disastrous for them as for their owners. It could mean that they would be sold again.[58] The gruesome system meant that from the labor of the enslaved came vast wealth for the few. British traveler Thomas Ashe described the final eighty-mile stretch of his downriver journey from Natchez to New Orleans in 1806 as a scene of "uninterrupted" plantations bearing the names of the Deep South's richest white men: McDonogh, Villiers, Pitot, Boré, McCarty, and Poydras.[59] These plantations, like those across the Caribbean, consumed people—sites of physical, social, and spiritual death.

As plantations grew larger and more industrial in scale, where would labor be sourced? Since its French beginnings in the early eighteenth century, Louisiana had always depended on African labor. During the Spanish period from 1763 to 1801, Louisiana's planters imported about 12,000 enslaved Africans, mostly men and mostly from Kongo. When asked, white Louisianans said they preferred to purchase African-born slaves: not only were Africans cheaper and more abundant than Creole slaves, but many were also expert hunters and anglers, had experience cultivating rice and raising livestock, and were seasoned boatmen—an essential skill in Louisiana, where so much time was spent on water. There is also some evidence that Louisiana planters, drawing on the same racial-immunity "common sense" as planters in Martinique and Saint-Domingue, preferred to purchase people from regions where yellow fever and malaria were endemic. When given the choice, Louisianans opted to enslave people from Fernando Po (present-day Bioko, off the coast of Equatorial Guinea), an island "more detrimental to health than any spot in the known world," which was thought to produce a "healthy and athletic race of people." Louisiana's enslavers also appeared to prefer Krumen people (from present-day Liberia and Côte d'Ivoire), known for their "fortunate exemption from . . . deadly fevers," making their "service invaluable" across tropical zones.[60] Indeed, the vast majority of Africans sold on the Gulf Coast (or in Charleston to be re-shipped to Louisiana) originated from the Bight of Benin, Senegambia, and West Central Africa, areas where yellow fever was and is endemic. People from these regions had probably developed immunity as children or acquired it at the cramped slaving depots of western Africa—Ouidah, Lagos, Elmina, and Agoué—awaiting the Middle Passage.[61]

Above all other reasons, white Louisianans preferred African-born slaves because they were the most socially isolated people in the Americas. Unfamiliarity with European or other African languages diminished an African's ability to plot, a reality that took on new urgency following the revolution in Saint-Domingue. Consumed by stories of Saint-Domingue calamities, Louisiana planters began to take stock of their position within the larger transatlantic slave trade. Some began expressing doubt about how "African" the slaves for purchase in New Orleans actually were, worried their "harmless African[s]" were, in fact, "the wretches of St. Domingo Martinique & Jamaica" fraudulently foisted upon them. There may be some truth to this. After a long transatlantic passage, marked by disease and doldrums, captains usually made their first port of call in Rousseau, Cap Français, or Kingston and reprovisioned. But as the crew refilled water casks and restocked the ship's larder, some captains did side deals, selling their "best" slaves to cash-rich West Indians, buying low-cost replacements from the port jails to sell in Louisiana, and papering over these transactions in their ledgers. This, some captains argued, was the only way to make it economically feasible to travel the additional 1,100 miles to New Orleans—a journey that gave the cargo an extra week to revolt or die from disease.[62]

Even if such practices were rare, the Cabildo (New Orleans's colonial-era, planter-run city council) considered "trans-shipments" of slaves an existential threat, even part of an international conspiracy to topple Spanish power in North America. Soon their paranoia extended to *all* Caribbean slaves, who potentially carried the contagion of revolt. Louisiana's last Spanish attorney general claimed, "Our enemies will go to Jamaica to look for slaves, because there they will cost them only forty or fifty pesos each." These slaves would infect Louisiana's bondspeople "with the pestilence of rebellion . . . blow into the hearts of Negroes and mulattos the seductive venom and place in their hands iron and fire with which to destroy the whites."[63]

Like slaveholders everywhere, white Louisianans spoke of revolt as if it were an imported contagion, as if something external was needed to infect their otherwise contented slaves to want freedom.[64] And a slew of well-publicized, seemingly Saint-Domingue-influenced slave revolts in the 1790s (or rumors thereof) seemed to confirm the contagion theory. In 1791 Pierre Bailly, a free Black man in New Orleans, was tried on hearsay evidence for inciting an uprising modeled on Saint-Domingue. In 1795 an alleged conspiracy took place in Pointe Coupeé, a rough frontier area about 100 miles from New Orleans. As there was "no doubt that such insurrection could spread to all the populated areas of this province"—especially New Orleans—"and envelop it like a whirlwind," retribution was swift: of the fifty-seven slaves convicted, twenty-three were hanged, and the rest were whipped and exiled; syndic Juan de Castañedo paid the city hangman 430 pesos for his services. More plans for insurrections were allegedly discovered at Opelousas (150 miles northwest of New Orleans) in February 1795, in Point Coupeé again in 1796, and on the German Coast just northwest of New Orleans, also in 1796.[65]

In ultra-reactionary mode, the Cabildo banned the "introduction of Negroes of any kind" in 1795. But it loosened these restrictions the next year following heavy lobbying from planters. Enslavers, many of whom had just spent thousands of dollars building sugar works and were leveraged up to their teeth, proved very able to suppress their fears of slave revolt when their economic interests were at stake. As French traveler C. C. Robin concluded in 1802, the perennial thirst for slaves in Louisiana was "higher . . . than in any other French colony." With "so much land to cultivate," planters overwhelming priority was securing a continual supply of human property, Black and predominantly male. They would cross the revolt bridge if and when it came.[66]

For most of the eighteenth century, Louisiana's planters spent little time defending racial slavery as no one was attacking it. But their rhetoric shifted in the 1790s following the outbreak of unrest on Saint-Domingue and Louisiana's subsequent agricultural boom. Now, white Creoles claimed, their ability to tame Louisiana's wilderness and transform it into a productive agricultural region *required* the labor of *enslaved Black* people. White laborers were not an adequate substitute, because they died too quickly. Planters urgently appealed to Madrid, Paris, and Washington that no one would voluntarily do this work—clearing old-growth forests, draining swamps, and cutting cane. Sugar, in fact, required "long and hard work, expensive equipment, and such a quantity of men," planter Joseph Dubreuil de Villars told Jefferson, that "anyone undertaking its cultivation by day-laborers would be ruined within a year."[67] The cotton planters of Natchez made their position clear in a 1797 petition to Congress. Without the labor of enslaved Black people, they argued, "the farms in this District would be but of little more value to the present occupiers than [an] equal quantity of waste land." Before departing on his great exploratory mission in 1803, Meriwether Lewis related that white Louisianans would never relinquish the "right which they claim relative to slavery" in its "present unqualifyed [sic] shape."[68]

Unqualified meant just that: unlimited, unregulated, and especially unencumbered by international slave trading laws. Meanwhile, senators back East began debating the terms of Louisiana's governance in 1804. Everyone knew that slavery was the biggest question on the table. Over months of debate—and looking for a way to say yes and move on—many senators uncritically echoed claims about Black slavery's epidemiological necessity in Louisiana, summoning gothic descriptions of the Gulf Coast's climate. New Jersey Federalist Jonathan Dayton, one of the few senators who had actually been to Louisiana and survived yellow fever, argued that 1804 was not the right year to meddle with slavery as "our government is not yet established there." Moreover, he insisted, slavery protected fragile white constitutions. "Gentlemen from the north and east," Dayton claimed, "do not know that *white men* cannot indure [sic] the heat of a vertical sun."[69] Having "traversed a large portion" of the Deep South, Dayton believed that prohibiting slavery would "bar the cultivation & improvement of that extensive territory." His colleague James Jackson, Republican of Georgia, explained why free Black labor, abundant in New Orleans and Louisiana, was an unacceptable middle ground. "It is unfortunate that we have slaves," Jackson stated, "but having them we cannot with safety or policy free them. A very few *free negroes* in Louisiana would revolutionize that country." One free Black person, he added, was more dangerous "than . . . 100 slaves."[70]

Most congressmen appeared to accept wholesale Dayton's claims about Black bodies, though good-faith observers should have arrived at the opposite conclusion. The politically expedient path for most senators was to use these scientific "facts" about Black people and immunity to elevate the economic position of white Americans in Louisiana while also undercutting the Creoles. This was the motivating principle behind the Breckenridge Bill, sponsored by the Kentucky senator and secretly authored by Thomas Jefferson. It provided that after 1804, only white American citizens venturing into Louisiana could bring in or purchase enslaved people. These slaves had to be "safe," meaning they had to be either American-born or imported into the United States before 1798, and the "bona fide" property of their masters. Creoles would hereafter be cut off from obtaining more slaves, and thus, apparently, the growing cotton and sugar industries. Without access to slaves, the Creoles would watch their fortunes—and power—diminish.[71]

The Creoles Strike Back

Creoles were apoplectic. In December 1804 three Louisiana planters traveled to Washington to present the "Remonstrance of the Louisiana People" to Congress. This petition was signed by hundreds of Creole residents of New Orleans and ghostwritten by Edward Livingston (a. YF 1803, NY), a disgraced former mayor of New York who had risen to prominence in Louisiana and allied himself with the Creole community (into which he had recently married). All three delegates to Washington—Jean Noël Destréhan, Pierre Derbigny, and Jean Sauvé—were sugar planters or merchants. All three were major slaveholders. And all three knew that matters of epidemiology were as terrifying as they were ostensibly apolitical. The Remonstrance had been drafted at the height of the dreadful 1804 epidemic, after all, so the petitioners had Louisiana's diseased environment, one deeply "unfriendly" to "the labouring class of whitemen," on their minds.[72]

The Remonstrance is linguistically telling: the petitioners masterfully appropriated the political vocabulary of the American Revolution, using key phrases like "taxation without representation." Intermixed with revolutionary soundbites were complaints about Claiborne and the imposition of English as the official language. The petitioners' greatest concerns, however, were the impending ban on the African slave trade, the precariousness of white Creoles' continued access to slaves, and a potential outright ban on slavery. Descriptions of Louisiana's promising yet perilous climate—a place of unlimited, though as yet throttled agricultural potential—set the mood of the Remonstrance. Without Black slavery, preferably African slavery, the petitioners threatened, the land would descend into an untamable, swampy deathscape, and all of America could follow its decline: "This labor is great, it requires many hands, and it is all important to the very existence of our country. If, therefore, this traffic is justifiable anywhere, it is surely in this province." Should the Breckenridge Bill be enforced, they warned, so many white people would die that "the improvements of a century [will] be destroyed, and the great river resume its empire over our ruined fields and demolished habitations."[73]

Thomas Paine, America's most famous pamphleteer and propagandist, derided the Remonstrance as an arrogant assertion of rights; he cast Creoles as an American minority who claimed democratic rights only to enslave others. Paine feared their stupidity would "renew in Louisiana the horrors of Domingo." But by the early nineteenth century, white Americans were primed to accept the petitioners' claims about Louisiana's exceptional climate and Black people's exceptional immunity. Indeed, American planters and slave traders had become well versed in arguing that Black people of any origin were protected by God and nature from yellow fever; that Black immunity was not individual but intergenerational, passed down from parent to child through some alchemy of blood and skin.[74]

Back in Louisiana, matters were tense. Newspapers in every state reported that Louisiana's Creoles were on the brink of rebellion, with many reprinting the Remonstrance in full. One editorialist in the *Connecticut Gazette* related, "The people (I mean the ancient inhabitants) are extremely jealous of the American government . . . The night before last, a placard was posted in different parts of the city, calling on the people to revolt . . . They were told to recollect that the blood of the Gaul and the Castilian flowed in their veins, and that the present moment was the only one that would ever offer itself to assert their ancient dignity."[75] Even recently immigrated American farmers, slaveholders, and speculators—"men of no country"—worried about the precedent of federal intervention in what they claimed were local slavery issues. Whites in Louisiana seemed suddenly, and vocally, united on one issue: they would rather live under *any* power, even a European power, that would guarantee slavery than under an American government whose commitment to slavery seemed halfhearted. As John Watkins, Claiborne's confidential agent, urgently conveyed, a repeal of any restrictions on slavery "would go farther with them, and better reconcile them to the Government of the United States, than any other privilege."[76]

Congress understood it had to accept and endorse racial slavery in Louisiana now, or risk losing control over the territory altogether. As the epidemic raged across New Orleans in September 1804, Congress quietly divided Louisiana into two territories at the thirty-third north parallel (essentially creating the modern outline of the state of Louisiana) and ended its restrictions on the interregional slave trade, giving all white Louisianans legal access to *American*-sourced slaves. Congressional sanction for a domestic slave trade was not everything white Creoles wanted—they would have preferred a vigorous African slave trade too—but it was enough to satisfy their basic needs and maintain the racial status quo. And Louisianans had until 1808 to import as many African slaves as they could through South Carolina (the only state that still elected to have an open Atlantic slave trade). Between 1804 and 1808 alone, 46,648 Africans disembarked in South Carolina, many of whom were marched or shipped directly to New Orleans. For some white politicians back East this was a calamity. But most others easily assuaged their consciences, justifying that expansive Black slavery in Louisiana was better than the alternatives: mass white death from yellow fever or the loss of the territory altogether.[77]

Death and Tariffs

Early on, Anglo-Americans were genuinely scared that yellow fever would throw a wrench in the wheels of American government. The disease killed so many migrants that it embarrassed American authority. Those who would gamble their lives by moving to the Deep South for a *government* job were often at the end of long lists: people with good connections but few qualifications, many of them very young, disgraced, or otherwise unemployable. And in a place like New Orleans, an urban island in a sea of sugar and cotton fields, most white men saw public sector jobs as a steppingstone, a quick way to gain the necessary capital, prestige, and connections to parlay into a lucrative plantation. Many American politicians in New Orleans during Louisiana's territorial period were risk-seekers by nature, men of erratic judgment—bankrupts, criminals, hotheads—not the even-keeled bureaucrats required. Even when able candidates were identified from established political families—Clays, Monroes, and Adamses, for example—few were willing to relocate to this subtropical outpost to fill dead men's shoes. Kentucky congressman John Adair wrote to James Wilkinson (a Revolutionary War hero who had taken possession of Louisiana with Claiborne in 1803) that he would have liked a position in Louisiana but was afraid to go to such a diseased place until the government was more stable.[78] Adair's friend Henry Clay had also been interested in moving to New Orleans in 1806 to join the nascent government. But he was warned against it on disease grounds by his close friend US attorney James Brown (a. YF 1804): "I cannot *yet* advise you to change your establishment . . . I beg of you remain where you are." Disease created such a lack of viable candidates that when, in April 1806, Virginia congressman John Randolph proclaimed that "the antechambers of our great men were crowded with applicants for offices in Louisiana . . . for every office there were at least one hundred and fifty applicants," it was news to those actually trying to build an administrative state in New Orleans.[79]

Nowhere was disease a more obvious problem than in the all-important Customs House. In every American port city, customs collectors stamped out smuggling, tracked immigration, and controlled erratic foreign shipping. Most importantly, the collector levied customs or tariffs on foreign imports, the primary mode of federal funding prior to the Sixteenth Amendment, ratified in 1913, providing for an income tax. With the immense flow of goods and people into and out of the port of New Orleans, Claiborne believed the port's collector was "one of the most desirable jobs in the United States government"; emoluments for the position could reach thousands of dollars per annum.[80] In 1803 Jefferson appointed his friend and protégé Hore Browse Trist to the job. This ticked a lot of boxes for Jefferson. As the collector for Mississippi District, just eighty miles upriver in Natchez, Trist was already close by. And as a young man, Jefferson had known Trist's grandmother, Mary House, and boarded in her Philadelphia home during the 1780s. Trist's mother, Elizabeth, was wary of Hore Browse taking the job—her husband had died from yellow fever at Natchez twenty years before, and she was sure New Orleans was even more unhealthy. But nearly bankrupt and newly married, Hore Browse jumped at the opportunity. He begged his wife, Mary (described by many as the most beautiful woman in America), to leave Virginia and join him in Louisiana, which he insisted was healthy. He told Mary his job in government could provide a springboard to lavish wealth, perhaps even a sugar plantation to call their own. Trist boasted that he knew "upwards of 60 enumerated" individuals in New Orleans "whose annual *cash* revenue exceeds eight thousand dollars." Mary did join Hore Browse in New Orleans in August 1804, but their reunion was short-lived. He was dead from yellow fever within the month.[81]

In a high-risk place like New Orleans, where "talents [we]re as scarce as republicanism," yellow fever made it difficult to replace men like Trist.[82] Trist was succeeded by his brother-in-law, the dashing twenty-one-year-old William Brown (a. YF 1807). Jefferson agreed to the appointment partly because he hoped Brown would financially support his newly widowed sister. But Brown lived expensively, entertained disreputable friends, and frequented gambling halls. In 1808 Brown became the director of the Louisiana Bank on top of his government job. Then he purchased a plantation he could not afford and eloped with a teenager. In 1809 he absconded with $150,000 in federal notes, a huge sum considering that the Customs House in New Orleans raised just over $700,000 in revenue annually. Brown timed his escape well, fleeing at the height of the chaotic 1809 yellow fever epidemic while the government was dispersed and people were dying "without almost any warning." It took days for anyone to even notice he was gone. A communiqué, a type of all-points bulletin, was circulated around the Caribbean calling for Brown's apprehension. He was arrested and made partial restitution. But Brown's embezzlement and "fraudulent elopement," as the Bishop of Louisiana William DuBourg described it, were deeply embarrassing to the new American government.[83] After the Brown scandal, multiple candidates rejected the job of customs collector. Writing to Madison about the vacancy, Claiborne grumbled, "I know not another Citizen of this Territory, whom I would willingly recommend." Claiborne proposed headhunting a capable outsider of "sterling Integrity" and "pure Republicanism," suggesting that with a salary increase and the ability to "reside only one mile without the City of New-orleans" in a more healthful setting, they might secure a candidate who could rely on "enjoying health."[84]

Across government, yellow fever created so many sudden and prolonged job openings that giving a single person multiple full-time posts became standard practice. After the untimely death of John Ward Gurley (attorney general of Orleans Territory, aide-de-camp to the governor, and registrar of the Land Office) at the hands of Mary Trist's second husband in a duel, Claiborne appointed the French-born Revolutionary War hero Benedict Van Pradelles, already a notary public, as the new registrar of the Board of Land Commissioners in 1808.[85] This was no ceremonial title. Stabilizing land claims across thousands of acres claimed by Indigenous and colonial peoples, packaging it for sale to eagle-eyed cotton planters, and creating a standard system of ownership in fee simple was key to making American sovereignty an operational reality and a prerequisite for statehood. But as Congressman John Breckenridge of Kentucky described, land claims from the Spanish period were dubious, incomplete, and "dispersed over a great part of that extensive country several hundred miles . . . from the bank of the Mississippi." Few settlers had proper documentation, and in some parishes around New Orleans, registrars faced fifty or sixty competing claims to the same property. Each claim took commissioners weeks—if not months—to investigate, which led to problems with squatters. Van Pradelles was required to trek through miles of swampland, climb steep ravines, and traverse numerous cane breaks. As if this were not enough responsibility, Claiborne also appointed Van Pradelles a justice of the peace for Orleans Parish in the summer of 1808. Stretched impossibly thin, he held all these positions for only a short time, until he died from yellow fever in December, just six weeks after the birth of his son.[86]

Van Pradelles's death stalled the operation of the Land Office, underscoring the fact that effective governance required either acclimated personnel or multiple staffers with redundant capabilities. US attorney for Orleans Territory Philip Grymes (a. YF ca. 1811) took over as chief land commissioner at the beginning of 1809 while he was preoccupied with the high-profile prosecution of William Brown. Grymes wrote to the Treasury Department in May 1809 to explain why the land commission had completed so little work and would need until July 1810, a year and a half past deadline. "The failure to finish the business assigned to the Board within the limited time, is attributable," Grymes wrote, "to the death of Mr Gurley in the first instance, and Mr Van-Pradelles in the second." In the interim between their incumbencies the office had closed. The board therefore "ceased to act definitively upon any claim."[87] But the land commission was again delayed when its clerk, Mr. Dean, died from yellow fever in July 1810. Dean was the commission's sole repository of institutional knowledge and was "very much behind in his business," so the board was left in an "embarrassed situation." Then the commission ran out of money. Dean's replacement from Kentucky, Columbus Lawson, worked without pay for over a year, personally employing two secretaries to shave eighteen months off the project. It took the commission until June 1811—a further year past the already extended deadline—to stabilize the thousands of land claims in Orleans Territory and ready it for statehood.[88]

Judicial Immunity

Claiborne was most distraught about Louisiana's lack of judges and the instability of its court system as it shifted from civil law, an immensely complicated process often "betray'd into little Irregularities." On October 1, 1804, all colonial judicial authorities lost their positions and a new American Superior Court consisting of three judges was installed. But Louisiana had no written laws, let alone a settled system of precedents and procedures.

Instead, courtrooms were an "awful cacophony" of linguistic and judicial confusion. Litigants and lawyers often could not understand each other. The court of pleas, thrown together by Claiborne to handle disputes between residents, was an almost comical "confusion worse than that of babel." Most concerning of all, there were no judges to head up these lesser courts. Judicial candidates seemed especially sensitive to the prospect that a stint in New Orleans might result in "sudden Death," a risk that dimmed the allure of the $2,000 salary.[89]

Jefferson had initially appointed three men to fill the Superior Court bench. The first appointee, French-American jurist and Revolutionary War veteran Peter Stephen Du Ponceau, declined. The second, Ephraim Kirby—a many-times-wounded Revolutionary War veteran, many-times candidate for Connecticut governor, and first general high priest of the Royal Arch Masons—died of yellow fever in early October *en route* to New Orleans, a "Serious misfortune" to the territory, as well as to his widow and eight children.[90] The third, John B. Prevost—a lawyer holding a minor judicial position in New York City, and stepson of Aaron Burr—was the only American judge to actually make it to New Orleans. He did not arrive until late October 1804 and had to rule immediately on a complicated case concerning Spanish property claims. Soon, he was "labour[ing] under considerable difficulty" and so overwhelmed with cases that he resorted to one-line decisions. Then he fell sick with yellow fever, reportedly ailing from the bench as he plowed through the cases before him.[91] Prevost survived. His wife did not. He remained the lone Superior Court judge for over two years, and soon quietly refused to hear many cases concerning prominent merchants and planters. Then he bought Laurent Sigur's sugar plantation about a mile below the city with its sugar works and thirty-five slaves following a bankruptcy adjudication he had ordered. Prevost transitioned out of Louisiana public life, now a wealthy man.[92] The politicking-to-plantation pipeline had worked—at least for him.

Understandably, future candidates for the Superior Court expressed apprehension about New Orleans, leaving Jefferson "very much puzzled to find judges who can speak French." Jefferson appointed George Duffield of Tennessee, but he resigned for health reasons in July 1805. Rufus Easton of New York was then offered the slot but became so embroiled in Aaron Burr's conspiracy that Jefferson never submitted his name to Congress. It took until 1806 for the Superior Court to reach three members: George

Mathews of Mississippi Territory (a. YF childhood), William Sprigg of Ohio (a. YF ca. 1807), and Joshua Lewis of Kentucky (a. YF ca. 1809). Mathews himself admitted that he was not particularly esteemed, but "in an unhealthy Climate & with a moderate Salery [sic]," he was "determined to accept" the job for the sake of the nation.[93]

The chaos inflicted by yellow fever on Louisiana's legal system caused justice to be delayed and thus denied on multiple occasions. The most colorful incident, later satirized by Washington Irving, involved a military tribunal convened in New Orleans on July 1, 1805, to try Colonel Thomas Butler for disobedience and mutinous conduct. Butler had refused to cut his long hair, enraging his superior officer, the famously tempestuous General James Wilkinson. The trial proceeded in great haste because of the mounting epidemic. All three judges fell sick mid-trial; Judge Richard Sparks heard most of the testimony from bed. Immediately after the trial ended, on July 10, the courtroom scattered. The judgment against Butler was not issued until September: he was found guilty and sentenced to a year's suspension from duty, rank, and pay. But it was too late. Butler had died of yellow fever the month before. On his deathbed Butler apparently begged his friends to drill a hole in the bottom of his coffin to let his long hair hang out, a final insult to General Wilkinson.[94]

The obvious solution to the government's disease problem was to hire Creoles. That started to happen more often, though quietly. In the spring of 1807 Claiborne recommended that either Julian Poydras (a French-born sugar planter) or Jean Baptist Macarty (a Creole planter) be appointed as territorial secretary, the second most powerful job in Louisiana. The first three customs collectors had been American-born (and largely disastrous), but their successors were Creoles with strong commercial interests in cotton, sugar, and New Orleans, including the Saint-Domingue-born merchant Pierre Francois Dubourg de St. Colombe (1813 to 1814), the Creole planter Pierre Le Barbin Duplessis (1814 to 1816), and the Virginia-born but New Orleans–raised merchant Beverly Chew (1817 to 1829). Creoles might have questionable morals and politics, but at least they did not die.[95]

Another solution adopted from colonial and Caribbean precedents was to effectively shutter government during the fever season—roughly July to November—hoping to prevent Louisiana's "most useful citizens" from falling victim "to this fatal disease." Even acclimated Americans like Claiborne worked during the summer from Point Coupée or Mandeville, spas and "watering places" a few dozen miles from New Orleans considered *just* safe from yellow fever. And it was not as if the territorial or city governments were stepping back from fervent activity. During city government's most active period, from November to May, its function whittled down to three essential matters: maintaining a "very active surveillance" over the growing Black population, protecting white people's private property, and ensuring the smooth movement of goods and people through the port.[96]

Boom Times

The continual attrition caused by yellow fever was demoralizing to those in government. But for those whites at the top of the private sector—*anciennes* and an increasing number of acclimated Europeans and white Americans—business was booming. Merchants and planters complained when disease disrupted their activities or killed off their clerks. But most also recognized that death was not a structural problem *per se* as long as people—whether lured by the prospect of cotton wealth or forced through slavery—kept coming to replace those killed in the previous epidemic.

And come they did. Free and enslaved people from points north and east flowed in. In 1809 a sudden influx of about 9,000 French and Spanish-speaking Saint-Domingue refugees landed in the city by way of Cuba, more than doubling New Orleans's free population of color. These boats carried so many people that New Orleans became the fifth-biggest city in the nation by 1810, with a population exceeding 17,000 that included 5,000 free people of color, 6,000 slaves, and about 6,500 whites. There was plenty of work as more and more goods poured in from the vast stretches of the Upper Mississippi Valley, all the way up to Pittsburg. New Orleans's precise rate of growth is difficult to determine before 1815, but the value of receipts from the Upper Mississippi Valley alone increased from about $1.5 million annually, in 1801–1803, to $3 million by 1807. Staple exports rose from 5,000 hogshead of sugar and 18,000 bales of cotton in 1802 to nearly 10,000 hogshead of sugar (and molasses) and 42,000 bales of cotton in 1810. That year, thousands of flatboats, keels, barges, and ocean-faring vessels were so densely packed along the levee that a sailor could traverse the entire length of the city hopping from deck to deck. Soon steamboats would be docking there, too, propelling people and goods up and down the Mississippi faster than ever before.[97]

Strangers were everywhere. Some were wealthy men, the second sons of Boston businessmen or agents of European banks, seeking to invest capital in Louisiana. But a growing number of strangers were poor. They threw up crude lodgings, lived cheek-by-jowl in shotgun shelters, and crowded the levee looking for work. The influx of people changed the look, feel, and size of the city. Swamps at the "back of town"—land owned by Claude Tremé—were drained and subdivided for housing. To the east, Bernard Marigny, a fabulously wealthy Creole planter and real estate developer, sold his family's downriver plantation to the city for use as a new *faubourg,* or suburb. As the city swelled out from the original walled town, Canal Street became the unofficial divide between the Creoles of the French Quarter and the enterprising eastern transplants of St. Mary's.

Bigger was not necessarily better. As the city became more crowded, and more demand was put on already scant infrastructure, it also became filthier—and the gap between rich and poor grew starker. One astute visitor, Saint-Domingue physician Paul Alliot, observed that many homes in New Orleans were dilapidated, their roofs falling in, and displayed "a depth of poverty which is surprising."[98] Even rich families drank water straight from the Mississippi or else from wells dug next to the latrines in their backyards. There was no streetlighting or sewerage. The roads were so potholed that a clumsy or drunk passerby could fall into and drown in the deceptively deep pits.[99] There was no college or public library. The Charity Hospital was falling down. Butchers slaughtered animals in the streets, leaving blood, excrement, and offal to be fought over by packs of feral dogs.[100]

The Creole Strategy

The city was filthy and very unhealthy. But for Claiborne and others, the way to make Louisiana "safer"—for whites—was to make slavery more structurally and legally American. That meant suppressing enslaved and free Blacks in this majority Black city. Black people, who had been declared immunologically superior to whites, would be made even more legally inferior. White Americans in Louisiana never trusted *gens de couleur libres,* alleging that they were behind all manner of plots to topple American power in New Orleans. In October 1805, for example, a free Black man named Stephen alleged that "certain Creoles of Colour" had secretly met to "concert plans of hostility against the Americans."[101] These men were armed,

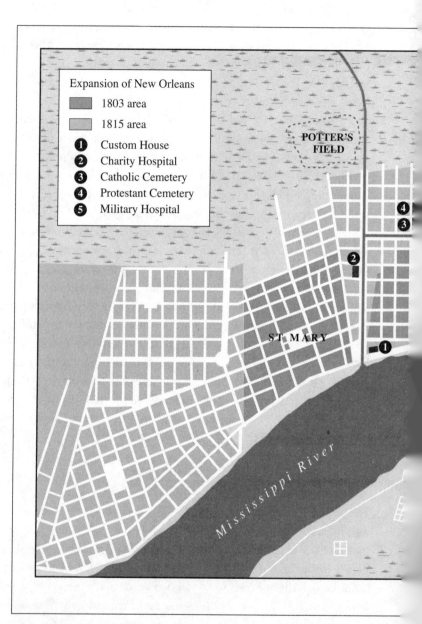

New Orleans, ca. 1815.

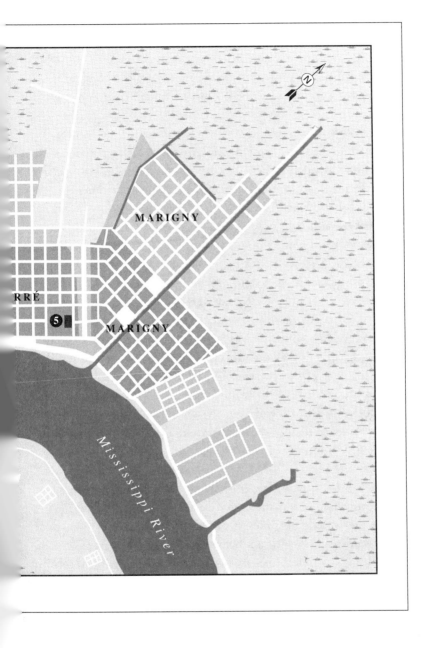

MARIGNY

MARIGNY

RRÉ

⑤

Mississippi River

organized, and would simultaneously attack the city at the call of a "WHOOP," aided by "one or two nations of Indians." Then two houses a few blocks from Place des Armes were burned to the ground, maybe from arson. The gendarmes made arrests, and a stockpile of arms was discovered. Around-the-clock surveillance was placed on the house of Mr. Mils behind the Charity Hospital, alleged to be a gathering place for free Blacks, runaways, and plotting slaves.[102]

Responding to events like this, in 1806 Claiborne invited the Territorial Legislature to address the alleged problem of slave crimes. Delegates pounced on the opportunity to redefine the entire master–slave relationship with a new Black Code, mixing colonial precedents with American enforcement. This Black Code—borrowing elements from far-flung sources like the 1724 *Code Noir*, the *Loi Municipale* of 1778, and even South Carolina's notoriously harsh Negro Act of 1740, promulgated in the wake of the Stono Rebellion—was the most repressive slave code in New Orleans's history. It classified slaves as real estate, defined now as the "passive" extension of their master. It also overturned the Spanish laws on slavery and manumission that were still in effect. Enslaved people could now expect no more than half an hour for breakfast, could not own property or carry weapons, could not ride on horseback, and could not drink alcohol. The Code even stripped slaves of their customary property rights to garden plots, chickens, and artisanal tools. Then, in 1807, the legislature ended the slave's right to self-purchase or *coartación*—which had been law across the Spanish Americas for three centuries—and banned the in-migration of any free Black person from any state or Caribbean island, with the penalty being (re-)enslavement. Notaries were instructed to insert racial markers after the names of free Blacks, "fcl" or "hcl" for *femme* or *homme de couleur libre*. The legislature also criminalized insults and physical assaults by free Blacks against whites, stating they should not "presume to conceive themselves equal to the white . . . [but] ought to yield to them in every occasion."[103]

White people in New Orleans had created a legal state that affirmed their power over Blacks. But how else could Anglo-Americans prove their worth to the white Creoles, in a place where the inadequacy of "Yankee" blood was on full display each fever season and where the public sector hemorrhaged personnel? The strategy the white American elite developed, ever more explicitly, was to embrace yellow fever; if Creoles held immunity as a matter of nature, white immigrants could earn it through rugged nurture.[104] All of the most famous and successful American- and European-born merchants and slaveholders of New Orleans's early years incorporated their acclimation into their genesis stories, staking their claim to status, wealth, and power on their triumph over disease. Each of the following in this guild of the immune had started out as "strangers": Irish merchant Maunsel White (a. YF 1801); merchant and customs collector Beverly Chew (a. YF ca. 1796); merchant and cashier of the Louisiana State Bank Richard Relf (a. YF ca. 1801); land speculator and purported richest man in America Daniel Clark (a. YF ca. 1801); Scottish-born merchant and land speculator John McDonogh (a. YF ca. 1801); future president Zachary Taylor (a. YF 1809), banker and insurance magnate Joseph Saul (a. YF 1804); and merchant Vincent Nolte (a. YF 1806).[105]

Acclimation—an invisible and unstable marker—could not be transferred to others. But these "intelligent old gentlemen" passed on the *knowledge* of how to become acclimated. Cotton factors offered their clerks tips on the best nurses, reminding them to stay temperate and eat a specific diet. Merchants told recent transplants that yellow fever was very dangerous to the newcomer, but on the other side of disease, Louisiana could be their oyster, the only place in America where "the true spirit of commerciality reigns supreme" and where, as German immigrant Johann Joachim Lagemann put it, the "right and moral value of a person is measured by the size of his moneybag."[106] Bankers told the ambitious that a paltry government salary was not worth their while—that smart men got acclimated, leaned on their connections, and went into cotton. By 1810, declaring oneself an "acclimated citizen"—like declaring oneself white or free—was a claim to an identity. These men effectively became New Orleans "natives," not to the manor born, but epidemiologically sound. Many white immune people classified survival as a patriotic act, a public demonstration of fidelity to the expansion of the Cotton Kingdom and America's westward project writ large. Some even redubbed yellow fever the "patriotic fever." Facing it down, they claimed, required no less bravery than that displayed by Continental soldiers at Yorktown. As James Brown wrote to Henry Clay from New Orleans in 1806, he had "every reason to believe" that he and his wife Nancy were acclimated. Now "fearless of the danger," Brown could look forward to "many happy days in the Country."[107]

With acclimation serving as the difference between obscurity and wealth for white people, Black people's alleged natural immunity increasingly had the opposite effect. It was used to justify slavery's permanence and expansion. But what would happen to this theory of racial immunity when it was explicitly tested and disproved thousands of times in Louisiana, just as it had been in Philadelphia in 1793? This sticky matter came before Louisiana's courts in 1809, when a seasoned slave-buyer and justice of the peace named William Dewees sued a planter named Morgan under Louisiana's redhibition statute, a Spanish legal concept with Roman antecedents that gave the buyer of a defective "product" recourse against the seller. Dewees sued for a full refund of the money he had paid for a man who had died from yellow fever ten to twelve days after purchase. Morgan's lawyer argued that at auction, purchasers took on all risks and that given "the lowness of the price, and the season of the year," Dewees should have known better and made his decisions with "an eye to the probable danger." Joshua Lewis (a. YF ca. 1805), the lone judge deciding the case, found in Dewees's favor and ordered Morgan to repay the purchase price.[108]

This case seemed to acknowledge what was probably a widely known fact: Black people could and did die from yellow fever. But *Dewees v. Morgan* was the first of only two lawsuits explicitly concerning yellow fever and Black people heard by Louisiana's courts. After 1809 yellow fever was reclassified from a "redhibitory vice" to a "curable disease"—therefore the evanescence of Black immunity was put outside the court's purview.[109] Slave owners would have to grapple among themselves with the contradiction between theoretical Black immunity and the reality of Black sickness. And by the end of the territorial period—with the number of slave-dependent plantations growing exponentially and the population of New Orleans doubling every three years—recasting racial slavery as a health imperative provided a veneer of rationality, even respectability, to its violence. Whites argued that domestic slavery—that is, "safe" slaves sourced from within the United States—had the happy effect of neutralizing Louisiana against the threat of Haitian ideology *and* local climate, paving the way to a full-blown, muscular Cotton Kingdom. The system, simply, was already too entrenched to bend to the terrifying epidemiological reality.

From Territory to State

According to the census of 1810, Orleans Territory had enough white people—more than 60,000—to petition for statehood. By this point it had stabilized most of its land claims, established a functional legal system, and developed a lean but operational government. There were still some white Creole naysayers unconvinced by American governance, but most had been brought on side by the federal government's commitment to increasing slavery, the booming cotton and sugar markets, and white people's now legally codified personal domination over Black people. In January 1811, however, cataclysm struck as Black people fought back. A few miles above New Orleans on the German Coast, the largest slave revolt in American history exploded. Led by a Creole slave driver named Charles from the plantation of Manuel Andry, the overwhelming majority of the 500 insurgents who slogged through knee-deep mud toward New Orleans were Africans from Kongo, Gold Coast, and Bight of Benin. Inspired by Saint-Domingue insurgents, they attacked the plantations of American and Creole planters alike, cutting a swath of destruction through the bayous. Many white Louisianans remembered 1804 and feared the rebels this time would successfully burn New Orleans to ashes. But whites counterattacked. Claiborne blocked the Bayou Bridge with twenty-five supernumeraries of the city guard, then the US army and planter militias surrounded the rebelling slaves. Sixty-six poorly armed Black people were mutilated, dismembered, and beheaded on the spot. Though only two whites died, a hastily assembled tribunal of planters condemned eighteen more enslaved men to execution by firing squad and twenty-one more to decapitation. Their heads were put on spikes along the Mississippi River as a warning. As was true in slave societies across the Atlantic world, brutality against Black people had become the chief function of the state, a state by and for slaveholders.[110]

And unlike the colonies of the British West Indies, which had refused to join with the mainland colonies during the American Revolution, Louisiana wanted to become an American state.[111] On the first Monday of November 1811, forty-three elected delegates were supposed to gather at a New Orleans coffeehouse to draft Louisiana's constitution. But "apprehensive of the Fever," it took until December for a quorum to gather. The document, drafted by three future Louisiana governors, five future US senators, a future congressman, and one future minister to France, sailed to unanimous approval on January 26, 1812. Louisiana's constitution broke with every eastern precedent. It gave the governor extraordinary power. It set very high bars to voting. A key provision concerned elections, set for the "first Monday in July every two years," a tactic Creoles had used to temper Anglo-American power, as that was the precise moment newcomers and strangers were most likely to be sick with or fleeing from yellow fever.[112] New Orleans's city government was hardly more democratic. City councilors were elected, but the franchise had been made so restrictive that they might as well have been appointed. To vote, a person had to own a quantity of bank stock, or possess a billiard table, or have paid taxes on substantial property, essentially limiting suffrage to the richest planters and merchants. Moreover, voters had to have been continuously resident in the state for two years, all but ensuring they had lived through a yellow fever epidemic. The armies of clerks, dockworkers, and draymen were *de facto* excluded, as were free people of color, all women, and the enslaved. Finally, the new state constitution was made essentially impossible to amend; it was never altered during its thirty-three years of existence.[113]

Louisiana's apprenticeship to liberty had come to an end. In some sense, its white Creoles had won. This was a racially and epidemiologically stratified society in which whites could achieve riches if they simply survived, and where a sea of Black slaves labored in perpetual fear of state-sanctioned violence and yellow fever. The consequences of this high-risk, high-reward system, and the repetitive slaughter it engendered, would radiate through Deep Southern society.

2

Danse Macabre

In August 1819, Sylvester Larned, the twenty-two-year-old minister of New Orleans's newly established First Presbyterian Church, faced the most difficult moral dilemma of his career: Should he stay or should he go? Did he, an unacclimated Northerner, have an obligation to remain in town during the city's worst yellow fever epidemic in memory? Or should he flee and protect his health but abandon his fledgling congregation in this moment of profound crisis?[1]

Like most unacclimated strangers, Larned had not sufficiently considered the threat yellow fever posed to his life and prospects. His professors at Princeton Theological Seminary had warned him about Louisiana's dangerous climate. But when he accepted the posting, they had also assured him that New Orleanians (about 41,000 strong by 1818) craved his "Bible truth": that death was the consequence of original sin, that a retributive God saved some and damned others, and that no human action affected one's chance of salvation. Larned was cheered to see a crowd of 7,000 people turn out that January of 1819 to witness the completion of his new church, built in plain gothic style. But the peoples' religious enthusiasm seemed to dissipate. Larned attracted few Catholic Creoles to his congregation—they had their own churches and seemed uninterested in his message anyway. And while he had initially believed his "usefulness" among New Orleans's Protestants would be "literally boundless," he found few Anglo-Americans absorbed the tenets of Presbyterianism either. Townspeople seemed more interested in cotton prices and debating Missouri's pending statehood than in salvation. By spring Larned came to feel as many did, that in New Orleans "Death and the Devil" held "undisputed possession of the souls of men."[2]

Then yellow fever arrived in July. These were not "good deaths." At bedsides, Larned saw no affirmations of faith, no serene goodbyes to gathered family. Instead, jaundiced victims screamed at God, hallucinated, and wept for mothers through tears of blood. Exhausted by the endless stream of funerals and terrified of dying, Larned made the quiet decision to pack a bag and leave town on August 10, telling those who asked that he was attending to urgent business upriver at the St. Francisville Presbytery.[3]

In late October Larned returned to a city transformed. Between 2,190 and 6,000 people had died from yellow fever, the majority of whom were "as usual . . . emigrants from the northern states, and different parts of Europe." At least 501 registered Protestants had died, including Methodists, Episcopalians, and Presbyterians.[4] At Potter's Field, bodies of the poor and enslaved that had been interred in September had started to literally "reappear." Bloated, half-decayed corpses—propelled upward due to the inexorable power of buoyancy—were sticking out of the ground, and errant limbs were being eaten by dogs, crawfish, and birds. As the sun beat down, the corpses released such a putrid stench that the city council hired enslaved men to fish out the dead and burn them on massive pyres. Conditions and morale in town were so terrible, in fact, that one person declared New Orleans "the most wretched hole in the universe," wherein a person "has one third the number of lives of a cat—for in the first place he is *murdered* by the yellow fever, in the second he is *drowned,* and in the third he is *burnt.*"[5]

Demoralized, angry survivors searched for a scapegoat and Larned fit the bill. Newspapers castigated him as a coward in English and French, questioning whether his escape was "consistent with the character and obligations of a *Protestant* clergyman." Some mused whether a man who would "desert his people in periods of calamity and general suffering" believed in God at all. In contrast, the press hailed Catholic priests like Father Patrick Walsh (d. YF 1806), the vicar general of Louisiana, who had remained in town despite the risk, continued to perform last rites, and died a veritable martyr.[6]

Larned stood chastened before his considerably thinned congregation and apologized. Adopting the soldier's motto *"Victory or death,"* he promised to never again leave town during an epidemic. He kept his word: the following summer of 1820, he maintained his services even as a larger yellow fever epidemic ripped through the city. He visited the sick at their bedsides, baptized newborns, and performed dozens of funerals. He also made calls at the Charity Hospital, an institution that, despite recent renovations, barely had any medicine or food for patients. How could God condemn any of these poor and frightened folk to damnation, Larned wondered? Were they not already living in hell on earth in New Orleans?[7]

By July there was a marked shift in Larned's sermons. He now emphasized God's unconditional love, not damnation. He preached benevolence and universal salvation. By August he stopped talking about original sin. And on Sunday, August 27, he delivered an unusually impassioned sermon on the glory of everlasting life. Red-faced and giddy, he did not linger after services but instead hurried home. Within hours Larned developed an intense headache, weakness, and diarrhea. His new wife, Sarah Wyn (whose two merchant brothers had just died from yellow fever and whose mother and infant child would soon die from it), panicked and sent for the doctor, who dosed him with a constant stream of castor oil and mercury. Larned hung on for days. As he grew more anxious and delirious, he repeatedly asked the doctor if he had yellow fever and if he was going to die. At ten o'clock Thursday morning, he began regurgitating black vomit. By 6 p.m. the doctors could not detect his pulse. And at 10 p.m.—on his twenty-fourth birthday—Larned was declared dead. His last words were from Philippians: "To me to live is Christ, to die is gain."[8]

Larned's rejection of traditional Calvinism at the end of his life might have been part of a larger religious journey cut short—during the Second Great Awakening, the Protestant religious revival of the early nineteenth century, many Americans' relationship with God had changed. But yellow fever certainly catalyzed his theological transformation, just as it would for many men of God in New Orleans. His replacement, a Massachusetts-born man named Theodore Clapp, started off as a strict Calvinist, emphasizing punishment, the doctrine of the holy trinity, and spiritual election. But in 1834, following a dual yellow fever–cholera epidemic, he abandoned the teachings of Presbyterianism and resigned his ministry. From his new "Stranger's Church," Clapp developed a more ecumenical style, frequently lauding Catholics, celebrating their charity, and declaring that only Trinitarianism kept him from converting.[9] Eventually Clapp formally became a Unitarian, believing it was the only way to be a godly man in sickly New Orleans. According to Clapp, the city's mainstream religious tradition—as generations of priests, rabbis, rectors, and parsons would also discover—was morbid and simplistic. Catholics and Protestants here wanted their priests to offer a set of clearly defined rules. Obsessed or oppressed by cotton—and constantly nervous about their health—the people had little capacity for messages beyond God's forgiveness for their sins and the promise of eternal reward.[10] Whether "Jews, Gentiles, Pagans, Mahometans, Protestants, Catholics, gold worshipers, [or] disciples of mammon," as abolitionist Philo Tower mused, all New Orleanians became "lovers of pleasure more than lovers of God" in the end.[11]

Living among the Dead

By 1820, most Americans were well aware of New Orleans's unusual sickliness. Tourists routinely commented on the city's many beautiful, if expansive, cemeteries; obituaries and articles about yellow fever in New Orleans were nationally syndicated; in letters and travelogues, visitors took pains to vividly capture the strangeness of life amid an epidemic. Often, outsiders expressed shock at the locals' complacency toward mass death and many balked at the fatalistic culture yellow fever fostered. British traveler Henry Tudor remarked that yellow fever gave New Orleans "a character . . . totally different" from that "of every other in the United States." When asked how New Orleans compared to Richmond, Virginia, one immigrant responded, "not half so well," due to its "black legs" and "black vomit." Traveler Adam Hodgson also was unimpressed with New Orleans: "When I think of the moral pollution which pervades New Orleans, and the yellow fever which annually depopulates it," Hodgson wrote, "or of the intermittents and slavery which infest its vicinities, the rocky shores of New England have a thousand times more charms for me." Noting how disease kept people suspicious and indoors, British abolitionist Harriet Martineau called yellow fever "a serious evil to sober families."[12] Other visitors were disgusted by the grotesque comingling of life and death and the nonchalance with which everyone—even children—eventually approached death. Several visitors expressed horror at seeing children "engaged in the most joyous merriment" outside cemeteries while old women sold ice cream, everyone seemingly unconcerned by—or numb to—"the gloomy spectacle within."[13]

Yellow fever did make every second or third summer in New Orleans gloomy. But epidemics were events so convulsive that their aftershocks rippled across the whole calendar year, impacting the pace of business, corrupting the region's culture, and creating a sense of impermanence that was impossible to miss. There was little good information about yellow fever to give people comfort. Though doctors debated the disease's transmission, etiology, and pathology with "theological dogmatism," even these experts could not answer basic questions about the scourge. How did yellow fever spread? Was it carried by persons, spread in the air, or transmitted through water? Was it contagious? Was it imported or native to the region? What were the most effective treatments? Were Black people and Creoles naturally immune? Was it a discrete disease, or a mixture of fevers? Did a doctor's attention actually help?

In the absence of answers or reliable mortality data, New Orleanians developed crude systems—cultural, medical, and commercial—to live with yellow fever and manage their fears. Some turned to God, others drank. Some dueled, others composed songs, ballads, and poetry to "Bronze John."[14] Still others resorted to gallows humor. The opportunistic found ways to monetize the disease, figuring out "how to make money from filth"—so much money, in fact, that health became New Orleans's third major industry, behind cotton and slavery. Doctors charged extortionate "yellow fever rates." Gravediggers upped their prices in August. Lawyers charged high premiums during the fever season. Shopkeepers hiked up their prices and sold all goods—flour, shoes, wood, candles—"at northern prices." Indeed, all products came to "bear an enormous price" during epidemics, making both dying and living "extremely dear."[15]

When the first frosts descended and yellow fever abated, the market refocused its attention on cotton. The dead were quickly forgotten. But as Baron Ludwig von Reizenstein, a minor German noble, offered in his sprawling 1854 novel *The Mysteries of New Orleans,* this city "is the spring from which so many thousands have drawn their wealth, but it is also a bitter cup of suffering, misery, and despair." Inhabitants knew that if anyone could die, *everyone* was replaceable; if no one could plan ahead, *everyone* lived reckless for the future—speculating wildly, risking fortunes, and inuring themselves to an incredibly high level of violence. New Orleans, Reizenstein concluded, was "the whore insatiable in her embraces, letting go of her victims only after the last drop of blood has been drained and their innermost marrow of life sucked dry." Everyone sank into this *danse macabre* eventually—living, spending, loving, worshipping, and dying according to yellow fever's rhythms.[16]

A Disease Sui Generis

Though antebellum New Orleans contained thousands of self-styled yellow fever experts, no person actually knew much about this disease—or, at least, not much more than had been established two centuries earlier.[17] Yellow fever was custom-built for confusion. Not only did its victims die quickly and violently, but it also killed with seeming randomness. Doctors were flummoxed by how it spread. "Fifty *times* have I had my hands and face besmeared with the putrid blood, black vomit, or the foetid slimy matter of perspiration," Dr. Dupuy De Chambery wrote in 1819, but he had never, to his knowledge, been infected by the disease. Dr. Ashbel Smith, surgeon general of the Republic of Texas, wrote that during postmortem examinations he regularly handled "every organ without squeamishness; immersing [his] hands freely in the black vomit and other fluids; smelling and viewing them closely." Smith added that he had "*repeatedly tasted black vomit,* when ejected from the stomachs of the living; and I am not aware of ever having experienced further inconvenience or effect than fatigue."[18]

Heeding the prevailing "environmentalist" framework of disease communicability, most antebellum physicians argued that yellow fever—unlike smallpox, yaws, plague, and syphilis—was "noncontagious," meaning it was not spread between humans through microbes. Instead, it was "miasmatic," the organic result of the city's heat, filth, climate, soil, and meteorology.[19] Drawing on the theories of Greek philosopher Galen, Dr. Daniel Drake attributed New Orleans's acute yellow fever problem to foul "airs"—the result of local filth and poor sanitation. He wrote, "from the dwelling houses, taverns . . . oyster-sheds, sugar wharves, and cotton-presses, a vast quantity of filth, and organic recrements, find their way into the water's edge." When "subjected to solar influence," this waste produced dangerous, fever-causing miasmas.[20] Densely packed with people, animals, and garbage, cities were especially dangerous. But nowhere in the Lower Mississippi Valley was entirely safe from yellow fever, and many approached swamps and cane fields with caution. Margaret Brashear (d. YF 1834), a sugar planter in lower Louisiana, recounted the death of her overseer in 1830 at plantation Belle Isle, about fifty miles south of New Orleans. "Poor Mr. Priel is dead," she lamented to her son. After Priel "went into the swamp with a number of our Negroes for the purpose of getting timber, firewood, and hoop poles," he returned with a fever, and "after a long and painful illness found his grave."[21]

Antebellum Southerners did not connect mosquitoes with yellow fever, though some got close. Geographer William Darby noted that the year 1811 was "remarkable for the great numbers of the mosquito" and for "the existence of the yellow fever in New Orleans." He warned readers that when "June and July usher [in] uncommon quantities of these creatures," it was best to prepare for danger. Austrian journalist Karl Postl likewise drew a connection between mosquitoes and fever in 1828, noting that New Orleanians were generally "forewarned of the approaching disease" by swarming mosquitoes, bugs that were present every summer but were infinitely more abundant prior to epidemics. However, most Louisianans saw mosquitoes more as an omen of a bad night's sleep than as a harbinger of death. Landscape architect Benjamin Henry Latrobe (d. YF 1820) observed that in New Orleans, mosquitoes "furnish a considerable part of the conversation of every day and of everybody; they regulate many family arrangements . . . and most essentially affect the comforts and enjoyments of every individual in the country." At times, mosquitoes could swarm so densely that they blocked out the sun and blackened white walls. One writer joked in 1824 that if the "Pharaoh had felt the New-Orleans' moschetoes, he surely would have let the Israelites go the first time."[22]

Today between 75 and 85 percent of yellow fever victims suffer only briefly before improving, and only 20 to 50 percent of people with serious cases die. This places the modern fatality rate somewhere between 3 and 13 percent. Two centuries ago yellow fever was much more virulent, for reasons modern epidemiologists do not entirely understand. Historical mortality estimates range broadly, from 10 to 50 percent on the low end, to 85 or even 95 percent on the high end. The modern and historical fatality gap cannot be explained genetically—the virus has not mutated significantly over the past four centuries in a way that would explain its decreased virulence. Rather, the explanation probably lies in the broader determinants of human health. Many Caribbean dwellers and antebellum Deep Southerners had several comorbidities. The journey across the Atlantic was terrible for everyone, especially the enslaved, and most people disembarked ships immunosuppressed and malnourished. Tobacco and alcohol use were widespread; malaria and sexually transmitted diseases were commonplace. As Steven Stowe writes, it was routine even in elite circles to consume a monotonous diet of near-rotten meat, just-turned milk, and microbe-laden water. Many people who died of yellow fever in New Orleans, living in cramped and buggy conditions, likely had very high viral loads. J. R. McNeill accounts for the discrepancy between modern and historical mortality by suggesting that the risk of exposure has drastically decreased in recent years: rarely, if ever, do large numbers of nonimmune/unvaccinated people (armies, refugees, laborers) travel to destinations where yellow fever presents a risk.[23]

In the nineteenth century, people did not understand how yellow fever spread or why it was so lethal. But most agreed that yellow fever did not treat all people equally. Many observed that it tended to kill young adults, especially those between the ages of fifteen and forty, rather than the very young or old. Children often experienced milder, flu-like cases of yellow fever, becoming acclimated around the same time they survived bouts of chicken pox, scarlet fever, and measles.[24] Likewise, many believed that women were less likely to die from yellow fever than men and pointed to death registers as proof. In 1817, for example, yellow fever officially killed twelve times the number of men (760) as women (63); during the last week of September 1841, eighty-five men were interred at city expense in Lafayette Cemetery compared with just seventeen women. Their sex did not provide women with any innate protection against yellow fever, but gendered circumstances probably did. New Orleans' antebellum population skewed male, and men generally spent more time outdoors performing manual, sweat-inducing labor, making them attractive to *A. aegypti.* Men were also more often in yellow-fever-prone spaces—docklands, warehouses, ship hulls—where they were more likely to come in contact the virus.[25]

Southerners also associated yellow fever—like most disease—with "free livers" or alcoholics, especially those in lower classes. Poverty and alcoholism did not cause disease *per se,* but they did increase the risks. Mobile, Alabama, a port city about 140 miles west of New Orleans, suffered an especially fatal yellow fever season in 1819, when 21 percent of the population died. A special committee, formed in the epidemic's aftermath, found that the majority of the 500 people who remained in town all summer were "those of the poorer class of people, who either lived in small, crowded filthy dwellings, or even without any, frequenting the grog shops near the wharves." Among this "intemperate" class of people, "the fever was observed to be dreadfully mortal—almost all of them died." Landscape architect Benjamin Henry Latrobe put this connection simply: "The sober lived; the drunk died, with few exceptions."[26]

The Stranger's Disease

Like elsewhere in the tropical and subtropical Atlantic, yellow fever's strongest association in Louisiana was with foreigners, especially poverty-stricken, recent white immigrants from the Northern states and Europe. This association was so strong, in fact, that yellow fever earned the moniker "stranger's disease." During bad epidemics, overstretched Charity Hospital administrators would yell out "name, age, and country?" to those hobbling to the gates. If the response was "Wörte," "Bruntz," or "Mahoney," the patient was ushered to the yellow fever ward with no further consultation.[27] Stories of unacclimated Scottish sailors, German weavers, Pennsylvania farmers, and Swiss stevedores abounded as a kind of reverse bildungsroman—of promising young men cut down by yellow fever in their prime. Many such people sickened and died alone. Dr. Benedict, for example, discovered a boy from Liverpool in an attic room during the epidemic of 1858, "entirely alone with a high fever on him"—so high that he sent the boy to the Charity Hospital. Benedict did not note the boy's name or what happened to him. Most likely he died, just like thousands of other immigrants that summer. To this day, tombstones and placards across New Orleans stand as memorials to unlucky foreigners, bearing inscriptions like "Died of yellow fever, 17th Oct., A. L., a native of Hamburg, aged 28."[28]

Sympathy for friendless strangers easily slipped into disdain. The first cases reported by city officials were always dissolute Irishmen, drunken Dutchmen, or Italian seafarers. Dr. J. S. McFarlane, a city councilor, stoked this nativist antipathy. "Go and survey the seats of impurity," he wrote in 1853. "Who are their conductors? who are their occupants? who are their supporters, and who their frequenters? Strangers." Not only could New Orleans thank strangers "for the principal portion of our crimes and disease," but McFarlane blamed them, as well, for diminishing the morality of the city's population overall. Dr. Charles Caldwell put it even more sharply: yellow fever was "more attributable to the faults of the sufferers, than to those of the place."[29]

Diseases plagued immigrants in every nineteenth-century American city. But foreigners faced especially grim odds in New Orleans, primarily because of yellow fever. Using mortality data compiled by doctors in the wake of the epidemic of 1853 (this data is incomplete, as we will see), modern statisticians have determined that white American-born migrants died from yellow fever at four times the Creole rate; British and French migrants at ten times the rate; and Irish and German migrants at twenty times the rate. In total mortality terms, yellow fever accounted for 20 percent of all deaths among native New Orleanians, but between 75 and 90 percent of deaths among immigrants. Thus, while as many as 8 percent of all New Orleanians died annually—making New Orleans America's deadliest major city by far—deaths could reach 20 or even 30 percent in certain predominantly immigrant neighborhoods like Marigny and Irish Channel. In 1853 at least 29,120 people contracted yellow fever in the city and about 12,000 people died from it, though estimates range from lows of about 7,000 to highs of 15,000. Conservatively, this means that one in twelve New Orleanians died from yellow fever that summer, but one in five Irishmen died.[30] One life insurance company calculated that Irishmen were fifty-seven times more likely to die from yellow fever than native-born Louisianans, and that people from Holland and Belgium were over ninety-one times more likely.[31] One estimate suggests that of the 60,000 Germans who made their entry into the United States through New Orleans between 1848 and 1858, about half died from yellow fever and cholera. If the seventeenth-century Caribbean was, in historian Richard Dunn's words, the "white man's grave—and the black man's, too," statistics suggest that New Orleans was nineteenth-century America's equivalent—the white strangers' graveyard, and everyone else's, too.[32]

Racial Immunity, Again

Antebellum white Southerners took it as axiomatic that all Black people were less affected by yellow fever than all whites. By this logic, enslaved Black people who were generations removed from Africa and the Middle Passage, had been born in temperate Maryland or Massachusetts, or had some white ancestry were considered naturally immune or at least extremely resistant to yellow fever. This logic of racial immunity also applied to *gens de couleur libres,* a group generally lambasted by whites for immorality, sexual deviance, and drunkenness, qualities that—according to the prevailing medical orthodoxies of the time—should have increased their vulnerability to the virus. But white people insisted that all Black people, free or not, possessed a racial immunity so powerful that it protected even the most serious alcoholics from sickness and even the most depraved from death.[33]

Like everywhere in the Atlantic world, official data published in New Orleans presented a veritable chasm between Black and white yellow fever deaths. In 1820, for example, when city officials determined that the "black" and "white" populations were exactly balanced (total population 27,176), one professional association for American doctors categorized 84 percent of that year's 863 yellow fever victims as "white." In 1841 a prominent Scottish physician claimed that only three Black people (two of them children) were among the 1,800 people who died in that year's epidemic. Another doctor insisted that only three Black people died from yellow fever in 1849 compared with 766 whites.[34] An 1853 commission found that out of 7,849 total deaths (a vast undercount) during that year's epidemic, only forty-three victims were "colored" people. And in 1858, health officials noted that of the 390 people who died during the first week of September, only nineteen were Black, ten of whom were enslaved.[35]

Even if certain doctors conceded that Black people did fall ill with yellow fever, they always insisted the disease was milder among them, "usually tedious, but seldom fatal." Dr. Fassitt, for example, tended to Judge Baker's plantation in 1854, about sixty miles west of New Orleans on Bayou Teche. During the epidemic, Fassitt claimed that 130 of the 190 people enslaved at Oaklawn fell sick with yellow fever and only six died, including a young child and a "mulatto."[36] Dr. Josiah Nott, one of the South's most famous medical proslavery thinkers, insisted that yellow fever was highly sensitive to skin tone. He wrote that "a Mulatto, from the healthy parts of Virginia or Maryland, however small may be the proportion of Negro blood" will "face yellow fever with impunity." Nott claimed that in ten years of practicing medicine, he had seen only two exceptions to this rule while "Whites [died] by hundreds." By the 1850s almost the entire medical community of the Deep South publicly agreed with Dr. Samuel Cartwright that Black people were "perfect non-conductors of yellow fever." This, in fact, became a kind of dogma, amplified by doctors, repeated by slave traders, and echoed unquestioningly by planters across the Cotton Kingdom.[37]

There were some white apostates who, in private correspondence and confidential doctor's ledgers, challenged the theory of racial immunity, conceding that "whites, mulattoes, negroes, Indians, indigents, old residents, and strangers were all sufferers . . . equally obnoxious to it." For every Dr. Fassitt, there was an Armand Duplantier, who noted in 1799 that all the people he had enslaved fell ill with the disease and many died from it (as did his wife). One Natchez-based physician listed multiple Black patients in 1817, noting "black vomit" and "sallowskin" among their symptoms and that "the negroes upon the plantations suffered severely."[38] And after the devastating 1853 epidemic, Dr. William Holcombe conceded that Cartwright's claim of perfect Black immunity was "as baseless as the fabric of a vision." Black people themselves were also acutely aware of their vulnerability. Escaped slave and abolitionist William Wells Brown wrote in his most famous novel, *Clotel,* that outbreak after outbreak in New Orleans proved that "the negro . . . was not proof against the disease."[39]

As the racial mortality gap is so striking and consistent in the historical record, and because whites at the time so fervently insisted on Black people's special immunity to yellow fever, the question of racial immunity has persisted among generations of scholars and biomedical statisticians. Today, most scholars agree that *in all probability* there is no racially specific immunity to yellow fever; that Black people died of yellow fever in the past, and die still. Modern epidemiologists have discovered no mechanisms for the intergenerational transfer of resistance to yellow fever as they have for other diseases like malaria—where immunity is transferred "passively" in utero from parent to child. However, it remains *possible* that people of African descent developed genetic adaptations due to selection pressures imposed by a high yellow fever environment in West Africa (as is the case with malaria) that allowed them to better fight off the virus. Simply, we do not know with full certainty whether hereditary resistance exists, and if it does, why it does.[40]

The answer to the racial immunity question, however interesting, does not fundamentally change the racialized nature of the immunity debate in antebellum New Orleans. Nor can historical data from New Orleans shed more light. Mortality statistics for Louisiana—consistent with those across the American South and wider Atlantic World—were, by design, structurally incapable of capturing an accurate Black death rate. Contemporaries rarely, if ever, provided data for categories of people outside "black" or "white." Data collection was decentralized, even hyper-local or plantation-based. Moreover, most statistics about Black deaths reflected the implicit biases of a white- and male-dominated medical profession operating in a slave society. If it was impossible for a Black person to die from yellow fever—as the logic of racial immunity held—then it would be ridiculous to mark a Black person down as dying from it. Even when the theory of Black immunity clashed with the fatal reality on the ground, white elites chose to construe yellow fever resistance in a racially specific manner. It was a means to justify the deeper immiseration of Black people, and especially the enslaved.[41]

Dead Reckoning

The manipulation of mortality data was not limited to Black victims. Rather, it was part of a much larger elite-led effort to suppress the seriousness of yellow fever in New Orleans and downplay the overall incidence of epidemics. Even "epidemic" was (and is) a contested term. Strictly speaking, a disease becomes epidemic when it deviates upward from individual and communal notions of "normal." But epidemics can take on metaphorical elements (we speak of suffering through "epidemics" of racism, loneliness, or disbelief). And, as Charles Rosenberg described, epidemics are inherently dramaturgical: they "start at a moment in time, proceed on a stage limited in space and duration, follow a plot line of increasing and revelatory tension, move to a crisis of individual and collective character, then drift toward closure." During the nineteenth century, when mortality and morbidity statistics were often inaccurate and not easily obtainable in any case, defining "epidemic" was even more arbitrary. New Orleanians gradually came to accept as "normal" an extremely high level of disease and death—higher even than residents of other large cities like New York or Charleston. Numerous observers were shocked at just how many people had to die from yellow fever in New Orleans before city officials took notice and declared it epidemic.[42]

"Official" data—promulgated variably by New Orleans's board of health, city council, commercial class, and press—reported that yellow fever killed about 41,000 people across the entire nineteenth century, ten times more than in Charleston, America's next most afflicted major city. But this data was incomplete at best or scandalously deficient at worst, capturing only a trivial percentage of cases in some years, and none at all for any year before 1817. The major obstacle to painting an accurate mortality picture is that, unlike in many other American cities, there was no central, disinterested body responsible for collecting or tracking health data in New Orleans. There was no "health police" and there was no actual "official record," though elites tried to present their data as accurate. In reality, mortality data was collected by churches, hobbyists, innkeepers, charities, ethnically stratified medical societies, and individual doctors. Sometimes this data was assembled and cross-checked by sanitary commissioners (often long after the fact); more often it was not.[43]

On paper, the task of tracking, defining, and preventing disease fell to the city's board of health, a body first established in 1804. But the board was *ad hoc,* generally convened after a bad epidemic and then dissolved before the next summer. It operated entirely at the discretion of the city council, which kept it so impotent that one doctor joked in 1855 that New Orleans's health authorities were as likely to declare war against a foreign power as they were to issue a sanitation order.[44] Most health officers had no medical or statistical training. In 1824, for instance, Messrs. Rousseau (lawyer), Méance (wood merchant), Abat (gentleman), Gainnié (gentleman), and Christie (lawyer) were the health officers of the city.[45] When New Orleans split into three semiautonomous municipalities between 1836 and 1852, health administration became even more decentralized and haphazard. And when the city re-merged, the reconstituted health board was designed to have no independence, funding, or authority. By then, the board had fully morphed into a propaganda arm for commerce, tasked with proving that New Orleans was actually healthy and that the port should remain open even as serious epidemics raged. Dr. M. Morton Dowler put a sharp point on his criticisms in 1854: "Never yet has any measure emanating from any Board of Health in this city, warned us of an approaching epidemic, prevented its extension, shortened its duration, or given the least idea of its origin."[46]

For many of the years that a health board was in existence (and most antebellum years the board was "literally *defunct*"), it did not track the deaths of the indigent poor and it arbitrarily removed whole sections of the population from its roster. Sometimes foreigners, newly arrived immigrants, and even, oddly, Californians, did not factor into the official record.[47] The board also made no effort to track or count the "floating population"—sailors, boatmen, and seasonal workers—who died outside city limits while fleeing epidemics. Because it received most of its information from churches and religious cemeteries, it often did not capture those without ecclesiastical ties. And—accepting the conventional wisdom that Black people were either entirely or partly immune—Black mortality, especially of the enslaved, was undercounted to an extraordinary, even conspiratorial, extent. Health officials also routinely changed diagnostic criteria, sometimes mid-epidemic. Abner Phelps (a. YF 1844), clerk of the city court and future mayor of Lafayette, noted in October 1846 that doctors had "changed their notions with regard to this disease much this season." It was not officially yellow fever "unless black vomit & bleeding at the gums & nose" took place. Phelps, whose first wife, Elizabeth, and two children, Leon and Leona, died of yellow fever in 1844, knew that such symptoms did not occur in all cases. Consequently, he believed, the actual count of yellow fever deaths was much higher than officially reported.[48]

Due to a complicated set of social and economic pressures, many health officers bent over backward to *not* declare epidemics, instead purposely misdiagnosing obvious cases of yellow fever as "relapsing" or "sporadic." The irony was not lost on laypeople. As Abraham Oakey Hall, a travel writer who later served as New York City's mayor, sneered, "Very fine logic all this, but one naturally asks what difference does it make whether one dies sporadically or otherwise!" Angry about the city's necropolitan reputation, some health officers vigilantly promoted the false notion that yellow fever was barely a problem. As the reform-minded physician J. C. Simonds argued in 1851, the health board "appears to think that its first duty is to assert the *healthiness* of New Orleans; and its second duty, to furnish such tables that none can easily controvert their position."[49]

Average New Orleanians, well aware the "official" data released each Sunday night was a lie, called this tactic a "city disgrace, and a crying shame." But with data collection so atomized, it was impossible for even the most intrepid statistician or hobbyist to assemble a truer picture. Landscape architect Benjamin Henry Latrobe (d. YF 1820) tried in 1819 but was quickly frustrated. "No exact register is anywhere kept of deaths and burials," he grumbled. Another writer noted in 1837 that even if an interested party made personal enquiries at all the city's graveyards, they would be frustrated as some cemeteries and churches kept no records at all. Most townspeople believed the rumors that the cost-cutting Charity Hospital piled the indigent dead three-deep into unmarked coffins (after rifling through their pockets for coins) and that those who dropped dead in back alleys were thrown into the Mississippi, without benefit of doctor, coroner, or clergy.[50]

Aware that they were being misled, city residents learned to trust their own eyes and ears. Lay estimates range from impossibly small ("no fever this year") to apocalyptic ("the entire city has been exterminated"), more reflective of an individual's emotional experience of an epidemic than a true record of mortality. Still, the observations of average people—triangulated with doctors' ledgers, hospital and interment reports, obituaries, diaries, letters, military dispatches, insurance filings, plantation books, tax and immigration records, as well as common epidemiological sense—appear more credible than official apologias.

According to townspeople, the disease appeared every summer, establishing the "normal" baseline; every second or third year, outbreaks tipped over into epidemics, some very serious. The disease killed as many as 1,500 people in 1804, hundreds in 1809 (nine out of ten strangers, according to one travel writer), at least 500 in 1811, 1,150 in 1817, and anywhere between 2,190 and 6,000 in 1819. During the epidemic of 1819, one doctor claimed to have witnessed fifty-four deaths in one day and that it was common to see "6 funerals within a few minutes."[51] Yellow fever likely killed tens of thousands of people during the 1820s; the outbreak of 1824 was particularly lethal. In July 1828, Dr. Perlu had already attended nearly one hundred yellow fever patients, though no epidemic had been declared and the city was officially fever-free that summer.[52] One conservative estimate placed deaths at 8,000 in the 1832–1833 season. In 1833, Maria Inskeep stood at her window and counted ten funeral processions in one hour. The Charity Hospital admitted at least 122,317 patients during the 1830s and 1840s, the majority during the fever months and the vast majority being from Ireland and Germany.[53] Dr. J. C. Simonds believed that between 1847 and 1850, 37,785 people died (an annual average of about 8,719), even though the city was officially fever-free during these years.[54] In 1853—the year of the city's worst epidemic—approximately 12,000 people died, followed by at least 3,000 the following year, 2,600 in 1855, and 5,000 in 1858. After the Civil War, yellow fever returned with a vengeance, killing approximately 3,500 people in 1867 and approximately 5,000 people in 1878, while a further 15,000 died across the Mississippi Valley. New Orleans's last epidemic, in 1905, saw 500 people die.[55]

We will never know precisely how many people yellow fever killed in New Orleans—or across the larger Yellow Fever South. But it is clear that the 41,000 "official" deaths represent the absolute lowest possible number. It appears reasonable to take seriously the conviction of contemporary New Orleanians, that yellow fever mortality was as much as double or even triple the official tally.

Carnival of Slaughter

Statistics can only hint at how people experienced life in such a deathscape. From January through Mardi Gras, the cotton and sugar industries hummed. But as the weather warmed in May, discussion of the fever topic was urgently resurrected: "Will it come this season? Do you stay and weather it?" By June, physicians became "characters for ocular interest," their nods and winks "scrutinized with great care." If a health officer "suffering under dyspepsia or any other complaint" should accidentally grimace in the morning, the whole town would know by afternoon. When cases of fever were reported in Veracruz or Havana in July, a race against the clock commenced: merchants frantically processed one last cotton shipment; brokers pushed to close just one more deal; enslaved women packed up their masters' townhouses. When an in-town case was confirmed, an exodus ensued. Luxury hotels that had bustled with foreigners and tourists were entirely vacant by nightfall.[56] Hundreds of rich white people piled into carriages with their precious valuables. Some went to nearby plantations, which they put under virtual lockdown, while others traveled as far away as New York or Europe. Other "truants" sojourned at the many luxury health spas closer to home, at Mandeville or Sulphur Springs. But such a stay could cost upward of $400 for the three months of the fever season—an entire year's wages for a clerk—putting such a sojourn out of reach for most. Less affluent and unfree people had no choice but to hunker down in town, limiting their outdoor activity whenever possible. If the epidemic got really bad, some reckoned, they could walk out of the city or spend 25 cents to take the "Smokey Mary" railroad to breezy Lake Pontchartrain, if only for the night.[57]

For the uninitiated, the transition into the fever season was jarring, like landing amid Defoe's plague-stricken London or Boccaccio's Florence. The unacclimated, acutely aware of their vulnerability, lived "in fear and trembling, not knowing what moment [they] may be attacked." If they met an acquaintance on the street, they refrained from shaking hands lest the other be "contaminated," tried to stand upwind of them, and made every excuse to hurry home. An eerie stillness enveloped town, disturbed only by the mourning vehicles wending their way to the cemetery. Canal Street—New Orleans's busiest thoroughfare—emptied. Weeds sprouted waist high on major roads.[58] Schools shuttered. The editors of the *True American* lamented in August 1839 that with so many employees sick, it was "exceedingly difficult to get our paper out." By August the color black was everywhere. People of means who remained in town dressed in full or half mourning, donning black veils, armbands, caps, and cravats. Badges of death—rosettes of black crape—hung motionless from every other door and portico. Black-margined placards announcing the local dead studded every street corner. The black was so pronounced, it popped even through the thick smoke enveloping the streets, produced by flaming black tar barrels lit by the city to dispel the miasmas.[59]

By the epidemic's midpoint in early September, all commodity-based activity ground to a halt. With the disease eating through town "like worms in a cotton field," stores shut up and the post office opened only for two or three hours a day. "No sort of business is going on," wrote Bohemian immigrant Carl Kohn, and "scarcely any body [was] to be met with in the streets."[60] One Rothschild agent likewise informed the London office that the past week's "business has been limited," with yellow fever throwing "business back very much." Commission houses sent their clients regrets, noting that "no favorable change has taken place" in the markets because of disease. As business stagnated, commodity prices dropped. During particularly bad years, warehoused food and goods began to rot and non-perishable goods would not sell, even at a discount, because there were no customers. "The Levee is dull, dreary and lifeless at this time. No business doing," wrote the *Picayune* in September, "and the few ships in port are losing money for the want of cargoes. Steamboats arrive but seldom, and bring neither news, money or goods." The only activity was at the apothecary—where "applicants for physic" were so numerous, people had to wait half an hour or longer to be served.[61]

For those engaged in cotton and sugar, epidemic-time New Orleans could feel like an economic desert, a port suspended in time. Yellow fever played a large role in regimenting the timing of New Orleans's commodity market. In 1829, for example, the New Orleans Customs House exported nearly $21 million worth of cotton and sugar (and a small bit of tobacco). According one Barings Bank agent, nearly $15 million of this was exported in the first two quarters, between January and July, when the crops came in. Exports dropped precipitously to $2.6 million during the third quarter between July and October—the fever season—ticking up slightly to $3.3 million between October and year's end.[62] Planters complained that even in years when the cotton crop was good, disease compromised their ability to sell. Cotton planter Thomas Gale wrote in 1817 that his business had been "extensive and profitable" enough to "secure an interest that will be sufficient to settle me for life." But yellow fever had "swept off great numbers and put a stop to all business whatever." Planters could not sell their crops, nor would they venture into the city. "Perhaps," Gale mused, "no disease has ever been so fatal in any of the seaports of the U.S." William Kenner (a. YF 1801), a wealthy planter and merchant, blamed the fever-mediated

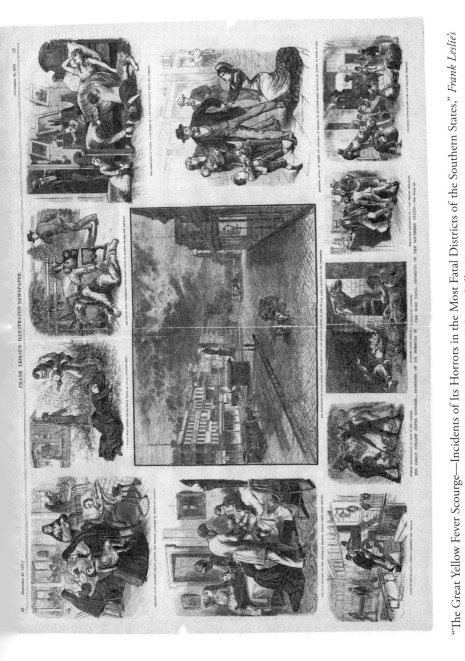

"The Great Yellow Fever Scourge—Incidents of Its Horrors in the Most Fatal Districts of the Southern States," *Frank Leslie's Illustrated Newspaper*, September 28, 1878. The Historic New Orleans Collection.

schedule for hamstringing his business, writing in 1820, "Cotton is selling at 16 cents cash. Something more could be had in Bills on the Eastward, but negotiations are difficult. Our Banks decline buying drafts for the present." Compounding the problem, widespread disease meant that "demand from casual purchasers is extremely limited."[63]

By September, an anxious monotony had set in. We "bury our dead, drink juleps, or brandy toddies, as mint is stale and out of date," wrote one townsperson. "Thus we are and thus we go." Mentally exhausted and claustrophobic, everyone felt like "sleeping or running away for the next three weeks and a half," wrote another editorialist, though most knew they were "bound to stay, to fulfil engagements, live or die."[64] Yellow fever haunted waking hours and spawned nightmares. Every headache, chill, or toothache was suspicious. Fear kept some people from sleeping. Many reported being so consistently frightened they could not urinate. Survivors remained in houses that constantly reminded them of dead loved ones, slept in beds once shared, and ate meals at tables whose empty chairs conjured the departed. *Everybody* knew someone who had died, probably many. Merchant William Crenshaw summed up the dire feelings about town: "It is an awful time here," he told a friend. "You can not imagine the distress that exists. Think for one moment of eight of our neighbors dying in 10 days . . . within a stone's throw of us." Crenshaw concluded, "Wherever I turn sickness and death stares me in the face. And now whilst I pen these lines, the thought strikes me that I may not be spared to meet you again."[65]

Stagnation in town stretched outward. An unhappy convergence of agricultural and epidemiological calendars meant that the cotton-picking and cane-cutting seasons overlapped substantially with the fever season. Just as the epidemic was at its most serious point, planters needed their slaves to commence picking—and vigorously. Sickness often thwarted their plans. In 1819, for example, the cotton crop was "remarkably fine" due to the best summer rainfall in a decade. But with yellow fever raging and so many enslaved people sick, "when or by whom it would be gathered, no one can conjecture," mused one editorialist.[66] One cotton planter worried about worsening fevers among his slaves in late September 1830. "More sickness," Zachariah Philips wrote in his diary. "Green down for a week or ten days; Jack and Eliza had chill and fever today . . . James with high fever today, unlucky boy, has been down three times." With two to eight enslaved people out of the picking rotation each day, Philips's progress was delayed by a month.[67] Sickness made some planters desperate. Overseer John North urgently wrote to his employer Eliza Lyons in 1850, "Twelve hands have been sick and some of them are not well yet." But if the health of the enslaved did not improve and Lyons did not send more people immediately, North warned, "you will be bound to lose all the cane that has had water . . . I need all hands."[68]

Epidemics were disorienting for the enslaved—times of increased mental and physical anguish. Working in swampy, cramped, and exposed conditions—and unable to flee—planter Moses Liddell conceded that "negroes here have not a full half chance for good health. They are too much crowded in the cabins and the mosquitoes are violent."[69] According to William Wells Brown, a formerly enslaved man, many plantations around New Orleans had to suspend their activities during epidemics, "for want of slaves to take the places of those carried off by the fever." A massively diminished workforce at peak harvest was a major concern for white planters—a bottleneck to building a plantation and making it profitable. Most planters, it seems, dealt with epidemics by forcing acclimated slaves to work harder and faster, extracting as much labor as possible from the sick, and allowing scant time for convalescence. Brown penned a stanza about life on fever-stricken plantations, encapsulating the horrors bondspeople faced:

Where the slave-whip ceaseless swings,
Where the noisome insect stings,
Where the fever demon strews
Poison with the falling dews,
Where the sickly sunbeams glare
Through the hot and misty air.[70]

Working through illness was miserable and dangerous. For some it was impossible. During his second or third summer in Louisiana, Solomon Northup, a free Black man from New York kidnapped into slavery, fell sick. He became "weak and emaciated, and frequently so dizzy" that he reeled and staggered "like a drunken man." Edwin Epps, his sadistic new master with a reputation as a slave "breaker," forced Northup to hoe the fields anyway, instructing the overseers to whip him if he fell too far behind the others. Soon, Northup collapsed and even the "sharpest sting of the raw-hide" could not rouse him. He remained deathly ill and confined to his cabin for days. By September, with the period of most intense cotton picking approaching, Northup had still "received no medicine nor any attention" from Epps, a man who considered all Black people "mere live property." But when "it was said that I [Solomon] would die," Epps sent for Dr. Wines of Holmesville, "unwilling to bear the loss, which the death of an animal worth a thousand dollars would bring upon him." Northup survived his fever, though he was given no time to recuperate. "One morning, long before I was in a proper condition to labor," he recalled, Epps thrust a sack at him and ordered him back out to the fields. During the harvest, the economic health of the enslaver, not the physical (or emotional) health of the enslaved, was paramount.[71]

By early October, the roads to city cemeteries—Girod, St. Louis, Cyprus Grove, and Lafayette—were rutted with foot-deep grooves, leading conveyances to gravesites like train tracks. C. C. Robin, a French traveler, noticed that white people's funerals were sparsely attended, but Black funerals always attracted large crowds. As Joseph Roach has described, Afro-Catholic burials were distinctive moments affirming the "semiautonomous but discreetly submerged existence" of Afro-Caribbean ritual and traditions.[72] One twilight in 1819, Benjamin Henry Latrobe witnessed "at least two hundred negroes—men and women" in a funeral procession. First marched a man in military uniform with a drawn sword, followed by three boys in surplices and pointed caps, two with candlesticks and one with a large silver cross. Next came the priests carrying urns and crucifixes. Father Anthony, the greying eighty-year-old Catholic priest, followed the coffin, chanting in Latin. Then came mourners, women and men "dressed in pure white" holding candles—white, the color associated with mourning and burial ritual in many African cultures. The crowd chanted, punctuated by intermittent "noise and laughter." This laughter was an expression of grief, according to the Trinidadian-Creole proverb—"dents pas ka pôté dëî," that *teeth do not wear mourning*. Behind this parade, a short distance away, was a surreptitious group of enslaved people carrying their own coffin. Without means, money, or mourners, this group sought to "take advantage" of the resplendent ceremony being performed ahead.[73]

Latrobe followed the procession to its destination and discovered that the deceased was a hundred-year-old "African (Congo) Negress belonging to Madam Fitzgerald." As children played among human bones disinterred by the gravedigger's shovel, the pallbearers lowered the coffin into the shallow grave and the candle-bearing women pressed in close. One woman—the deceased's granddaughter—threw herself upon the coffin with "very loud lamentations," until she was forcibly carried away by the gravediggers and other mourners. Latrobe asked why this woman was so distressed. A mourner shrugged her shoulders and responded "Je n'en sçais rien, cela es tune manière"—*I don't know about that, that's the way it's done.* Before leaving the graveside, the women in white picked blades of grass.[74]

Deliverance

By October's end, when the weather chilled, the region awoke from hibernation. One morning there would be frost on the ground. By afternoon, New Orleans's streets would be jam-packed with "girls, boys, men, and women . . . exchanging congratulations and compliments" on getting through another season. Now the "dead old year, with all its sorrows and disappointments, seems almost to be forgotten." Merchant John Dunlap told his wife that after the cold snap no one talked about fever, and that "in a few brief weeks the dead will be forgotten," with the "living plunging in hot haste into the deep vortex of dissipation, reckless of the past, and forgetful of the future."[75]

For the entire month of October, grave wares and artificial flowers were peddled outside cemeteries. Goods were balanced "on the heads of bright quadroons . . . sold to all those who desire to render attractive, for a day at least, the narrow dwellings of departed relatives." In a "rival geography" outside the city walls and adjacent to the Catholic cemetery was a marketplace called Congo Square, once a site for the corn feast of the Poucha-Houma Indians. Here, slaves, *libres,* and Native Americans mingled in relative freedom, hawked their goods, danced, drummed, and were possessed by spirits.[76] Shop windows along Canal Street displayed "curious circlets" with inscriptions such as *A mon bon ange, Eternal Regrets,* and *Tears for the Dead.* Cotton sales once again became "very brisk." Shops and schools reopened. Widows started courting. Hundreds of steamboats docked at the levee. Job-seekers knocked on every office door. Slave auctions recommenced, with buyers seeking to replenish their thinned workforces. Capitalists had hopes for a profitable winter.[77]

November 1, locally celebrated as All Saint's Day or *La Toussaint,* was the day Catholic mourners decorated the graves of the departed, rendering the city one "vast funeral assemblage." Every second servant wore a black armband, the customary mark of a lost master, boss, or employer. Most people dressed in full mourning, complete with cloaks, mantillas, bombazines, parasols, and veils. Outfitters Michon & Desportes on Royal Street sold imported French garlands of pearls, feathers, and velvets, as well as tomb vases and rustic flower baskets. Townspeople put in orders for *immortelles,* artwork made out of a dead person's hair woven into designs like "ici repose mon père" (here lies my father) or "souvenir, 5 août" (memory, 5 August). Others fashioned macabre cufflinks and bracelets from the hair of dead sisters, uncles, or sons. Whitewashers and painters brightened the tombs and mausoleums of St. Louis Cemetery so that "when the fete day comes round everything will be prepared for goodly celebration." Those with disposable income—whatever money was left after an already expensive fever season—paid stonemasons to make additions to the funerary art on family tombs. Canadian visitor William Kingsford explored these ornate mausoleums, remarking, "As you walk among these last homes of your fellows, you feel indeed that you are in the company of their remains."[78]

By the Christmas season, "Grief in her sable garments [had] taken her flight to other regions." One editor wrote that "sorrow for departed friends is, in some measure, assuaged by the joyful meetings of the living." Presbyterian minister J. B. Warren told his Massachusetts family in November 1847 that though thousands had "just been swept to Eternity," including many of his friends, "the voice of health is now heard." The dead were forgotten, said Warren, "and the streets are swarming with multitudes—who are as busy and gay as though nothing had occurred." Planter Mary Copes likewise noted how easily New Orleanians suppressed sad memories of the recent past, willing themselves to return to normal. "Where one died . . . ten have come to fill the place," she told her husband.[79] No one seemed to want to talk about the epidemic, or the dead, anymore.

Ghost Stories

Seasoned Louisianans came to accept the yearly rhythms and ravages of yellow fever as part of God's plan. As New Orleans native Nancy Brown Phelps wrote in 1858, she would rather live in a deadly place like New Orleans than "in a place where people seldom die, for it is what we all have to come to, Death." Phelps felt the more a person accustomed themselves to death, "the less dread we have of it." Maybe so. But not all had the strength—or perspective—to return to normal after epidemics, especially children. One young German girl lamented that "[when] all you can see are dead-carts and coffins . . . in the end one becomes convinced one must die." A mother bemoaned that her "little Leila asks so many strange questions for a child of her age that it makes me sad"; Leila spoke of nothing but dying and going to heaven to become an angel.[80] Some were so consumed with grief they lost the will to continue living. Creole sugar planter Valcour Aime—locally known as "Louis XIV of Louisiana" for his immense wealth—lost his only son, Gabriel, to yellow fever in 1854. Overcome with sadness, he wrote in his diary, "Let him who wishes continue. My time is finished." Following "Gabie's" death, Aime withdrew from society and became a recluse.[81]

Young fever orphans struggled to understand and accept their parents' deaths. William L. Robinson, a volunteer for the Howard Association—the largest health-care-providing charity in New Orleans—met a ten-year-old boy in 1853 in a temporary asylum. The boy was writing out the words, "My dear father I love you of all my hearth [*sic*]. And you did Died so quick. And I think that I see you always. And I which [*sic*] that you would live. You was so good." Robinson inquired about the rest of his family. "They all died too," replied the boy, before breaking down in tears. New Orleans's many orphanages, segregated by religion, race, and sex, struggled to keep up with demand and to keep surviving siblings together. Robinson also recalled meeting an "interesting-looking girl" of about ten years. When she discovered she would be separated from her younger brother and not be allowed to visit him at the Boy's Asylum, she screamed "*No!* No! NO! . . . I promised my mother on her death-bed never to leave my brother Sammy, and, if you take him away from me, I will kill myself."[82]

Adults had difficulty coping, too. Some tried to drink away the blues. Others gambled. Some danced to songs about defeating "Saffron John" and sang along to lyrics like "Yellow Jack, with us, is said to be / Making this great cheverie; / At his approach every body is in awe—/ Let's give him a touch of old 'Lynch Law.'" Others tried humor. An oft-repeated joke was that man checking into the St. Charles Hotel was greeted by the proprietor, who "immediately took his measure for a coffin" and asked him to note down his preferred cemetery. In another joke, a man landing on the levee was approached by health officers, who "immediately took his name and entered it in their books as *deceased,* to save all trouble in calling upon him again!"[83] The lower classes got to the punchline quicker: "Die!—No; it's too d——d expensive to get buried here! Bless your heart, sir, I couldn't afford to die!"[84]

Some sights and experiences were simply too tragic to be joked away. Clerk George Fennell recalled seeing a crestfallen father in 1848, unable to pay for a coffin, carrying his son's stiff body to the graveyard under his arm. The following day, Fennell saw the same man, now conveying his wife's frozen body in a wheelbarrow to the cemetery. The next day, Fennell noticed an enslaved porter carting the man's dead body to the cem-

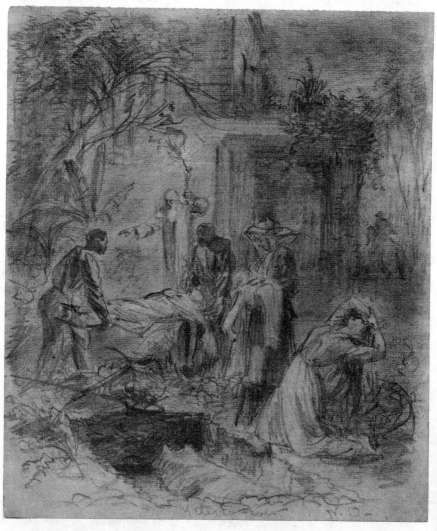

Alfred Rudolph Waud, *Yellow Fever, N.O.,* 1870 or 1871. The Historic New Orleans Collection, The L. Kemper and Leila Moore Williams Founders Collection.

etery, the last member of a whole family cut down by yellow fever in just three days.[85]

Some told ghost stories. Such stories were almost always once-removed—something that happened to a neighbor's cousin or a seamstress' old master, in the manner of an urban legend. Many involved a live burial. Olivier Blanchard, a formerly enslaved man, recalled a local white woman, Colene Bonnier, who was to marry on Sunday but fell sick with yellow fever on Friday. On her intended wedding day, Colene died. Her body was placed in a coffin and hastily buried in the ground. Weeks later, the family disinterred Colene to place her in the family mausoleum. Colene's father opened the coffin to find that she had not been dead at all, just in a deep coma—fairly common in late-stage yellow fever. She had awoken in the ground, panicked, and ate "her own shoulder and hand away." When her sweetheart saw the corpse, he was so repulsed and heartbroken that he fled. Then he sickened with yellow fever and died. Stories of live burials were especially common among the enslaved, perhaps because this was one of the most feared punishments an enslaver could inflict—a means of physical death and spiritual cataclysm. Whether true or not, such stories come up again and again in the historical record. Recalling her experience of yellow fever in Memphis long after the Civil War, Lizzie Barnett related with horror, "When they got to looking into the coffins, they discovered some had turned over . . . and some had clawed dey eyes out and some had gnawed holes in dey hands. Dey was buried alive!"[86]

Mercenary Bias

High epidemic casualties combined with the seasonal exodus gave New Orleans a feeling of perpetual flux. Only half the white population, wrote Reverend Clapp, "looks upon New Orleans as his home." The remainder were intent on fast fortunes, on fulfilling "their respective personal schemes of profit and independence." Nearly every New Orleans visitor remarked on this feeling of impermanence and frantic bustle, with each person staying just a little bit longer, to accumulate wealth and spend it elsewhere. The city's "palaces of abode have been hotels; its exchange has been in the strangers' bar-room; its churches have been like missionary stations on the edge of barbarism," declared one editorialist. Some commentators argued that yellow fever checked economic development and industrialization; that the region could not attract the factories and railroads that increasingly defined industrial regions in New England and the mid-Atlantic. Instead, as a seasonally driven and "emphatically . . . commercial town," with a geographic position that seemed to mandate its cotton market dominance, New Orleans was dependent only to a "small degree . . . upon manufactures."[87]

Critics noted that a pass-through, services-based economy in a city with a high death rate did little to foster "the right kind of public spirit" for a republic. J. D. B. De Bow (a. YF 1847) believed it was unfortunate for New Orleans that "the men who create and direct her commerce are strangers, who have no permanent stake in her future destiny . . . Capital does not accumulate, because its resources are drained by a ruinous absenteeism." De Bow continued, "Our city has been considered a great depot of merchandise, one vast warehouse in which every inhabitant is a mere transient adventurer, without any kind of local feeling or bond of union." He believed that "Something higher must be aimed at than mere trade or commerce, high as these may be . . . A society must be formed."[88]

James Robb, one of the Cotton Kingdom's leading capitalists and railroad boosters, agreed. In a controversial speech delivered in 1852, he said, "The annual flight and dispersion of our citizens is a great drain upon the prosperity of New-Orleans." "You may talk of receipts of cotton, sugar, and tobacco," Robb bellowed, but what New Orleans needed most was "an active and industrious population, that would become permanent and progressive"—an impossibility in a place so scourged. As disease increased the risk of coming to New Orleans, it also increased the white population's mercenary bias: getting rich quickly was their *only* goal. As C. C. Robin, a strong critic of Creole culture, put it, "The universal desire to acquire wealth insures that no profession is despised as long as it makes money." No wonder, Robin mused, that gambling halls were filled each night with people risking their fortunes. What else was there to do? Discuss philosophy? No, Robin conceded, instead "they play, and play heavily . . . They are disgusted by a game in which the stakes are too low."[89]

When the frame of reference for a white man's risk tolerance was literally life and death, it affected the way he approached everything else. He drank and gambled more and lived hedonistically. He was also more violent—inclined to brawl, whip, and duel. As one traveler put it, if a man "wishes only to be rich, and to lead a short life and a merry one," New Orleans was the place for him. Some found fast living in a dangerous city exhilarating. Others found it exhausting. "I don't like New Orleans," commission merchant James Wyche commented in 1857, "and only remain here because I think I can in a few years be able to say that I am independent of the world in regard to pecuniary concerns." Cotton planter William Lafayette Gunnels likewise wrote of his exasperation. Not only could he not sell his land during the epidemic of 1855, but his brother Andrew would also not lend him money, thinking Louisiana too risky, and because the "two last crops [had] been so short," he was now compelled to sell some of his slaves. "I am getting in the notion of leaving the river," Gunnels wrote. "My family runs such risk of yellow fever & cholera that I feel constantly uneasy about them." Debts and disease had driven him crazy: "I am so much altered since you saw me," he ended. "My beard has become as white as cotton."[90]

Making a Killing

Not everyone felt the same degree of stress about yellow fever and cotton market stagnation. For white doctors, the fever season—when the market's attention shifted from commodities and slavery to preserving health and processing death—was the busiest and most lucrative time of the year. Many physicians and nurses performed their jobs with integrity. Some risked their lives to help others, and many died in the course of their duties. Others volunteered their services gratis for the poor and enslaved, through charities like the Howard Association. But the Deep South also had its share of medical professionals who made vast sums off scared people in their most vulnerable moments. Many then invested their earnings in the cotton economy, buying plantations and enslaved people, and perpetuating the system of disease, enslavement, and exploitation. Unlike the cotton and sugar industries, the size of which can be gauged by export tonnage and price currents, the health industry was nebulous, spanning a variety of formal and informal economies elusive to both the historian and the governments that occasionally sought to tax them. But given the amount individuals spent on their health, the immense wealth of certain doctors, and the ubiquity of health-related businesses, the Cotton Kingdom's third industry—health—was worth many millions of dollars annually.[91]

Adopting the mantra "[the] sickl[ier] the country the better of course for the physicians," entrepreneurs of a medical bent saw New Orleans as a great opportunity. There were "doctors" everywhere: men with varying degrees of medical training, and often none at all—so many, in fact, that the city council cracked down on the "great number of individuals recently arrived in this city" in 1804, who were practicing medicine and surgery without obtaining permission.[92] Getting licensed in Louisiana was not especially difficult. A white man had to be over twenty-one, hold a diploma from an American or European medical school (this included two years of classes and a practicum), undergo a brief examination in New Orleans (before a committee of doctors and nondoctors), and establish his good moral character.[93] There was some wiggle room on these qualifications, at least early on. Black men, for example, were barred by the Cabildo from practicing medicine after 1801 and the Americans made it a felony for any slave to "administer any medicine whatever" if not told to do so by their white master in 1808—the punishment execution without benefit of clergy. But in 1805—and for a time thereafter—a formerly enslaved man from Philadelphia named James Durham was practicing in the heart of the French Quarter, with the full knowledge of the city council. In these early epidemic years, with so much sickness and not enough doctors, the council found that Durham's activities were in the "interests of the community," especially as he had a good yellow fever reputation. Durham boasted to his correspondent Benjamin Rush that in 1794 he had lost just six patients to yellow fever out of fifty, fewer "than all the other doctors here." In 1800 Durham reportedly lost only eleven out of sixty-four patients, treating them with a concoction of garden sorrel and sugar.[94]

In 1809, New Orleans counted eighteen doctors and surgeons, five apothecaries, and two dentists. But by 1823, fifty-three registered physicians practiced medicine in New Orleans, many of them refugees from Saint-Domingue, or their descendants who had not been formally trained in medical schools but had learned their arts in tropical medicine during Caribbean wars. By 1858 there were 217 licensed doctors working in private practice, 117 druggists pedaling medications, and hundreds of "steam doctors," advocating homoeopathic remedies, roaming the city. Elites who could afford it convalesced in their mansions under medical supervision or in one of seven private hospitals. In the well-furnished Circus Street Infirmary (costing $2 to $5 per day), nurses and esteemed doctors like John Ker—a self-proclaimed fever specialist—attended patients around the clock with expensive medicines, billed on top of the cost of admission.[95]

In New Orleans especially, a doctor's reputation—and expense—was proportional to his success in treating yellow fever. But there was little consensus about how to do that. Before 1845 there were only five medical colleges in the entire South. Yellow fever pathology was not routinely taught at most medical schools until the end of the nineteenth century so physicians facing the disease simply improvised. Where one doctor bled, another blistered. Some dosed their patients with mercury; others offered quinine only. One doctor might give patients Sydenham potion or Blue Mass, while another dunked them into ice baths. One cure patented by Dr. J. Shecut involved dissolving two ounces of "Rochelle or Epsom Salts" with three or four grains of "Tartar Emetic" in half a pint of warm water, and dosing the patient every fifteen to twenty minutes. If that failed, Shecut called for "Jalap, half a drachm," and ten grains of Calomel dissolved in molasses. The concoction produced an immediate bowel movement, allegedly ridding the body of noxious poisons. Some doctors developed cult-like reputations for their proprietary methods. Dr. Pierre Lambert, for example, was famous for his opium and coffee cocktail. We now know that none of these therapies worked. But scared New Orleanians paid handsomely for such cures as nothing else was on offer.[96]

White physicians fell into two rough camps, delineated by ethnicity. European-born and Creole patients patronized "French" physicians, men who claimed to have trained in Paris or had gained direct experience with tropical disease as military surgeons in Martinique and Saint-Domingue. These physicians typically advocated "passive" procedures like baths, bed rest, hydration, and a dash of hope-inducing medicine. For example, one English visitor related he had seen a French physician sit an ailing man in a lime juice bath "as hot as he could bear," bringing "instant relief" to yellow fever symptoms.[97] American-born patients, however, sought out American-trained doctors. These physicians were known for their "heroic" or "energetic" interventions, like blistering, purging, bleeding, and pepper rubs. Some bled so copiously that their patients fainted. Others, following the advice of Benjamin Rush, used excessive amounts of calomel.[98] Powerful and poisonous, calomel was a violent laxative, causing the breath to become fetid, gums and tongue to ulcerate, teeth to fall out, and jaw to corrode. And because it was mercury-based, calomel could also be deadly. In 1812 one doctor lamented that most of the soldiers posted in the city had died not from yellow fever but from the calomel given to them as its remedy. Conscious of its dangers, physicians frequently called for the administration of calomel only until the patient was "salivated," the first symptom of acute mercury poisoning. Laypeople generally did not perform heroic interventions: too much bleeding or mercury could kill a patient. A doctor's skill was mapped by his ability to identify the critical therapeutic point.[99]

Doctors of all ethnicities agreed that patients should seek physicians "acquainted with their mode of life"—that is, a physician of their religion or ethnicity. But in cases of yellow fever, any medical care was considered better than none at all as there was no disease to which the adage "a stitch in time" applied "with greater force." For this reason, epidemics were exhausting and stressful for doctors, who were called on at all hours of the day and night by an unbroken stream of sick, dying, and desperate people, many of whom did not speak English or French. Dr. E. B. Harris cared for about eighty patients in 1833 during the dual yellow fever–cholera epidemic. One night in late August, Harris went to see a twenty-eight-year-old man at 7 p.m. who lived in a windowless and offensively dank basement. He remained with the patient until well past midnight, returning at 6 a.m. the following day. He then spent two days constantly attending him. Nearly every day for the next month Harris had a new patient.[100]

Doctors bragged endlessly about their yellow fever numbers—those they saved versus those they lost. One pundit joked that when many of the city's most prominent physicians met after the 1853 epidemic, they compared their stats. Barton bragged he had saved 900 cases and lost only eight; Hunt had 1,300 saves to seventeen losses; Fenner saved 700 to lose only six; Rushton had 600 saves and not a single loss. Dr. Warren Stone interrupted the doctors: "Gentlemen, you must have been wonderfully successful. But as the records show nearly 10,000 deaths, I suppose I must have killed all the balance!" These comically inflated numbers veiled the uncomfortable fact no doctor wanted to admit—they bore some responsibility for cases being so numerous in the first place. Essentially no doctor would diagnose yellow fever in a patient before July, fearing a backlash from the business community (of which many doctors were members), concerned about being wrong, and weary of inciting panic. Physicians' hesitation to diagnose cases early in the season might reduce alarm in the short term. But it could also spark a public health disaster.[101]

This happened in 1847. On June 21, an Irish drayman visited a friend at his crowded boardinghouse on Adeline Street, three blocks from the Charity Hospital. He was attacked with fever, and soon became so ill that his friend called for Dr. Mercier, who found the feverish patient experiencing searing pains in the head, small of his back, and neck—clear signs of yellow fever.

Mercier, however, said it was too early in the year for that disease. Instead, he bled the Irishman copiously and left. When Mercier returned, the drayman's affliction "began to look so much like yellow fever" that he sought a second opinion from Dr. Landreux, who concurred with his diagnosis. Yet even then, they remained silent. Mercier and Landreux did nothing for two weeks, worried to look foolish before their colleagues. The drayman died. So did most of the boarders in the house. And so did 6,000 other people across the city that summer.[102]

Many doctors died, too. Medicine was an unquestionably dangerous vocation, especially for the unacclimated. Just a few weeks into the epidemic of 1833, seven city doctors had already died of yellow fever, leaving the remaining physicians so busy that it was "a hard matter to procure" a doctor "even now at this early stage." In 1855 two medical students in the Charity Hospital, Thomas M. Neal and P. O. Tête—natives of Louisiana but new to New Orleans—died of yellow fever while completing their residencies. Most long-practicing doctors likely developed immunity through exposure, but they could never be completely sure. Few committed the ultimate professional *faux pas* of fleeing during the sickly season along with other elites. Not only was truancy a reputation killer, but the fever season was also doctors' busiest and most lucrative time of the year.[103]

Yellow Fever Rates

Yellow fever influenced the economics of the entire medical profession. In 1824, doctors associated with the New Orleans Medical Society adopted a fee schedule: $3 for an initial visit, $1 for a subsequent visit, $4 for a nighttime visit, $10 to $30 for a written consultation, $20 to $40 for a simple syphilitic condition, and $5 to $30 for a simple operation. Fees were reduced by a third for enslaved Black patients, billed to their owners.[104] But doctors routinely disregarded the guidelines, instead charging what locals called "yellow fever rates," an opportunistic—and extortionate—risk premium for a physician's troubles that people paid because they had no other choice. Once the calendar ticked past July 1—the first acceptable date, according to businessmen, for yellow fever to appear—doctors were incentivized to diagnose "every little fever" as yellow fever. This benefited them in two ways: it allowed them to charge as much as double their normal rates, and it boosted their standing. Benjamin Henry Latrobe laid out the logic plainly: "If the patient recovers, the cure of that fatal disorder adds to the reputation of the physician; if he dies, his death detracts nothing from his credit, because the majority of such cases are fatal." One woman later put it even more pointedly, "As long as money is on hand," doctors will find "yellow fever is on hand."[105]

Abuse abounded. Some doctors demanded $30 up front as well as cab fare to convey them to the patient's home, ignoring desperate promises that "we will pay you double and triple later." Other doctors would not leave their offices for less than $50 in cash, sneering that "the most pitiful quack [would] not accompany you" for anything less. And doctors' fees were only the beginning. As one newspaper described it, a physician's bill usually ran to $50, but then came the "Cupper's bill, $20; nurse's bill, usually about six days, $30; medicine, about $5; contingencies about $5 more." This came to "a cool hundred" in *cash,* "besides the wear and tear of conscience, and the loss of some 40 pounds of flesh and bloom."[106] This meant the total cost of sickness could be equivalent to many months' wages.

Then there were other add-ons. There were medicines to speed convalescence: Indian Vegetable Pills (25 cents a box), Radway's Ready Relief (a $2-a-bottle cure for "pestilential diseases or organic derangement," the most successful mail-away patent medicine of the nineteenth century); and Stillman's Sarsaparilla Syrup ($3 a bottle, and an apparent favorite of presidents Martin Van Buren and Andrew Jackson). There were also Epsom salts, levigated antimony, pulverized licorice, powdered resin, and flowers of sulfur. Then there was the question of lodging. Many boardinghouses demanded a yellow fever premium on tenancy during convalescence. Mary Campbell cried to her brother in 1847 that she was deathly ill with fever and had to borrow $40 to pay supplemental house rent, a sum she could not afford even in healthy times.[107]

Some people, in fact, bankrupted themselves in the process of trying to get better. Territorial governor W. C. C. Claiborne spent half his salary on doctors in 1804, and his wife and child still died from yellow fever. German immigrant Johann Joachim Lagemann fell ill in Natchez in 1806 and spent his life savings on doctors and medicine. In 1853 a professional gambler named George Devol agreed to pay his doctors and an "old colored woman" $25 per day. At the end of his twenty-three-day convalescence, Devol passed over all the money he had in the world. In anticipation of yellow fever rates, newcomers were encouraged to save as much as they could from the old country—between $50 and $100—for their inevitable medical expenses.[108] A $2 box of medicine, after all, was equivalent to a day's salary for a skilled clerk, two to four days' wages for lower- and middle-class white men, and a whole week's wages for white and free Black women. Travel writer Charles Lyell noted in 1849 that the "Irish servants in the hotel assure us that they cannot save, in spite of their high wages, for, whatever money they put by soon goes to pay the doctor's bill, during attacks of chill and fever." With no health insurance or reliable safety net, such massive financial outlay proved an impediment to social mobility unique to New Orleans. Max Neubling, an immigrant from Ulm, Germany, wrote home to his family in 1824 about this predicament, stating "I would have saved some money already, had it not been for the misfortune of contracting the prevailing fever, and spending nearly all of my savings"—$55—"to pay the doctor." Neubling concluded, "A man can surely earn money here, but it is hard earned money, in this hot climate, especially, if one contract the fever."[109]

If the doctor was unsuccessful, the expenses continued. The whole process of mourning, burial, and settling estates also cost money. Lawyers were busiest in the early summer, with people crowding their office to write up wills, establish executors, and notarize documents. Merchant William Crenshaw wrote to his friend in September 1841, when at least eighty people were dying per day, "I have made my will to prevent trouble in the case of my death. You will find it in our iron chest. It is very short leaving everything to Ma and you my executor." Crenshaw signed off, "Should I not be spared to meet you all again, farewell, Farewell, Farewell!"[110] Certain attorneys made most of their money from estate management and successions. As yellow fever killed quickly and unexpectedly, sometimes attacking those who presumed themselves acclimated, many people died intestate. This too could be a boon for lawyers, since in the absence of wills, attorneys could make even more money as lengthy court battles ensued between heirs and business partners. In extreme cases settlements took more than a decade.[111]

Expenses often fell to surviving relations and acquaintances. A funeral could cost as little as $25 (body carting and grave digging only) but could easily exceed $100. If a free Black or white person could afford it, they used Pierre Casenave, a cabinetmaker by trade who became one of the richest free Black men in New Orleans through his undertaking business. As the only licensed embalmer in the city—he claimed he could preserve a body "for an indefinite period, perhaps forever"—he choreographed all the funerals of New Orleans's rich and famous. Some very wealthy people spent $500 and more on ornate Casenave-designed events, including mahogany coffins and ornately carved and draped hearses, drawn by caparisoned horses, and accompanied by a dirge-playing full brass band. Then there were the costs of gravediggers, normally Black men who could earn as much as $10 a day during non-epidemic years, and as much as $5 to $10 per coffin in desperate times. There were also payments to the priest. The Catholic Church earned most of its annual revenue during the fever season, charging $20 for last rites and about $100 for interments in the consecrated cemetery. Then there were the grave wares to decorate tombs. If a person could afford it, they contracted Florville Foy, a free man of color, to cut a bespoke marble tomb ornament in celebration of the life of the deceased.[112]

Some people fought back against epidemic price gouging. In 1855 Dr. R. T. Collins charged J. W. Graves $500 for medical services for Graves, his wife, daughter, son, and a "negro woman." When Graves refused to pay such a large sum, Collins sued. The jury agreed $500 was too much, awarding Collins only $150. But three years later Collins appealed the verdict, making a "reconventional demand" of $209.50 for the insult Graves had served him. Graves countered that not only were the doctor's initial fees far more than the accepted double rate of $100 for the head of household and $50 for each additional family member, but, as his lawyers said, the mere "existence of epidemics does not authorize exorbitant fees." This case illustrated that New Orleanians felt besieged during epidemics on two fronts: by fever and by economics. As the mayor put it during the 1832 epidemic, "The fact is, that even in our present unfortunate time, there is no dearth of Speculation, and there are some who speculate even on public misery." The mayor continued: "The sacrifices which the fear of death can induce the living to make on their income or credit" were many.[113]

Physician-to-Planter Pipeline

Most New Orleanians accepted that medical care was a necessity, albeit an expensive, inconsistent, and unproven one. Hiring an elite private doctor was a public statement that a patriarch had done everything in his power to save himself, his enslaved property, or a family member from death. But in a city where hundreds of thousands of Black people were sold at auction, some physicians saw medicine as a capitalist endeavor rather than a civic calling and yellow fever as "a money making scheme" as good as any other. With a constant supply of sick people, doctoring was an ideal mechanism to acquire capital that would eventually be invested in a plantation, the region's primary engine for wealth creation.[114]

One such medical entrepreneur was Christian Miltenberger, a white refugee of the Haitian Revolution. In 1796 Miltenberger apprenticed at a Cap Français hospital with the Parisian surgeon Dr. Arthaus. He doubtless saw hundreds suffer from yellow fever. After Leclerc's disastrous campaign to retake Saint-Domingue failed, Miltenberger lost hope that the old colonial order would be restored and in 1802 he fled to Cuba with his young wife, Marie-Aimée Mercier, leaving behind most of his possessions. When Napoleon invaded Spain, and Cuba expelled all Saint-Domingue refugees, the only option left for the Miltenbergers was New Orleans. They headed for the city in 1809 along with 9,000 other refugees—many of them free people of color—landing in Louisiana nearly bankrupt.[115]

With an epidemic brewing, the municipal medical examiners pushed through Miltenberger's certifications. He sold the slaves he had illegally smuggled into the United States from Cuba to fund a medical practice on Royal Street, establishing himself within the French medical community. Soon he developed a following as one of the best doctors around. Whether Miltenberger deserved his reputation remains unclear. He did not record how many of his patients died or with what frequency. But he did make money, and fast. His 648-page medical journal reads like a who's-who of New Orleans, though he also served marginalized and enslaved customers. In a given month, he might earn $3 for a home visit for a young Black man suffering from fever and convulsions, $3 from a Black woman who came to his office with a sore throat, and $8 for a home visit for an old man with tetanus. In April 1821 he made $93.50 in one day, much of it from smallpox inoculations.[116]

Fevers were his bread and butter. By 1821 Miltenberger was earning over $6,700 in his practice annually—most of it during the epidemic season. He invested the money in land and slaves, and by 1826 his sugar plantation earnings in Opelousas (and later in Plaquemine as well) exceeded his physician's salary. His medical practice funded the expansion of his sugar plantations. Those plantations required equipment for pressing and boiling that could run upward of $10,000, as well as an army of enslaved laborers. This required cash, and doctoring—unlike a great many professions—was mostly based on cash, not credit. Miltenberger's expanding plantation-based wealth subsequently propelled him into positions of social and political power. According to insurance records, by the end of the 1820s Miltenberger owned at least three properties in New Orleans, dozens of slaves, and a great many luxury goods. And his wealth trickled down through the generations.

Miltenberger's three sons—Alphonse, Gustave, and Aristide—became the most prominent sugar factors in New Orleans. In separate offices next door to one another, the sons held the controlling portion of the New Orleans sugar business, as well as thousands of dollars in real estate, slaves, and personal property.[117]

Though most rural practitioners in the South made significantly less than Miltenberger—between $500 and $2,000 per annum—Miltenberger was representative of his class in one important respect: most Deep South physicians owned (or aspired to own) plantations and slaves. Dun & Bradstreet's credit report for G. W. Campbell was typical: "Is a physician by profession & owns & runs two plantations near the city also owns fine R.E. [real estate] in N.O. Is undoubtedly wealthy & solvent & his notes are promptly paid." The report likewise described Dr. E. D. Fenner, editor of the *New Orleans Medical & Surgical Journal,* as rich though risky, noting that he "stands well in the profession—owns several slaves—single." Later the agent reported that Fenner "took the benefit of the Bankrupt Law to get rid of his old debts; made his slaves over to someone else . . . took back his slaves; continued to improve in his practice & must have made some money at it."[118]

Treating slaves, in fact, was the most lucrative business strategy for physicians in and around New Orleans. Several doctors made so much money off of slave sickness—in private practice and in providing services to slave marts—that Samuel Cartwright even conceded that "the most profitable kind" of medical practice was "that among negroes," allowing a Louisiana physician to stand "some chance of making his bread while he has teeth to chew it." In 1821 Dr. Sanchez opened a hospital for slaves where every patient would be "lodged, attended, physicked, fed and washed" for 75 cents per day—billed to the white enslaver. Another hospital, the Touro Infirmary, in 1855 cared for many Black people, some suffering from yellow fever. Among them was Mitchell, a twenty-two-year-old man from Virginia who had been sick for eight days before his owner, D. Madden, sent him to the hospital, paying $5 for his care. George, another twenty-two-year-old enslaved man from Virginia, had been in the state for only three months when he fell sick in June; his owner, O. J. Donnella, paid $17 for his stay. Donnella also paid $19 for the care of Ellen, a fourteen-year-old from Virginia, when she sickened with yellow fever.[119] Doctors could also make a lot of money in "country practice." Medical bills were one of the year's largest expenses on many plantations, accepted by whites as a necessary capital investment like any other. When planter Joseph Erwin paid $250 worth of doctor's bills in 1814 for his slaves' medical care, he hoped not only to recoup his losses but to profit much more in the future through these now-healthy people's labor.[120]

The potential for wealth in the Cotton Kingdom meant that for many doctors, medicine became less about protecting the health of individuals and more about financing the doctor-turned-planter's investment in the cotton and sugar economies. Perhaps physicians did not perceive any conflict of interest in amassing fortunes from failure and death. But many certainly avoided taking substantial steps to improve the public's health more generally. Most doctors, even fever specialists with government affiliation like Miltenberger (city councilor) and Pierre Lambert (president of the board of health), spent the majority of their energy on their private practices and plantations.[121] In an era predating standardized medical ethics or germ theory, epidemic disease was simply good for business.

Alternative Medicine

Not all people could afford licensed doctors or believed in their methods. British journalist William Chambers claimed that the "nursing of a creole negress, accustomed to the disease, is considered better than any of the usual modes of medical treatment." Many New Orleanians agreed, deriding doctors as licensed quacks who made it up as they went along. Chambers scoffed, "If you were to call in, one after another, six of the most eminent physicians in New Orleans . . . it is probable that they would prescribe six different modes of treatment," with the patient's chance of recovery "not improved by any."[122] If a doctor or nurse was too expensive, a steamer might do. As early as 1804, steam doctors roamed the Deep South, employing homeopathic remedies like hot steams and herbs to cure yellow fever as well as many other ailments. Derided as empiricists and charlatans by licensed physicians, steamers were popular with the masses for their affordability and less frightening interventions. Mississippi governor Hiram Runnels estimated in 1835 that almost one-half of the state's inhabitants followed steamers' homeopathic advice.[123] Doctors repeatedly tried and failed to use their political clout to regulate steamers into oblivion. In turn, steamers hated the medical establishment, claiming (truthfully) that licensed physicians poisoned their patients with mercury and bankrupted them for the privilege. Why, one steamer's journal asked, were the vendors of "carnage and death" protected by their licenses, while steamers who provided "inoffensive and efficient remedies" were declared illegal?[124]

But even a cheaper steamer was out of reach for some, as was the dignity of medical choice. Many enslaved and poor people were forced to rely on the charity of individual physicians, their masters, or institutions like the Howard Association when they fell sick. Few could afford expensive medicines or cheaper steams, and even fewer could afford the exorbitant rents demanded outside the city during the fever season. The Baton Rouge *Comet* suggested a self-help regime for those unacclimated people without friends or money: "Get a flask of Gin," the paper instructed, "and place an ounce and a half of rats-bane in it—and then go out into the country some where and die comfortably."[125]

Craving some kind of solution—or perhaps spiritual autonomy—many turned to the heterodox and the supernatural. This was especially true of Black people, who had less money and whose religious and ritual traditions had deep Haitian and African roots. Mariquita Orfila boasted that she cured

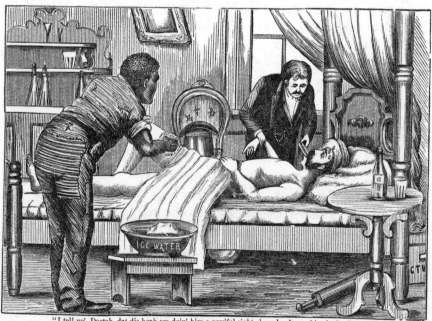

"I tell yo', Doctah, dat dis heah am doin' him a pow'ful sight o' good. It am fo' a fac."—Page 54.

James Dugan, *Doctor Dispachemquic: A Story of the Great Southern Plague of 1878* (New Orleans, 1879), frontispiece.

many people who had been declared "quite hopeless" by doctors; she administered the juice of verbena, in small doses three times a day or by injections twice a day, until the bowels emptied. Orfila supplied the juice and syringe for a cost. Marie Laveau, the famous "Voodoo Queen," was said to have healed thousands suffering from sickness with charms, gris-gris, and herbs, dancing at Congo Square with "a snake called Zombi, the Snake God." Necromancers, fortune-tellers, and phrenologists all found takers in New Orleans. Madame Virginica, the "Great Russian Prophetess and Healing Medium," was willing to look into the "hidden mysteries of the Past, Present, and Future" and predict the outcomes of lawsuits, disease, travels, and even "prize numbers in lotteries." Virginica also provided medical services with "fully guaranteed" remedies "for healing all manner of disease." Madame Caprell, billed as "the greatest Clairvoyant, Seer and Spiritual Physician in the known world," treated all diseases.[126] Nelson Desbrosses, a native of New Orleans, studied vodou under J. B. Valmour, a well-known practitioner from Haiti. When Desbrosses returned to New Orleans, he gained fame as a healer and medium—as well as for his poetry in *Les Cenelles*.[127]

While white doctors, healers, and a few Black priestesses like Laveau enjoyed high status and esteem—as well as high pay—for their work, most health-care work was far less glamorous, falling on neighbors, mothers, enslaved women, and children. In cases of yellow fever, nursing was "very laborious." Cotton planter Horace Smith Fulkerson insisted two nurses were required at all times. He remarked that he had saved a patient who was "entirely pulseless" by feeding him milk toddy all night, the "total quantity of which would make half a dozen well men drunk for a time, with, apparently, little effect upon the patient."[128] Margaret Brashear (d. YF 1834), who owned fifty people at the sugar plantation Belle Isle on Bayou Teche, complained in June 1824 that the slaves were unusually sick. Because the plantation was "so remote from all Medical aid," she fretted that not enough slaves would be well enough when the harvest commenced. So she treated these people herself. Louisiana governor Thomas Robertson (a. YF ca. 1807) said in August 1823 that almost all his slaves were sick, but that he and his wife had experienced "great success" with their home remedies. Planter J. E. Craighead wrote to his father about the growing fever cases on the family plantation in 1847. Thirty-five enslaved people had been stricken. And after his overseer died, Craighead said that he "had to act as Doctorer, overseer, and everything for awhile."[129]

Women often butted heads with the white male medical establishment and openly questioned men's expertise. When Dr. Mordica, the "oldest and best doctor" in Mobile, saw the dire situation of Mr. Woods, suffering from yellow fever, he prescribed beef tea and champagne. As Woods's condition worsened, Mordica deemed him beyond medical care. Woods's neighbor Elizabeth Hart, an Irish immigrant, believed Mordica was a quack and told him so, loudly. Years before, she yelled, Mordica had killed her daughter by misdiagnosing her yellow fever as worms. With tensions running high, Hart mixed French brandy, allspice, and mint, and forced Woods to drink the "julep." She put a poultice on his stomach and throat and rubbed red pepper and vinegar down his body until her hands blistered. Soon, Woods's pulse normalized. Later, Mordica tried to take credit for his recovery but was again rebuked. "Had I been depending on you, I would now be a dead man," Woods sneered. It was "to Mrs. Hart alone I owe my life, she saved me when you gave me up." Thereafter, Mordica always called on Hart when he had a particularly bad case, monetizing her remedies and using them to his professional advantage.[130]

Most nursing fell to Black women. This was sometimes paid work. The Howard Association, for example, employed many free Black women during epidemics, with patients, apparently, preferring their skill and steadiness to the services of aloof white doctors. Though the usual pay for a twenty-four-hour nursing shift was $2 to $3, two nurses of color in 1853 demanded $10 per day and got it.[131] Most Black women's health-care labor, however, was unpaid, with enslaved women developing a pharmacopoeia of remedies for yellow fever, often without money or sanction. One woman recalled that she gave charcoal, onions, and honey to babies sick with fever, and camphor to adults. She also made red oak and cactus weed tea, but believed the best remedy was to tie a rabbit foot around the neck of the victim. Creole slaves prepared a variety of tisanes of sassafras and orange-leaf. Ceceil George recalled that when her mistress, Mrs. Jerry, fell sick, Mrs. Jerry implored George to make her some tea and give it to her secretly because she did not think the doctor's remedies were working. Discreetly slipping out of the room, George boiled the guts of a pumpkin with whisky, and fed it to Mrs. Jerry, who quickly improved.[132] Alice Douglass recalled that while many slaves wore amulets, beads, and charms to protect their health, all "wore asafedida," an herb that threw off a fetid smell, to keep diseases away. Such were the small ways people sought control over their lives amid a terrifying disease environment.[133]

To Acclimation

Yellow fever was deadly and expensive. And no matter what a doctor said, it was incurable. In fact, the only defense against yellow fever was to get acclimated. Most white people faced this risk willingly, though sometimes naively. Enslaved people did not have a choice. Though fearful of the disease like everyone else, few slaves could take any prophylactic measures against infection. They could not flee, afford doctors or medicine, or convalesce sufficiently before returning to work. Those were the privileges of white, free, and wealthy people—the antecedents to immunocapital. If an enslaved person died, their owner would mostly have lamented it as a financial loss, not a human tragedy. But when an enslaved person survived yellow fever, the *enslaver* benefited twice over: not only did the slave recover, gain immunity, and live to generate more capital in cotton (or potentially children); the capital that person embodied was now "safer," and worth considerably more.

3

Immunocapital

On Easter night 1806, a twenty-seven-year-old, Italian-born, French-speaking German stranger named Vincent Nolte sailed into New Orleans harbor. Nolte was initially unimpressed with the quality of the local townspeople and business opportunities, thinking the Creoles philistine and remarking that "there was not a single [merchant] house there possessed of any capital worth mentioning"—just a handful of French, Scotch, and new American concerns. But *anciennes* were likewise skeptical of Nolte. Who was this risk-taking "merchant prince," they asked? Nolte stoked this mysterious persona, telling stories of his obscure beginnings in Leghorn, his connections with the Parisian banker Gabriel-Julien Ouvrard, and his acquaintance with Napoleon and Charles IV of Spain. He sealed his dominance over New Orleans business with one dramatic stunt, arranging for three schooners to sneak past the British blockade into New Orleans carrying half a million dollars in Mexican silver—the capital to back his new venture. Now, once-skeptical Creole planters—*motif de plus!*—embraced this "stranger," and there was not a town soiree to which he was not invited.[1]

Over time—and with a few false starts and failed schemes along the way—Nolte became one of the most powerful merchants in New Orleans. By 1819, Vincent Nolte & Co. was worth millions, responsible for shipping about a quarter of the cotton that passed through New Orleans—4 to 8 percent of US exports—on its way around the world. As historian Edward Baptist describes it, no man did more to transform the early New

Orleans cotton market into a global behemoth than Nolte, who in the process accumulated a level of power that "few who were not absolute monarchs had ever felt before." Collectively leveraging his various forms of capital—whiteness, maleness, connections—Nolte was instrumental in underwriting the cotton revolution sweeping across the Deep South.[2]

But Nolte possessed one form of capital more important locally than his boatloads of Spanish silver or high European connections. Three months after his arrival in New Orleans, he fell sick with a serious case of yellow fever. On the first day of his illness, Nolte developed a headache so intense he believed his brain was on fire. The following day, a French doctor named Raoul dosed Nolte with so many emetics and purgatives that he lost consciousness. On the third day, Nolte was dying. Worse, he was dying intestate, thus exposing the funds entrusted to his care to "extremely unsafe hands." "I need not tell you that you have the yellow fever," cashier of La Banque de la Louisiane Stephen Zacharie (d. YF 1807) told Nolte, "and it is more than probable that you will die to-morrow." Zacharie begged him to write a will and save his capital from pillage. But Nolte insisted he would not "leave the world [for] yet awhile." He did not wish to "bother [his] head" with money matters as he ailed.[3]

Nolte got lucky and survived his acclimation. And now what had made him sick made him strong. He possessed "immunocapital": socially acknowledged lifelong immunity to a highly lethal, incurable virus. Assured of his acclimation, Nolte could use his immunity to gain the confidence of associates in New Orleans and abroad. He could gamble ever-greater sums, restart quickly after frequent financial panics, and move first in new investment opportunities. He could command the labor of increasing numbers of other people, both Black and white. Confident that Nolte would not drop dead in October, bankers across the Atlantic World—including the Barings and Labouchères—were happier to deal with him. In turn, he could loan large sums to individuals, and even the cash-strapped municipality, at high interest rates.[4] He could remain in town year-round or travel safely to other tropical ports when epidemics raged. His social position also improved: now he could marry more advantageously, father children, and rub elbows with the political elite. Generals Andrew Jackson and Marquis de Lafayette, banker Nicholas Biddle, naturalist John James Audubon, and Austrian finance minister Carl Friedrich Kübeck were among Nolte's acquaintances. And demonstrating his commercial and political dominance,

Benjamin Henry Latrobe (d. YF 1820), the man who designed the US Capitol and the porticos of the White House, built a grand house for Nolte on Royal Street, one block from the Cabildo.[5]

Nolte considered his episode with yellow fever important enough to include it in his autobiography, written almost fifty years later. In memory, *he* had made the *choice* to survive, having "not at all [felt] like dying," taking his acclimation as proof that God and nature had sanctioned his entrepreneurship. Though he officially became an American citizen around 1811, by attaining immunity in 1806 this immigrant became "*of* a different country"—an acclimated citizen who had been naturalized and *legitimized* in the Atlantic's torrid zone.[6]

Six Easters later, forty-three-year-old cotton planter John Palfrey (a. YF ca. 1804) contemplated how to avoid financial ruin for the third time in a decade from his aptly named cotton plantation Forlorn Hope. In 1803 Palfrey had left his family in Boston for New Orleans, seeking commercial advantages "tenfold to what they are in the Northern States." He first found work as a ship chandler. Then, with a small bit of capital, he established one of those American-backed commission houses Nolte so disparaged. But Palfrey, Shepherd, & Company failed in 1807, leaving him indebted to the tune of $10,500. Next, Palfrey tried his hand at sugar planting. But a poor crop in 1810, combined with the British blockade, drove him further into debt. His obligations mounted. He lost sleep and his health deteriorated. Before creditors could repossess all his property—the sheriff had already seized some slaves and silver candlesticks—Palfrey fled west to try his hand at cotton planting.[7]

With a loan from the commission house of Beverly Chew (a. YF ca. 1796) and Richard Relf (a. YF ca. 1801), Palfrey purchased 900 acres of cotton land in the frontier region of Attakapas and twenty people for $7,750. As a security, Chew and Relf held the mortgage on Forlorn Hope. Right away, Palfrey's slaves worked to transform this "piece of land without a fence, house, or any thing of the kind" into a profitable plantation. They cleared forest, hauled fence rails, threw up buildings, plowed land, and grew food. The women and children cultivated cotton, through hunger, inclement weather, and disease—producing 37,000 pounds that first year. But even this was not enough to meet Palfrey's debts. In 1812 he defaulted. Chew and Relf threatened to sue.[8]

Like many white men in Louisiana—highly leveraged, property rich, and cash poor—Palfrey laid out his position to Chew and Relf in terms he thought they would understand. He assured them he would immediately send them 25 bales of ginned cotton (12,500 pounds) as a gesture of good faith. But, he pleaded, "in addition to my crop I have no other resource but the disposal of some of the negroes" and selling slaves would be financially "ruinous" to him in future years. After some consideration, Chew and Relf agreed to a compromise: they would drop their reputation-damaging lawsuit if Palfrey sent them the cotton and half his slaves. Their clerks estimated that these people were collectively worth about $2,200, or—with the cotton—enough to cover about half of Palfrey's debt.[9]

As luck would have it for Palfrey, the War of 1812 caused such disruption to the New Orleans market that the debt issue was dropped until 1815. And by then, as he told Chew and Relf, the situation had changed. The ten enslaved people were "now season'd to the climate" and only now "beginning to be useful" and were thus "intrinsically more valuable than at the time of purchase." Palfrey elaborated on this theory about disease risk, slavery, and acclimation to his attorney, insisting that *he* should be compensated for the risk *he* had adopted in taking on unacclimated property. The "risqué was mine," he wrote, "& has cost me loss, expense, & a great deal of trouble & anxiety." To prove his point, he wrote out a "very modest" back-of-the-envelope calculation demonstrating how the value of a nine-year-old girl named Maria had increased:

Maria cost 250
Keeping 4½ years—54
Clothing—22.50
Taxes—4.50
Risque 5 per cent 56.25
387.25

If his 5 percent per annum risk calculation applied to all ten enslaved people, their collective worth would be $3,500 "and more"—a sum significantly larger than Chew and Relf's "unfamiliar" clerks had estimated back in 1812. In 1815, Chew and Relf acquiesced to Palfrey's logic. Maria was one of eight slaves reverted to the firm for a lot-price of $2,628.[10]

For men like Palfrey, Black people's acclimation was a risk reducible to a numerical value and it was his prerogative, as a white enslaver, to leverage it for his gain. In essence, he held financial ownership of their risk. We do not know what Maria—or Adam, Daniel, Eloy, Ephorim, Leticia,

Mississippi, or Phetis—thought about this speculation. It must have been horrible to know that even their sickness and suffering could be monetized, another cruel twist in a system where all value generated by enslaved Black people—forged, picked, or embodied—transferred to whites. Palfrey never used such dispassionate and actuarial language when discussing his white family. When his sons Edward and Henry died from yellow fever in New Orleans in 1817 and 1824, he was overcome with grief.[11] Nor could he find consolation in his eldest son, John Gorham Palfrey, who refused to move to Louisiana, became an antislavery Unitarian minister, and joined the faculty of Harvard Divinity School. Shortly after Palfrey Sr. died in 1843, John Gorham freed the slaves he had inherited and wrote a pamphlet laying out the series of calculations underwriting slavery in the Yellow Fever South: "The advertisements of prime negroes in the more southernly slave States constantly describe them as *acclimated*," he wrote, "Why? Of course with a view to a better price."[12]

Generating from Sickness

One mosquito bite put Vincent Nolte and Maria on two very different paths. For a white man like Nolte, surviving yellow fever helped propel him into society's upper echelons. For an enslaved girl like Maria, acclimation increased her value to her white owner, becoming one more matter for speculation in the debt and credit markets underwriting the Cotton Kingdom. While their bodies' immune responses were identical, this society—inundated by yellow fever and filled with risks—responded to their acclimations differently, using assumptions about epidemiology and race to justify yet more inequality and create yet more wealth for some.

Nineteenth-century Americans were highly attuned to "risk": identifying it, quantifying it, and mitigating it. Once narrowly associated with maritime insurance, risk by the nineteenth century seemed to span just about everything: distant markets, private fortunes, harvests, fires, and life and limb. Risk, in fact, became so consuming and pervasive that it was "all but impossible," as historian Jonathan Levy describes it, for Americans to disentangle it from the "modern condition."[13] New Orleanians organized their daily lives according to what levels of risk they deemed acceptable and unacceptable. The steamship carrying a person down the Mississippi River was risky—it might explode. Securing a loan was risky—banks might over-speculate and go bust, as many did following the panics of 1819, 1825, 1837, and 1857. Buying people was risky—they might run away, die, or become injured. Planting cotton was risky—periodic droughts, hurricanes, or caterpillars could destroy an entire year's harvest and leave the richest planters suddenly insolvent. Some people found these risks unacceptable; others sought to mitigate them through insurance, collateralization, or other financial instruments.[14]

Yellow fever was New Orleans's most widely distributed and considerable risk of all. Creditors might default, the levee might break, and row houses might burn down in a freak fire. But yellow fever was a near certainty. By the 1830s many treated disease risk as indistinguishable, linguistically and practically, from all other mortal and market risks. But disease was different in key respects. Unlike other uncertain catastrophic events, like steamboat explosions or bank failures—events that *might* happen and *could* be mitigated—yellow fever risk was "uninsurable." There was no vaccine or inoculation, and there was no way to truly avoid it. The *only* means to mitigate against this risk was to survive a (hopefully) mild case in childhood, avoid the city during epidemics, or publicly embrace disease and get acclimated as an adult, a highly risky act in and of itself.

The risk of *not* embracing yellow fever, however, was also perilous. Here, the "necessities" and "temptations" of business—wealth through cotton, sugar, and slaves—made risking death and gaining immunity to yellow fever indispensable for whites who wished to climb the ladder.[15] All white newcomers understood that until they were acclimated, they would be regarded "with suspicion . . . considered a bird of passage only." They would have few acquaintances and would "never [be] positive of [their] place in society." But once they took on the "risqué of acclimation" and became "*creolized,*" friends flocked in. As the *Commercial Bulletin* put it, "One soothes him by pleasant words—another solaces him with the candor of intimacy—a third gives him business, and all extend confidence." The rewards of taking on acclimation risk were so wonderful that a true New Orleanian never "regret[ted] to hear that one of our friends is sick with fever. If he die, we are sorry, but if he live, the wealth of the reward is far paramount to the danger."[16] Taking on disease risk became locally linked with white legitimacy—a stranger had gambled his life to attain "native" status, a form of social capital that Creole planters, free people of color, and French grandees were apparently bestowed as a birthright.

Risk was ubiquitous, but so too was the notion of choice. Self-made white men in Jacksonian America picked their political leaders, chose their civic and ecclesiastical affiliations, selected from an array of consumer goods, and opted to succeed in business. And rejecting the Calvinist orthodoxy about election and predestination—as many Americans did following the Second Great Awakening—men in this age of "the first person singular" even chose not to sin.[17] Predictably, acclimated whites narrated their personal yellow fever stories as if survival had been a choice, too; they had *chosen* to vanquish yellow fever. Ipso facto, lesser men—immoral weaklings, failures, probably drunks—chose to die.[18]

Such thinking was absurd, even perverse. And despite pious fidelity to this hierarchy of immunocapital, all self-made, acclimated men harbored private doubts. Was the disease he survived back in 1837 actually yellow fever? Was his Creole wife safe? What about his children? And that "fully acclimated" Virginia-born slave he purchased—was that guarantee just one more slave trader's lie? Because immunity was invisible and all too easy to mistake, at best one could be quite certain but never positive of anyone's acclimation status, including one's own. But whether genuinely immune, mistaken, or recklessly faking it, all New Orleanians played the game. Mastering the performance of immunity—by remaining in town during epidemics, speaking of acclimation like an "old-timer," producing credible witnesses, or boasting of surviving a particularly serious case—was crucial to local legitimacy. As the *Picayune* urged in 1841, "If a man intends to make himself a citizen of New Orleans, his first duty is to become acclimated. He owes it to himself and to society."[19]

For enslaved Black people, yellow fever immunity opened no such doors. As embodied capital, they could possess immunity but not immunocapital, a perversion of the principles of risk and choice that whites used to enrich themselves, justify racial slavery, and reinforce their social and political dominance over Black people. By definition, enslaved people were not free to choose which risks were acceptable. That choice was made for them by whites who insisted they owned the disease risk of the people they enslaved, adopting it along with the deed of sale. The Cotton Kingdom was structured such that any rewards for taking on disease risk through acclimation—longevity, promotions, social advancement, power—accrued to the master class, not to the enslaved people who built their wealth.

Vaguely Acclimated

By the mid-eighteenth century, the idea of "acclimation"—a "remarkable idiosyncrasy" of nature where humans, animals, and plants could adapt to the heat, climate, and moisture of the tropics—existed across the Atlantic world.[20] At first the concept was disease-agnostic and couched in vague environmental terms to do broadly with the air or climate. But as yellow fever epidemics grew more frequent and ferocious in the first few decades of the nineteenth century, New Orleanians came to see acclimation as disease specific. By the 1820s the word was adopted into everyday conversation and used as a strict binary: a person was either "acclimated" or "unacclimated," a valued insider or untested outsider. By 1830, acclimation had clear economic value and had infused the logic of the cotton and slave markets. By 1840, a white "acclimated citizen" was considered superior in all ways to an "unacclimated stranger." Indeed, every Atlantic society gave preference to *criollo aclimatados* or *de geacclimatiseerde*. By 1850, talk of acclimation had become quite varied linguistically: It could be a noun (*the process of acclimation*), a verb (*I am acclimating this season*), an adjective (*an unacclimated bookkeeper*).[21] Acclimation, in fact, was so closely connected with local success and value on the eve of the Civil War that even animals like cows and horses and inanimate products like seed and wood had to be expressly described as acclimated if they were to sell in New Orleans.[22]

Everyone valued acclimation. But if you asked a dozen people on Bourbon Street in 1830 to define what exactly acclimation was, you would get three dozen different responses. One clerk might tell you that acclimation was simply the body's years-long reconciliation to the "peculiarities of soil, climate and noxious effluvia." Another might respond with the words of South Carolina fever specialist Philip Tidyman, that an immigrant could consider himself "safe after a residence of six years." His friend might agree in principle but suggest that Bennet Dowler's claim that "long urban residence (with or without having had yellow fever) is, in a sanitary sense, an equivalent to nativity" was more correct; that acclimation was "a kind of naturalization, or rather creolization."[23] Another passerby might insist that acclimation to yellow fever was a one-off event, like a vaccination or inoculation. A Frenchmen would tell you that only acclimation "stamped" a person with "the seal of naturalization," giving immigrants "the title of citizen" in their adopted homes. An old-timer waxing poetic might ask you to look at the picture more holistically—to consider acclimation as an "initiation" to the climate *and* the culture. A slave trader might laugh at your ignorance and tell you acclimation was a gut feeling, an instinct one learned through years of experience.[24]

Finding those definitions unsatisfactory, you might ask follow-up questions that would elicit a more hostile reaction. Was acclimation reversible? Were the children of Creole parents acclimated from birth? Did mild cases of yellow fever lead to full acclimation? Was a "Gibraltar seasoning" to the *vómito negro* sufficient in New Orleans? Would a Louisiana acclimation protect against a "Panamanian" fever? And did people retain their acclimation if they left the region for long periods?[25] Hopefully, you would not commit the ultimate faux pas of challenging these men on their own acclimation status—that might put you in the hospital. You would likely leave these conversations agreeing with the wisdom of novelist and Mississippi River pilot Mark Twain, that acclimation was a highly sensitive and deeply personal topic on which "no two persons exactly agree[d]."[26]

In an age before serology or vaccination, yellow fever immunity was impossible to prove. Unlike smallpox, yellow fever does not leave physical scars. Not everyone exhibited the telltale symptom of black vomit. Some people experienced only mild symptoms, perhaps a headache or some nausea, or were entirely asymptomatic. Longer-term effects like poor vision, chronic exhaustion, and muscle weakness plagued many nineteenth-century Americans, especially those in malaria-endemic regions. Even leading physicians did not agree that yellow fever was a discrete illness, and debates about the disease's etiology remained heated across the European and American medical communities until the twentieth century.[27] Many physicians considered malaria, a so-called country disease symptomatically similar to yellow fever, just a different manifestation of the same illness. Some believed that yellow fever was one dire end of a fever spectrum: "[In] some seasons," physician Andrew Ellicott wrote in 1814, the fevers "are little more than the common intermittents, and remittents, which prevail in the middle states; but in others they are highly malignant," approaching "the genuine yellow fever of the West Indies."[28]

Accurate diagnosis could be almost impossible, especially in a stressful sickroom or hospital. And sometimes doctors lied to patients about the nature of their illness as contemporary medicine held that inciting panic could put sick people into even more danger. One man named Joseph, for example, told his sister in November 1847 that he had taken seriously ill earlier that summer with a "congestive fever"—at least that is what his friends and Dr. Charles McCormick, an assistant surgeon in the US army, had told him. Joseph suspected his illness was more serious than his friends had let on. But as he "was too sick at the time to quarrel with [his] friends about the *color* of the disease," Joseph concentrated instead on getting better. Only when he was safely convalescent did McCormick apologize for lying and confirm that he had indeed survived yellow fever. And now thoroughly acclimated and confident, Joseph celebrated that he held a "passport" that his "Yellow Majesty must forever hereafter respect."[29]

Joseph's yellow fever saga had a happy ending. But what if his friends or his doctor had been wrong? One British traveler's sad tale from 1836—one more version of the "Unacclimated Stranger" story—captured the catastrophic consequences of false assumptions. The traveler had met a "fine young" German of "iron frame and florid health" who "considered himself acclimated, having had the fever in the previous October immediately after his arrival." Falsely confident in his safety during future epidemics, the German remained in town during the next outbreak, only to have his name appear in the "deadly catalogue."[30]

The fundamental unknowability of immunity ate away at people, especially those who experienced only mild symptoms during officially nonepidemic summers. Many asked themselves the same gnawing questions over and over: Had my daughter experienced a case of genuine yellow fever? If there was no black vomit or bleeding at the gums, was it merely intermittent fever? And the greatest fear: Had I made the whole thing up? When there were only "sporadic" cases of yellow fever in 1842, the *Picayune* sent its congratulations to those "who have been acclimated by the recent mild visitation of fever," wishing them every "advantage from it, both in business and health." But the editors cautioned survivors to remain temperate and vigilant. Perhaps their acclimations were not so thorough after all.[31] Many Orleanians also feared their hard-earned acclimation would evaporate if they left the region for long periods, thinking their bodies would readapt to more temperate climates. This kept many people in New Orleans from ever leaving. Newcomer James McMartin of New Jersey was scared of this, telling his brother in 1849 that he was "in a measure acclimated here now," thus "going to New York would do me no good."[32]

A second opinion from a trusted medical source could assuage some people's doubts. But just as it was easy for laypeople to misjudge their acclimation, doctors frequently erred, too—especially because doctors were financially incentivized after July 1 to tell a sick person that what they were ailing with was yellow fever. In September 1847, for example, one Irishman entered the Charity Hospital with unimpeachable symptoms of yellow fever, including a raging fever, violent pains in his head and limbs, bright yellow skin, and bleeding gums. "A better marked case of yellow fever was never seen," said Dr. Erasmus Fenner. But the patient insisted that he had come to New Orleans in 1824 and survived yellow fever in 1825—a diagnosis confirmed by Dr. John Ker, one of the most esteemed Irish-born doctors in the Deep South. This mistake was as embarrassing for Ker as it was dangerous for the misdiagnosed patient.[33] Many doctors thus tended toward diagnostic conservatism, thinking it better to disappoint a patient and tell them they remained unacclimated than anoint them acclimated and encourage reckless behavior. Physicians proved especially conservative in self-assessments. In 1839 Dr. Edward Jenner Coxe—namesake of Edward Jenner, inventor of the smallpox vaccine—described a "moderately severe" fever he had experienced in New Orleans. Upon recovery, Coxe wrote, "it was asserted that I had passed through the yellow fever" and he had been "congratulated upon the event." But five weeks later he was seized by the "pure" yellow fever, "in its most violent and dangerous form, such as few recover from." Coxe later avowed that *A mild attack as well as one occurring in a non-epidemic season* may be sufficient for acclimation, but every attack *should be cautiously and doubtfully recognized as certain.*[34]

If most patients deferred to doctor's opinions, Creoles—of all races— loudly rejected any claim they were not hereditarily immune to yellow fever *and* malaria. Social norms, in fact, forbade anyone from even mentioning the words "yellow fever" around an ailing Creole. As novelist George Washington Cable noted, a Creole held "an absurd belief in his entire immunity" from an attack of yellow fever: "When he has it, it is something else." Dr. Warren Stone, head surgeon at the Charity Hospital, insisted that unless "country Creoles" had been "acclimated in *New-Orleans*," they should consider themselves and their children in danger. Stone had the worst proof imaginable: his nine-year-old daughter had died from yellow fever even though she had been born in New Orleans and he was acclimated.[35] But outraged Creoles claimed Stone was a malevolent quack for even broaching the topic. Some said he was too deranged to practice medicine. Physician and city councilor J. S. McFarlane—a non-Creole North Carolina transplant himself—insisted that "congenital city creolism," where one was born a Creole to "thoroughly creolized parents," exempted individuals from yellow fever with "nearly the same uniformity that vaccination prevents the smallpox." Obviously Creoles were not immortal, McFarlane conceded, but "any effort to shake the confidence of the people of New Orleans in the prophylactic security afforded by birth-right and acclimation," he seethed, "I consider the most unpardonable and reckless" offense, "not to call it by a harsher name." On the next page, McFarlane called these people "terrorists."[36]

Harsh language like this was mild within the larger debate on creolism and immunity. Debate sometimes threatened to spill over into actual violence. When one New Orleans–born child of Saint-Domingue refugees, Dr. Charles Faget, posited that Creoles of any race and all Black people never contracted yellow fever but instead only *fièvre paludeéne* (malaria), Dr. Charles Deléry countered that Creoles were just as susceptible as anyone. Deléry then challenged Faget to a duel. Faget refused on the basis of his Catholicism, claiming that he was allowed neither to murder nor to commit suicide. Instead, Deléry and Faget dueled in pamphlets for twenty years, writing seven exchanges filled with ad hominem attacks. In 1877 the weary and beleaguered Faget penned his *Dernier République,* closing off their debate, but never definitively answering the question about Creole (or Black) immunity.[37]

By the 1850s, as the perennial interethnic squabbles between Americans and Creoles quieted and intersectional tensions between North and South were rising, most New Orleanians agreed with Dr. Edward Hall Barton that "*perfect acclimation is only to be derived from once having had the disease*"; that all *white* people, regardless of parentage or nativity had to fall sick with and survive yellow fever for themselves. By this time most people also understood that yellow fever was an urban phenomenon distinct from malaria and that surviving one disease had no bearing on the other.[38] Dr. Josiah Nott argued in 1847 that acclimated "citizens of Charleston, Savannah, Pensacola, Mobile, New Orleans, [and] West India towns . . . may exchange one city for another with impunity." But he also insisted that the "fact is so glaring, and so universally admitted" that there was "no *acclimation* against the endemic fevers of our rural districts." Nott continued, "Books written at the North talk much about acclimation at the South." But he maintained that Northerners were ignorant on this matter. In the South, true acclimation was never "alluded to *out of the yellow-fever cities.*"[39]

Within such a stew of (mis)information, white New Orleanians rightly remained nervous. Elizabeth Trist, a family friend of Thomas Jefferson who lost her husband and son to yellow fever, wrote in 1806, "I hope that my constitution has become creolized as they term it here, having had a very substantial seasoning." Still, she wrote, "I can't help being afraid as the summer approaches." Steamboat captain Robeson DeHart from Louisville was likewise concerned for his brother, who had landed in New Orleans in September 1839 when "the City was very sickly." DeHart was sure his brother would be fine but hoped he would "not rely too much on his former seasoning and venture on it as a protection." Ultimately, Deep Southerners had to make peace with uncertainty because there was no alternative. As Dr. M. Morton Dowler noted, individuals simply could "have no assurance."[40]

By the 1830s most Americans associated yellow fever almost exclusively with New Orleans and its environs. Philadelphia's staggering epidemic of 1793 had faded from memory, and fewer outbreaks seemed to occur in Savannah or Charleston with each passing decade. Meanwhile, reports out of Louisiana worsened by the year—epidemics that killed as many people, if not many more, than in Philadelphia. And because New Orleans was the United States' most afflicted city, Americans considered an acclimation received there the best, a gold standard of sorts. A New Orleans acclimation approximated one attained in the West Indies, Brazil, or Liberia—it was considered biologically thorough and portable to even the most dangerous diseased locales. After acclimating in New Orleans in 1853, French geographer Élisée Reclus told his mother that he could now safely work as a tutor in Rio de Janeiro or Veracruz, a fact he thought should bring her comfort and him riches. A New Orleans acclimation could even protect against the "African fever"—the most virulent form of yellow fever, it was said—that predominated in Sierra Leone and the Gold Coast.[41]

Treated with such reverence domestically and abroad, a New Orleans acclimation eventually took on local meanings far beyond epidemiology. Acclimation took place, as George Washington Cable described it in his most famous novel *The Grandisimmes*, "not in body only . . . but in mind—in taste—in conversation—and in convictions too, yes, ha, ha!" White immigrants initially clung to their eastern ways, but once acclimated to New Orleans "they open their stores on Sunday, they import cargoes of Africans, they bribe the officials, they smuggle goods, they have colored housekeepers," Cable wrote. After all, "the water must expect to take the shape of the bucket." Acclimation was therefore both a biological designation and a cultural marker specific to the Yellow Fever South. Dr. Barton perhaps captured the true meaning of it best: a white person was acclimated only when they embraced the whole of New Orleans society, willing themselves to climatically and *morally* adapt to the "condition of a country."[42]

The Perverse Incentive

Many Deep Southern immigrants sought acclimation sooner rather than later. Ironically, facing yellow fever was the only guaranteed way to survive and prosper long-term. This was especially true for young white men aged fifteen to forty seeking professional advancement in cotton factories, merchant houses, and wholesaling—jobs considered springboards to slave and land ownership.[43] Londoner John Oldham refused to leave New Orleans in summer of 1820, knowing that staying to "face the danger will in future give him additional confidence" with his new business partners. Lawyer Charles Watts related to his family on Long Island in 1825 that ambitious men in Louisiana "submit themselves to the Yellow Fever," committing themselves to "changing their constitution by the shock." One shock-seeking immigrant named Isaac Charles boasted in September 1847 that he was "certain" that "both [brother] Dick & I are *acclimated.*" Expecting to "reside here altogether," Charles figured it was better to get acclimation over with "at once."[44]

Delaying the inevitable—by fleeing the city—was expensive and posed long-term financial impediments like diminished access to well-paid, steady employment. Moreover, in a place where risk-taking was embedded within the value system, postponing or eschewing acclimation—a very public demonstration of risk avoidance—impeded one's social and civic acceptance. Still, it was hard to remain confident in one's chosen path, given all the mixed messages. Even as, in October, the *Picayune* told all strangers and unacclimated persons, and "all who hold life in account," to "*Keep out of the city,*" in November it gleefully beckoned strangers to come as quickly as possible. And what did Dr. Charles Caldwell mean exactly when he said that in order to achieve greatness through acclimation, a "man must not tremblingly take counsel of his fears, nor always calculate, with clerk-like precision, the chances of danger"? Was this advice to leave or remain? Most people understood that timing was everything. As one doctor put it to a wavering unacclimated friend in late June, "If you are not prepared to take all the risks and stay them through, you had better go at once."[45]

New Orleans's business schedule, however, made "responsible" acclimation essentially impossible. Townspeople implored unacclimated immigrants to stay away until the first frost, worried that their arrival not only was "simple *suicide*" but also would prolong epidemics, causing "citizens, as well as strangers," to suffer. But come November, when "Frosty Jack" had expelled "Yellow Jack," all well-paid, upwardly mobile positions were already filled. Even then it was considered foolhardy to assume that any sudden professional vacancy would not be "instantly filled by some acclimated resident of the city." With floods of applications—allegedly fifty per job—employers preferred bilingual or trilingual "acclimated young men of the first character and qualifications." One editorialist concluded, "There is no chance for any kind of a clerkship," or job in any other trade "at any season, for young men from other places." Indeed, the *Picayune*'s editors personally knew of "thousands who contemplate coming to New Orleans this fall, who feel sure of situations, supposing half our population to have died." But there were "hundreds out of employ now in this city, who are fully acclimated and competent to fill any situation." In New Orleans, opportunity existed for acclimated men only.[46]

Despite the risks, the "universal rule" was to get to New Orleans before the throngs of people descended. If newcomers waited, they risked missing the "exhilarating" onset of the season and languishing in social and professional purgatory for the rest of the year. Rents in well-ventilated and convenient neighborhoods, affordable in September, were extortionate by December. Unable to afford the return trip to Providence or Paris, and with few good options, the unacclimated huddled in crowded, tenement-like quarters adjacent to the docks or set up just outside the city, frantically scanning newspapers to determine exactly when the death count began to drop. Many waited for the weather to become "Octoberish"—the moment it became just safe enough from disease for them to stage their appearance.[47]

Such hedging was easier said than done. As rumors of yellow fever swirled one summer, Connecticut immigrant Ralph Roanoke ceded all his "chances of preferment in a staunch commission-house" and fled the city. Upon his return in November, Roanoke no longer had a job. He again had to search for employment, "with my chances materially lessened by the very knowledge that I had not the courage to face the danger." Roanoke asserted that good qualifications and references were "insufficient without the 'sine qua non' of an acclimated citizen." His savings dwindled. Soon he determined that he could either retreat into his "former insignificance in Connecticut, or risk all upon the chances of acclimation." Following a promise to his former employer that he would remain next year "or perish in the attempt," the firm rehired him. "Terribly frightened" but determined, he fell ill with yellow fever, but survived. Now acclimated, Roanoke "stood before the world with all [his] doubts and misgivings at an end."[48]

Wanted: An Acclimated Man

White New Orleanians described acclimation as a rebirth. The *Daily Delta* declared in 1853 that the acclimated man walked the streets with a "tremendously bold swagger," sneering at the unacclimated who darted about "timidly and nervously." The acclimated would "pooh pooh" yellow fever and call it a "mere nothing"—it was a "pleasure" to have it, as it resulted "in such a splendid appetite *when* you get over it." One old-timer described the incredible airs of convalescents, those who "only a week or two ago [were] glad to be able . . . to take gruel and lemonade," but who now would supposedly go to Lake Pontchartrain "for a fish dinner . . . [and] quarrel about what brand of claret is best." Some "heroes of acclimation" began "to seriously talk about the relative pleasure and advantage to be enjoyed next summer." Maybe they would stay in the city, or maybe they would travel somewhere exotic. This "spunky set of fellows" now bragged, "What do I care for the yellow fever?"[49] Later, these "heroes of acclimation" would boast of the year of their ordeal—'17, '33, '49—like a membership badge in a fraternity of survivors. Some would even celebrate their acclimations like an anniversary with a yearly feast, chanting, "I have no fear!" But above all, as Dr. Barton put it, acclimated men could now expect *additional compensation,* for the additional risk run!"[50]

Seeking to capitalize on their hard-earned immunity, job-seekers filled newspapers with implicit or explicit declarations of acclimation. One clerk enumerated his credentials in this order: "well acclimated, well educated, speaking five languages," with "the best of references," notable integrity, and business capacities. One clerk in the dry goods business, after enumerating his skills, added "N.B. Fully acclimated." A grocer from Philadelphia promoted himself as "acclimated" and "willing to remain in this city during the Summer." One "fully acclimated" man reassured his potential employer that he had lived in the Greater Caribbean for eighteen years, and in New Orleans for the last several without interruption. Another "acclimated gentleman, possessing business qualifications and habits of industry," sought a situation in a cotton commission house. A middle-aged man claimed that he was "well acquainted with this city" and also "well acclimated between the latitudes of 32° and the Tropics."[51]

Men invoked their New Orleans nativity to give them an edge over skilled men from other states. In 1846 a "Young Gentleman of this city, aged 14 years . . . anxious to obtain a situation in a Commission House," related that he was "well acquainted with the duties requisite, speaks French and English, and has been raised in New Orleans." The subtext (and often the text) of declaring acclimation was that a person would willingly remain in town during the summer, even if bosses chose to leave. One English-born cotton trader, "being acclimated," emphasized that he was willing to temporarily stand in for any of the firm's partners wishing "to absent themselves during the summer months on business or otherwise." A Kentucky-born bookkeeper with several years' experience seeking employment in "a commercial house, or as Clerk on a steamboat running in a Southern trade," added that he was both acclimated and willing to commence employment immediately in August, or any time up to October 15—the danger zone for the unacclimated.[52]

Employers often demanded proof of local birth or a physician's letter certifying acclimation. References were generally useless unless provided by a former tropically based employer. From the boss's perspective, it was a waste of resources to train someone for a detail-oriented job only to see him stricken or dead by autumn. Eliza Breedam related that in 1833 her Uncle Millard had heard of a young, skilled apothecary from Natchez. Millard hired him, but when the boy arrived in New Orleans, he was immediately stricken with "a very severe spell of yellow fever," a case so serious they did not think he would live.[53] Millard maintained he had made the right decision in hiring an unacclimated boy, despite the steep medical bills he had to foot. But most employers considered this an unacceptable risk. As the unemployed German immigrant Gustav Dresel lamented in the 1830s, "I looked around in vain for a position as bookkeeper," but "to engage a young man who was not acclimated would be a bad speculation." As the rejections mounted and the weather cooled, unacclimated job seekers were forced into making all kinds of concessions. One man was so desperate for any clerking position by November that he told employers "wages [were] not so much an object as to be employed." Unemployed people worried about homelessness and thus being criminalized as vagrants. One seamstress, an "acclimated European Lady, of respectable family, resident in this city," was so nervous that she would end up in the streets that she conceded, "Wages no object: principally for a home."[54]

The Losers

Applicants routinely lied about their acclimation status, considering it a required (though perfunctory) line on a resume likely filled with other padded credentials. This is clear as even after rigorous acclimation screening, employees still died in droves. One traveler noted in 1836, "Five perished out of one counting-house; another house buried their book-keeper, employed another, buried him, and employed a third before the dead season had passed." Such mortality among the allegedly acclimated suggests that clerks either misjudged their immunity or willfully lied about it. That was high-risk: false declarations of acclimation merited termination. But many apparently believed the lie was worth it: they would feign ignorance, then worry later about surviving the disease.[55]

Acclimation, in fact, was so universally claimed and notoriously untrue that it became a running joke. One prankster even placed a fake wanted advertisement in the *Picayune* poking fun at the practice. Seeking a job in a merchant house, the applicant's declaration started off normally. He said that as he had "resided in the city twenty years, winter and summer; had the yellow fever, cholera and small pox," he "flatters himself that he is pretty well acclimated, and that he can remain at his post the year round." But he added that "if it would enhance his value in the estimation of his employer," he would not "object to spending the summer months at Niagara, Saratoga, &c., without any extra pay beyond his travelling expenses." He concluded his advertisement by noting that he was unmarried but that, "should that prove objectionable," he could "change his state in fifteen minutes." He ended with a variance on the usual custom, noting "that salary *is* an object."[56]

Friends and family abroad had serious misgivings about their menfolk seeking sickness to show employers they were made of the right stuff. Stories of acclimation gone wrong—of bright young unacclimated strangers cut down in an afternoon—were a dime a dozen. During a particularly brutal epidemic in 1819 that had already killed over 2,000 people, cotton planter John Palfrey pleaded with his son Henry in New Orleans that he should "quit the City & come on here"—to the family plantation Forlorn Hope. Though they had had cases of yellow fever on the plantation (Palfrey's other son, William, was convalescing and "all the negroes have been sick"), Palfrey Sr. still thought the city was too dangerous. "I am really astonished that you should continue in New Orleans surrounded as you must be by pestilence & death," Palfrey chided, continuing that just because "you have escaped thus far you must not think yourself invulnerable." Palfrey's remonstrances fell on deaf ears: quitting town was simply not an option for Henry.[57]

Henry managed to avoid yellow fever in 1819, but died from it five years later. Palfrey Sr. was distraught but was still luckier than many: he recovered his son's body and knew what had killed him. Sarah Hughes of Boston—and countless others—did not have such closure. Hughes posted an enquiry in the *Picayune* in 1842, begging for news of her husband, Patrick, who had not returned home to Massachusetts as promised. Having heard a rumor that the 1841 epidemic had been especially devastating, she implored *Picayune* readers that "any information" would be "most gratefully acknowledged by his disconsolate wife." The friends of Frederick Prigg from Suffolk, England, made a similar inquiry. They knew Frederick was employed in a drugstore in Louisiana, and last they had heard, he had fallen sick with yellow fever in October 1837. Was the news that he recovered false? Any information about their friend Frederick would be welcome, they pleaded.[58]

Many young white men assumed they would defy the yellow fever odds, only to be shocked when they fell seriously ill. More than one boy choked back bewildered laughter as he coughed up blood. Reverend Theodore Clapp recalled, "Often I have met and shook hands with some blooming, handsome young man today and in a few hours afterward, I have been called to see him in the Black Vomit, with profuse hemorrhages from the mouth, nose, ears, eyes, and even the toes." In October 1858 the chief bookkeeper of the St. Charles Hotel, Zenas Blinn, died of the "prevailing epidemic"; this shocked his employers because Blinn had lived in the city for six years and had already acted as bookkeeper at the Verandah and St. Louis Hotels. Even Mr. Ward, an agent for the Rothschild-backed firm Lanfear & Co., who could have afforded to flee, fell into the confidence trap. Ward had "recently purchased a plantation in the neighborhood" and stayed in the city "with the express view of getting acclimated," only to meet his dismal, black-vomit end.[59]

Filling Dead Men's Shoes

Acclimated white men could parlay immunity into raises and greater responsibility. The managerial class of merchant houses, wholesalers, and groceries was composed almost entirely of white men who claimed immunity. George Fennell, an English grocer, noted that the 1837 epidemic had been "truly awful." When Fennell's boss, Mr. Hawley, and three fellow bookkeepers died from fever, Hawley's competitors moved to shut down his grocery. Fennell—the last man standing—had his choice of remunerative jobs among the surviving competition. Cotton clerk H. J. Masson likewise remarked that the 1837 epidemic was the worst in memory, ravaging the unacclimated and "thin[ning] the counting houses." Consequently, there was "considerable demand" for entry-level clerks. After a competing cotton factor, Mr. Stringer, lost his clerk to fever, he was "very anxious" for the acclimated Masson to quit and join him.[60]

Acclimation allowed entry-level employees to get a foot in the door, but it was a virtual requirement for bosses and business owners. It was an unwritten rule that all named partners in cotton factories, commission houses, and law firms had to be either Creole or acclimated. A partner's sudden death by yellow fever could ruin a company's reputation and credit. Credit reporters Dun & Bradstreet often emphasized the length of time a person had been physically present in New Orleans—or if they were Creole—in their ratings. Agents, of course, could not be sure about a man's acclimation status. But length of time and nativity were hedges against the effects of disease on business.[61] In declaring acclimation, a named partner was emphasizing stability, signaling that their business was here to stay. In his official introduction to the New Orleans business community in 1842, for example, John Rayburn of Nashville emphasized that he had decided to put his name on his commission house because "being acclimated I shall reside in the city *permanently*," all the better to give "strict and personal attention" to clients.[62]

White people in just about every industry found acclimation to be a necessary credential, as important as degrees or other professional qualifications. In 1847 many fever-averse public school teachers did not return for the opening of schools in September. An editorialist, noting that a teacher's presence in the city was contractually obligated despite disease, made a case that the only good educator was an acclimated one:

> What is the feeling of the community towards any minister of the gospel who deserts his post for fear of the epidemic? Certainly it is *not* one of confidence and affection. And shall the teachers of our children, engaged in a work next in importance and honor to that of the ministry, be allowed to shrink from *duty* voluntarily assumed because some risk attends its discharge? Is this moral courage?

"No," he replied; it would be better if a few teachers "should fall martyrs" to yellow fever for the sake of the children. Most underpaid public school teachers, of course, were uninterested in martyrdom. Acclimated educators, meanwhile, moved into the private education and tutoring sector, where rich families more generously rewarded their acclimation.[63]

Religious leaders were not exempted from the "duty" of acclimation. No minister, priest, or rabbi wanted to go the way of Presbyterian minister Sylvester Larned, who fled town in 1819. Pastor Joel Parker, who left town in September 1837 for St. Louis amid a terrible epidemic, was most reviled of all. Parker insisted that he had had every intention of returning to New Orleans by mid-October but had been unexpectedly "detained" for a month upriver; that he was not "afraid of yellow jack" and had rather "wished that he might take it." But the *Picayune*—along with every other city newspaper—raked Parker over the coals. The truth, said the *Picayune,* was that Parker had left the city at the time that "tries men's *souls,"* whereas all Catholic priests and "Mr. Curtiss, Mr. Clapp, and some other Protestant ministers" had stayed—"they never fled." That Parker was morally irredeemable was confirmed for the editors of the *Picayune* when Parker was defended by the *Cincinnati Journal*—a newspaper that, the *Picayune* declared, was "identical" to the *Alton Observer* "of Lovejoy notoriety," verging "on abolition" of the "rankest kind." Elijah Lovejoy—a Presbyterian abolitionist printer—would be murdered by a proslavery mob in Illinois in November 1837, his press ransacked; Joel Parker—an abolitionist by association and noted yellow fever coward—would be hung in effigy in the streets of New Orleans.[64]

Parker's ostracization was extreme. But most New Orleanians, who equated capacity to stand up to yellow fever with salvation, felt that only acclimated men of God could provide the consistency necessary in their volatile world. Unitarian minister F. A. Farley hoped no man would consider accepting an invitation to the New Orleans pulpit "who is not prepared to face the epidemic." A pastor must "entirely [commit] himself to the will of God" by "taking the risks of acclimation." Farley concluded: "I deem this absolutely essential." Essential perhaps, but costly too—both mentally and mortally. All religious leaders spent a great deal of time during epidemics in spaces filled with sick, dying, and dead people, performing last rites as well as a constant stream of funerals. Many burned out; many found they could not cope with so much community suffering; and many died. But like everyone else, religious leaders knew they had to remain in town until they had faced yellow fever. It was for this reason that preacher John B. Warren told his family in 1835 that he was unsure whether he would be able to return home to Massachusetts next summer. "If God spares my life so long I will do so, if possible," he wrote, but added, "I am much bound to Louisiana. My friends here are not willing that I should leave."[65]

Moral Hazard

Declaring acclimation did more than assuage employers or congregants. It became a catchall statement of character. One editorialist in the *Daily Delta* opined in 1854, "A poor man who comes here for employment, so far from avoiding, should boldly face the acclimating fever, and thus become really a citizen." When he was "thus initiated," he could "command much higher rates of service," because "acclimated citizens" were preferred to strangers "in all the departments of life."[66] In this marketplace, a successful brush with yellow fever became the quintessential demonstration of a white man's calculated risk-taking, proof that he had willingly gambled his life, had paid his biological dues, and could now justifiably pursue economic advancement.

Successful acclimations factored into the genesis stories of almost all of New Orleans's political and economic elite. Though he could have fled back to Kentucky in the summer of 1801, the eighteen-year-old Irish immigrant Maunsel White remained in his boardinghouse in New Orleans, realizing, "Alas! there was no help for it, but to take my chance." Reminiscing decades later, White recalled his acclimation as a major life turning point: with only an informal education, he progressed quickly from ship loading to bookkeeping to running his own cotton factory. In 1812 he was elected city councilor, spearheading a plan to make property owners pay for street paving. In 1846 he was elected to the Louisiana Senate, where he often served as president *pro tem*. He married a wealthy Creole woman, Celestine de la Ronde, and after her death he married her sister Heloise. On his largest sugar estate in Plaquemines Parish, Deer Range, White had enslaved 192 people by 1850. This financial and social success, White recalled at the end of this life, was rooted in his acclimation half a century before.[67]

White framed his acclimation as a choice. He had contracted yellow fever and willed himself to survive, with only a little help from "God, a good constitution, the Doctor and Nanny." Nanny, described by White as "a great stout, strapping Negro woman," probably deserved most of the credit for his survival. She tended him night and day, ice-bathing, swaddling, feeding, tut-tutting, and taking him "up in her arms as one might take a baby" until he was "cured." White did not mention if Nanny was enslaved or free, or how much or whether he paid her. But her presence as a named character in a white man's recollections about his sickness is rare. Despite having been fixtures in yellow fever sickrooms, Black women were seldom identified by name in acclimation narratives (a Black woman caretaker was usually referred to only as the "negro nurse" or *femme traiteuse*). Nor were they credited as medical experts in their own right. Instead, these women were described as instruments, implementing care as directed by white male doctors who were often less experienced, better paid, and abusive. All too often, women like Nanny were written out of the narrative entirely. Indeed, when physician Samuel Cartwright fell ill with yellow fever in Natchez in 1823, he attributed his and his family's survival to his upstanding morality, medical expertise, and prudence, giving only scant credit to "cleanliness, fresh air and careful nursing."[68]

If great men *chose* to survive, as the narrative went, then lesser men literally *chose* to die. They died because they were drunkards, effeminate, sexually deviant, indiscreet, cowardly, or unclean, or because they did not seek timely medical care. Distilling the randomness of life and death to a matter of individual choice fed into a myth of meritocratic capitalism: that all whites of sufficient moral and physical courage had the *potential* for survival and success in New Orleans, and that men like White and Cartwright were socially and economically accomplished as a direct result of their willingness to take controlled epidemiological risks. Dr. William Holcombe put it this way: Yellow fever was like a "mean yellow dog"—if a man faced the dog and defied him, the dog would "slink away"; but show the dog cowardice and "he will pursue and attack you."[69] Survival was possible for those who *chose* it; those who succumbed to disease did not possess the requisite personal characteristics for success.[70]

Of course, the notion that recovery was entirely a matter of human agency clashed with the fatal reality. But the cold facts of disease risk—that about half of all victims would die—mattered little; the myth of immunological reward prevailed. Thus, while epidemics raged, young white men routinely touted aspirational mantras about human agency over disease, insisting that yellow fever was a mild ailment—asserting, "The unhealthiness of the place" will have "no effect on me as I will live temperate," boasting that they had never enjoyed better health, and reassuring family that they would succeed where others had failed.[71] Such optimism may have been self-delusional. But most unacclimated migrants bought into immunocapital and the hierarchy it created, believing that the system would benefit them eventually. After all, immunological discrimination was just one more form of bias in a region premised on inequality.

The logic of immunological supremacy—that all acclimated white people were righteous and all unacclimated people were untested and disposable—could easily slip into exploitation and abuse. Recruited directly off the boat, thousands of Irishmen built the New Basin Canal in the 1830s. Working in ghastly conditions (and prime mosquito breeding grounds), most of these Irishmen were exposed to high viral loads, working shoulder to shoulder in the mud by day and living on top of each other by night. Between 6,000 and 10,000 Irishmen died of yellow fever while digging the four-mile stretch, their bodies tossed unceremoniously aside to be eaten by alligators or sink into the mud. The bosses remained unfazed because thousands of desperate men waited to replace the dead for a dollar a day—and, management claimed, only the virtuous survived, so mass mortality was not their problem in any case.[72] In 1835, British writer Tyrone Power rode out to the swamp to see the Irishmen digging the canal and asked a foreman why he was not using enslaved Black labor for such a difficult task. Power was told that enslaved people could not "be substituted to any extent; a good slave costs at this time two hundred pounds sterling, and to have a thousand such swept off a line of canal in one season would call for prompt consideration." Such a shocking statement suggests capitalists *preferred* a labor model that focused on replacing the dead rather than keeping people alive. High turnover in a society with a legally fixed Black underclass *and* so many willing and desperate immigrants meant mortality cost them nothing. It also impeded menial laborers' ability to organize and demand better pay, conditions, and rights. Thus, immigrants' vulnerability to yellow fever helped the commercial elite keep its white workforce desperate and docile while still underlining racial slavery's implicit value to all white people and society at large.[73]

Yellow fever was seen as the friend of capitalists in other ways, too. A constantly cycling population of white workers and a permanently enslaved population of Black laborers meant that relatively few people survived long enough to leverage immunocapital, enter the commercial-civic elite, and compete against those already at the top. With undeniable nativist overtones, *anciennes* openly celebrated yellow fever's destruction, feeling "friendly to the scourge, as, in their opinion, it checked that tide of immigration which, otherwise, would have speedily rolled its waves over the old population." If acclimated white immigrants were allowed to become demographically dominant, thought the elite, they would sweep "away all those landmarks in legislation, customs, language and social habits" to which the elite "were fondly attached."[74] Expressing another kind of nativism, some Creoles felt that the "terrific slaughter of aliens" was socially beneficial as it demonstrated "the survival of the fittest." Unworthy Irishmen and Germans were culled, but a "parent stock" of worthy immigrants survived, those with an unequalled "reputation for vigor and enterprise."[75]

Yellow fever compounded poverty and its worst effects. Without acclimation, white people were shut out of well-paid, steady work. Unable to afford rents in healthy buildings and neighborhoods, they were forced to live in "fever nests," "fever manufactories," and "plague spots"—cheap, filthy spaces out of sight of the rich, and close to the swamps and docks where they were in constant proximity to disease. Considering the city's impoverished communities, Dr. Barton opined that the "poor are the greatest sufferers always," living in "crowded, filthy, and uncomfortable dwellings." He added that those who "constitute this class, are the *hands*, the *machinery*, that make the wealth of a community, and give it its power." Hence, they were the "rightful claimants of its fostering care."[76]

Most elites wholeheartedly disagreed, believing they held no social responsibility for the health of the masses. Rather, the extremely high death rate among the poor from yellow fever was evidence of their innate depravity, not some self-fulfilling prophecy aided and abetted by the actions of capitalists. This system was brutal, yes, but it worked, claimed the elite. The masses had to face yellow fever alone and the worthy would survive, just as they had. There was no *structural* problem within immunocapitalism that elites had to acknowledge or fix. And if pressed by a stranger on the virtue of this system, the businessman "threw up his palms and eyebrows—nobody asked [immigrants] to come to New Orleans."[77]

It is unclear how elites reconciled their conviction that poverty, intemperance, sexual looseness, and general moral decrepitude caused the lower classes to die of yellow fever with the fact that elite white persons also sickened and died from it. Elite men did not blame their wives' or children's deaths on intemperance or sexual deviance. It was almost as if the rich and the poor died from two separate diseases. When the elite died from yellow fever, it was God's will; when the poor perished, it was due to their own regrettable, despicable, often alcohol-related choices. This belief was, in many respects, one more iteration of the simplistic theologies that dominated New Orleans's mainstream religious tradition: sometimes a man was saved by works, sometimes by grace, though God was inscrutable in how he calculated election. Providence was invoked so liberally and predictably, in fact, that God must have grown bored of it.[78]

Virginia-born Thomas Gale moved to the Deep South in his early twenties and worked as a physician for the American armies fighting Creek Indians in Alabama. By 1817 he had established himself as a cotton planter in Mississippi, owning many slaves. Numerous members of his family and close friends died from yellow fever. But he survived. Gale explained to a friend what he understood by this: "I am willing to ascribe the little success I have met with in this inhospitable world in which it has been my lot to live. I believe not one act of my life has been produced by accident. On the contrary it has been from cool design." As his survival and success was God's will, Gale wrote, "I therefore shall never have occasion to apologise."[79] In Louisiana, a man might have to make callous calculations, but that was just how one got by in this risky world. The best anyone (or any white person) could hope for was to come out on top. And once at the top, surviving yellow fever—a fundamentally luck-based feat—was repackaged as a tale of individual determination and just rewards.

The Marriage Plot

Beyond its business and class implications, the immunity calculus factored heavily into all interpersonal relationships. New Orleanians emphatically believed that white men could not fulfill their patriarchal duties to their wives, children, and slaves until they were acclimated. As one editorialist asserted, "We conjure all the *interesting young gentlemen,* to become [acclimated] as soon as possible," for they "ought to recollect how cruel it is to visit among Creoles, or families acclimated, before they are so themselves." This rule applied to people of all races and classes, from wealthy *hommes de couleur* to firemen to skilled clerks. Old-timers and Creoles warned their daughters against "'linking [their] faith' with that of the unacclimated lover."[80] Not only were unacclimated men more likely to die, but they were generally poorer and less established than their acclimated counterparts. Indeed, the immunity differential may explain why it took many years for the Creole and Anglo-American populations to significantly intermarry, and why Creoles almost never married Irish and German immigrants, despite a shared Catholicism, even as late as the 1840s.[81]

To marry and reproduce without acclimation was considered irresponsible; it was not as bad as marrying across the color line, but it raised eyebrows. The *Picayune* noted, "We have known widows and children, left in sorrow and want by the death of the husband, from Yellow Fever." The newspaper laid out the stakes of this in a fable: A man comes to New Orleans, where he cannot help but fall in love. Marriage soon follows. In prosperous times, the man and his wife could quit the city during epidemics. But times changed with business, or debt, or something else compelling him to remain in town. Inevitably the man sickened with yellow fever and died. And though "the grave ends his trouble," his widow was now destined to a life of suffering. "Sincerely, as a matter of principle," the *Picayune* insisted, "we are opposed to the existence of any strong ties until acclimation has taken place."[82]

Yellow fever created many young widows. Every diary, newspaper, and letter seemed to tell some sad story, like that of Selina Jewell, whose husband Mr. Maltravers "is dead and buried. Taken sick at New Orleans of yellow fever . . . he died at a hotel, almost immediately." Selina "had but ten days experience of matrimony." Eliza Breedam recalled that when her children's tutor, recently hired from New York, died from yellow fever in 1833, he left behind a seventeen-year-old wife, now alone "in a strange place without a friend." When H. H. Smith, editor of the *Galveston Journal,* died suddenly of yellow fever in 1853, the paper noted that "his bereaved widow and helpless orphan child" were now without protection, "far separated as they are from all other kindred." If only he had been more prudent in get-

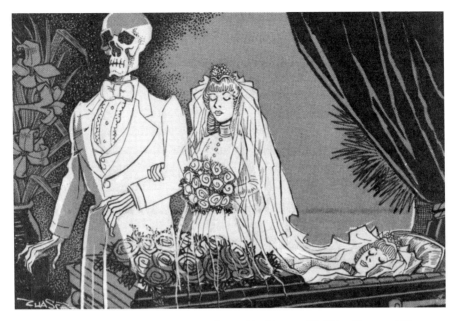

John Churchill Chase, illustration in John Wilds, "In 1878 We Were Here . . . When a Visitor Became the Bride of the Saffron Spectre," *The States-Item,* April, 1977. The Historic New Orleans Collection, Gift of Mr. John Churchill Chase and Mr. John W. Wilds.

ting acclimated before marriage, the suffering of his wife and daughter could have been avoided.[83]

Immunity was essential for would-be patriarchs, but it was also important for white women. Only acclimated women, it was believed, could reliably survive long enough to perform the feminine rites associated with marriage, especially childbearing. One newspaper put it this way: "The acclimated girl is a treasure," and though she "may not have yellow hair," "if she has had yellow fever she is worth a mint of money." Men screened their potential wives, asking: "'Miss—have you ever had the yellow fever?' 'Was it a typical case?' 'Are you certain your physician was correct in his diagnosis of your case?'" Courting men rejected unacclimated women, worried they would die young or else insist on spending hundreds of dollars to flee the city in style. Everyone knew women like poor Mary Dick, dead from yellow fever just nine months after marriage (one day after her mother died and two days after giving birth).[84] And no one wanted to see a once "proud, blooming, spirited beauty" become "a yellow, spotted, and ugly looking corpse." Elite yellow fever widows—assumed immune—held a powerful bargaining chip in a "widowocracy" like New Orleans. Mary Trist, a well-to-do fever widow, for example, parlayed her acclimation into a rich American second husband and an even richer Creole third husband.[85]

Lower-class white and free Black women found that their acclimation was not worth as much as men's. In the market of women's work, immunity often trapped women in an endless cycle of caretaking—for their sick families, employers, and neighbors, and for the city's thousands of orphans and foundlings in the aftermath of an epidemic. In 1853 a young, acclimated German girl named Lorie, though still "quite a child," was hired by a prosperous family after their previous maids had died, "one after another, of yellow fever." She acted, day and night, as the nurse to her boss and his two grown sons when they fell sick with the fever, and was paid quite well—$3 a day.[86] Black women could also make good money nursing during epidemics—as much as $10 a day.[87] This was an uncommonly large sum considering that women in New Orleans generally earned $8 to $10 a month in 1850, and sometimes as little as $5. Unlike these exceptional cases, most poor women of all races and ethnicities found that constant care work was unpaid, all-consuming, and thankless. And caretaking responsibilities effectively shut them out of independent employment, keeping them reliant on small handouts of money, wood, and food from the municipality, private charities, and the Catholic Church. Most philanthropic payments were one-time-only and thus did not address the structural problems yellow fever placed on womanhood, widowhood, and motherhood. Therefore, even though some Creole and acclimated women—Black and white—could demand higher pay as nurses and wet nurses, most found that the unceasing attrition of yellow fever left them overwhelmed, professionally insecure, emotionally drained, and poorer.[88]

Risk in the Slave Market

For centuries the profitability of the Atlantic slaving industry had rested on a cruel calculus: When exactly did an enslaved person create more capital, through labor or reproduction, than they embodied? Caribbean planters in the years of peak sugar prices—when the average enslaved person's economic value was about £56.76—recuperated their outlay in purchasing a person in a shockingly short period, a matter of years. Enslavers expected first-generation, African-born people to die within six years of landing. Some whites were willing to pay a small premium of about 6 percent for "seasoned" slaves, those who had survived their especially dangerous initial years. Evidence of surviving a deadly disease, especially smallpox scars, might increase an enslaved person's assessed value. But the smallness of this premium suggests that colonial-era planters were not much concerned with enslaved people's immunity to any disease; their model functioned on replacement rather than longevity.[89]

During the "second slavery," American enslavers approached slavery somewhat differently, if no less cruelly, than had previous generations.[90] Following the United States' African slave trade ban in 1808, whites could no longer rely on a stream of ships to supply them with an expendable, adult, and mostly male labor force. Now they worried about labor scarcity, fearing that the domestic slave trade could not sustain the labor force they believed was necessary to turn the vast lands of the Mississippi Valley into lucrative cotton and sugar fields. The price of enslaved people shot up following 1808, especially in Louisiana. One commission established after the War of 1812 to compensate masters who lost slaves to the British army set an average (artificially low) value of slaves in New Orleans at $474. This was significantly higher than in South Carolina ($317) or Georgia ($264). One of the last illegal cargos of slaves from Africa, seized and sold by authorities in New Orleans in 1818, went for an average price of $768 per person. By the 1820s the average slave sold for $617 in New Orleans, but prices regularly reached $1,000 or more. During the 1830s the value of the total domestic slave trade topped $143 million per year. Soon enslaved people were the Deep Southern planter's most significant asset, alongside the land itself.[91]

With so much disease risk in the Deep South from yellow fever (and also from cholera, smallpox, malaria, and measles), and with so much capital tied up in enslaved bodies foreign to the region, planters expressed anxiety that one bad epidemic could spell disaster. As the joint yellow fever–cholera epidemic "raged to a horrible extent" in 1833, for example, Captain Robert Proctor distributed opium and calomel to the 104 people he enslaved on Florisone, his sugar plantation, and then packed up his white family and left. Many enslaved people on Florisone ran to the lake and into the woods, seeking to escape the epidemic and the plantation. But eighty-two people died, including some of Proctor's "best ones." Proctor's neighbors—those who survived—believed he was ruined. So many enslaved people died, in fact, that by Christmas 1833 it was estimated that cholera had "erased" $4 million worth of human property across the South.[92]

Seeking to mitigate disease risk, some enslavers experimented with new securities and financial instruments. By the 1830s planters began taking out insurance on enslaved lives—particularly those people rented out, with specialized skills, or employed in dangerous professions like coal mining. Though often advertised as whole life, most of the policies lasted only for a term of up to seven years. This allowed, according to historian Sharon Ann Murphy, companies like Baltimore Life to respond to market conditions and take heed of an individual slave's evolving health status. To reduce "fraud"—a euphemism for the deliberate killing of an enslaved person—insurers wrote policies covering only two-thirds of the person's "actual value."[93] Dr. Josiah Nott was a critic of underwriting enslaved lives, seeing the potential for abuse, that the "Almighty Dollar" would "silence the soft, small voice of humanity" eventually. He insisted that "underwriters cannot expect fair play" if the insurance money was worth as much as the slave—then the enslaved person would be "regarded rather in the light of a superannuated horse."[94]

Nott was right about the perverse incentives (while inadvertently indicting the entire enslaving class). He was also right that the data underwriting these policies was incomplete, forcing agents into some strange guesswork when calculating premiums on Black lives. Most added place-specific premiums, suggesting that underwriters did not consider Black people's disease risk evenly distributed across the South. The one-year premium per $100 of insurance for a twenty-five-year-old man, for example, was $1.00 for a white person, but $1.47 for an enslaved person, from Richmond Fire & Virginia Life, and $2.00 for an enslaved person from a New Orleans–based insurer.[95]

Slave insurance never took off on a large scale outside of the urban, industrial areas of the Upper South. And as Louisiana planters saw it, the only way to fully mitigate *their* disease risk was to usher their slaves safely through acclimation—a process they knew could be "costly" to them. John Knight, a merchant in Natchez, for example, expected that the forty-nine enslaved people (including two infants) he imported from Maryland and purchased from traders in New Orleans for $19,027 would suffer at his plantation on the Red River in Louisiana. "My chief anxiety now," he told his father-in-law in June 1844, "is, to get them all safely acclimated . . . but I can hardly expect this without the loss of a few." Three people died that summer as yellow fever ripped across the region. Knight added, "I consider all my N. Orleans negroes will be well acclimated after two years," but "it is much more difficult to acclimate *old* negroes than young ones; and after their removal from their old homes to new ones, they seldom, if ever, become reconciled to the change."[96]

Valuing Immunity

Acclimation's precise monetary value was clearest in New Orleans's sprawling slave market—where over 100,000 men, women, and children were packaged, priced, and sold during the antebellum period. Health—both physical and mental—influenced many buyers' decisions as they strolled the slave lots on Esplanade. People described as "superannuated" or "blind and deaf" or "crippled" were less likely to be sold for a good price, if they sold at all. Those who had survived the great killers of smallpox, whooping cough, or measles, however, were more appealing.[97]

Yellow fever survivors were most attractive of all. Like "fancy" or "likely" or "choice" or "No. 1"—words used to capture a panoply of intangible qualities possessed by an enslaved person, as well as their fungibility— "acclimated" was much invoked. "A Choice lot of young Negroes, males and females," advertised one newspaper, which added that the people had been "here during the summer and therefore are partly acclimated." Another advertisement for "A valuable family of slaves" insisted that each was an "acclimated, willing subject and of obedient disposition." One typical flyer featured health front and center, advertising "Two Young, stout, likely negroes, acclimated and accustomed to work in a store house." Happily for potential buyers, these young men were "guaranteed free from the vices & maladies prescribed by law."[98] Travel writer Joseph Holt Ingraham witnessed a slave auction in Natchez and noted how the auctioneer marched people up and yelled, "Acclimated, gentlemen . . . a first rate carriage driver . . . Examine him, gentlemen—a strong and athletic fellow." Though many Orleanian buyers preferred bilingual slaves as a matter of course, advertisements often conjoined language skills with acclimation and guarantees. One ad for a "superior mulatto boy" was typical: "13 years of age, acclimated, speaks French and English; fully guaranteed."[99]

Whenever they could, slave traders asserted that the humans they sold were acclimated. But as immunity was invisible and the object of considerable definitional instability, there was no surefire test, no way to know for certain. Like everything else in the slave market, a declaration of acclimation was part boosterism, part lie, part speculation. But for white people, judging another person's acclimation status was part of the connoisseurship of purchasing a person. Indeed, the very act of asking the question *Is she acclimated?* demonstrated a man's savviness to other whites in the room; that he understood and accepted disease risk, and knew how to judge value in Black bodies. Thousands of people flowed into the New Orleans slave market from Virginia and Kentucky each year, and by the 1830s seasoned slave buyers and sellers came to adopt a loose though operational shorthand: an enslaved person was considered (or could plausibly be advertised as) "partly acclimated" or "partly seasoned" if they had been born out of state and had survived one summer in the Deep South; they were "fully acclimated," "guaranteed acclimated," or "thoroughly creolized" if they had survived multiple summers; and they were "creole" if they were native to the Yellow Fever South.

As crude and unscientific as these categories were, they pushed people into different price brackets. "Fully acclimated" and "creole" slaves commanded higher prices, costing 25 to 50 percent more than unacclimated slaves new to the region. Judge François Xavier Martin, who drafted Louisiana's 1808 territorial slave codes, wrote in 1818 that slaves generally cost between $750 and $1,000, but "if born in the country or seasoned thereto, a slave is worth from $1500 to $2000 in ready money; a genteel house servant $3000." In some instances, acclimation could more than double an enslaved person's appraised value. According to Ingraham, while most newly arrived enslaved people sold for about $800, acclimated slaves "often [sold] for eighteen hundred and two thousand dollars apiece, of either sex."[100]

With acclimation potentially worth so much to white people, the slave trade developed an entire subindustry concerned with moving enslaved people from unacclimated to acclimated status. Slave trader Walter Campbell maintained a "holding pen" eighty miles outside New Orleans where hundreds of enslaved people from the Upper South became inured to the new climate and diseases of the Deep South during the summer before their sale.[101] Campbell believed such stewardship would give him an edge in the New Orleans market, as "Virginia and Maryland negroes, with this advantage of acclimation and trained to plantation labor, offer inducements to purchasers." There were even services offered to owners of unacclimated slaves to push people through acclimation in a more "gentle" setting than New Orleans. William Grose from Harper's Ferry, Virginia, who eventually escaped to Canada in 1851, remembered that when he was sold south to New Orleans with his brother, his owner sent them "into Alabama to a watering place" as they "were not acclimated." There the brothers spent three months "till late in the fall—then we went back to him."[102]

Slave trader's gimmicks and schemes did little to remedy the fact that yellow fever killed many enslaved people, especially those who arrived in the Deep South after a long overland or sea journey, traumatized, exhausted, and immunosuppressed. Slave trader Joseph Hicks spoke for many in his business when he said, "We may calculate upon loosing [*sic*] some of them in becoming acclimated." Slave traders disagreed about what they considered an "acceptable" death rate. One writer in the New Orleans *Argus* estimated, "The loss by *death* in bringing slaves from a northern climate, which our planters are under the necessity of doing, is not less than TWENTY-FIVE PER CENT."[103] Such shocking mortality was attributable to an array of causes—including yellow fever—but it forced slave traders to adjust for disease risk in their business models. As with all commodities and goods, the pace and schedule of New Orleans's industry in human beings was controlled by disease. In 1830 only 2.6 percent of annual slave sales took place between July and October—the fever season—to lessen the already considerable risks associated with moving enslaved people south.[104]

Slave prices were routinely lowest in the late summer and early fall. Economist Lawrence Kotlikoff estimated that traders could obtain a price 10.8 percent higher if they waited from September until January to sell a person. This price differential was largely because slave prices were pegged to cotton—which was being harvested in the late summer and selling briskly by the early spring. But it was also because sickly summers drove off—or killed off—potential buyers. As one trader described this dilemma in August 1846, "It is hard to say at this season of the year what negroes are worth, for [during an epidemic] they will not bring their value." "Fall winter and Early spring"—when demand and therefore prices were higher—"is the proper time to bring them here," the trader continued, and "during the proper season of the year they would bring from 50 to 150 and in some instances $200 more." Moreover, for an industry that trafficked in both people and information about those people, epidemics could disrupt the flow of intelligence through the grapevine. Planter William Kenner told his business partner John Minor, "The person from whom we expected to get the information respecting your Negro . . . has died of the fever. We therefore cannot give you any account of them." In another instance, Kenner told a client, Mrs. Kerchival, that she should hold off on selling a man she owned "as most of the families likely to want a coachman" were absent from the city and would not return until health had been restored. Kenner recommended that Kerchival keep the coachman for a few more weeks because once white people returned "to their ordinary avocations," "a better sale" could be made.[105]

As early as the 1820s many whites considered New Orleans too risky for their valuable enslaved property. Even if a slave was declared acclimated, fraud was common, as traders fabricated backstories to enhance a person's value and hasten a sale. And with thousands of poor, famine-fleeing Irishmen pouring into the docks by the 1840s, the city's labor–capital calculus shifted completely. One stevedore claimed on the eve of the Civil War—in a manner reminiscent of how the bosses on the New Basin Canal described their preferences three decades earlier—that slaves were "worth too much to be risked here": "If the Paddies are knocked overboard, or get their backs broke, nobody loses anything!"[106] If a Black slave died, however, a white person's *capital* evaporated. The proportion of enslaved persons in the city thus dropped from close to 50 percent in 1806, to under 25 percent in 1840, to just 8 percent in 1860. Capitalist logic pushed acclimated bondspeople out of New Orleans and onto surrounding plantations—safer, less-diseased, and more efficient sites for Blacks to create capital for whites.[107]

Redhibition and Fraud

Louisiana's courts seldom became involved in defining acclimation or regulating it in the slave market. This is perhaps surprising, given that Louisiana had unique legal mechanisms for dealing with sellers who concealed or dissembled. Redhibition—a form of consumer protection that canceled a slave sale if a seller concealed "defects"—was a legal tool occasionally used by disgruntled purchasers of slaves during the antebellum period.[108] According to the *Civil Code,* slaves were legally considered defective merchandise if they were "diseased," and they could be returned as if under warranty. "Diseased" was definitionally broad enough to cover diseases of the body (like syphilis, leprosy, or consumption) and mind (madness, epilepsy, or serial running away). Of the 166 redhibition suits brought before the Louisiana Supreme Court for the concealment of a disease of the body, forty-seven involved tuberculosis. Only one case, brought in 1809, involved yellow fever, which was hereafter classified as a disease not "incurable by its nature" and thus not a redhibitory vice.[109]

Very occasionally, Louisiana introduced broad laws barring unacclimated slaves from being sold within the state. In 1826, for example, the state legislature passed a law prohibiting any *bona fide* citizen of Louisiana from selling or exchanging a slave who had been in the state for fewer than two years, "under the penalty of forfeiting the aforesaid slaves, one fourth to the use of the informer, the other three fourths to the use of the State."[110] A harsh punishment. But "A Creole" complained in the *Louisiana Advertiser* a year later that the law was being entirely disregarded by slave traders. "[By] reference to the paper of today, I find eighty Virginia negroes offered for sale," this Creole remarked. He asked if such a "barefaced violation of law" was to be tolerated. Should strangers "with impunity . . . be allowed to trample on and make [a] mockery of the institutions of our country?"—especially as the sale "of unacclimated slaves, one fourth of whom die during the first summer, has greatly impoverished the State." He concluded, "It was wise of the legislature to adopt a prohibitory measure, and it will be equally just, and wise, of some patriotic individual, to see that measure strictly enforced." That this 1826 law—and another law enacted briefly in 1834—went unenforced suggests the state was either incapable of or uninterested in establishing acclimation standards. How could such laws be properly enforced consistently and at scale? Instead, the legislature (like the courts) considered it a white individual's prerogative to determine which disease risks were acceptable when purchasing human property—*caveat emptor.* And most certainly, the government would not be in the business of compensating slave owners for the loss of enslaved lives during yellow fever epidemics—that would leave the state vulnerable to all manner of other financial obligations.[111]

How did enslaved people feel about living with so much yellow fever risk? From the few records we have that are written from the perspective of enslaved or formerly enslaved people, it is clear they were petrified by yellow fever, like everyone else. But they could not choose to avoid disease risk, save money for medicines, or flee. They had to work in dangerous swamps or accompany owners into town during epidemics if told to do so. Often they had to care for their sick masters. And enslaved people took no comfort in being told that because they were Black, they were safe. As one former slave named Peter Ryas said, "People die like dem flies. Dat fever pay no 'tention to skin color. White folks go. Black folks go. Dey die so fast dey pile dem in wagons."[112]

It is possible that immunity added to an enslaved person's sense of self worth and agency, as it did for free and mostly white members of this society. And certainly some leveraged their immunity for preference in the slave market, just as they leveraged other desirable skills and traits. But bonds people had no financial or social incentive to acquire immunity (beyond, of course, the massive incentive of avoiding death by a terrible disease). And as acclimation added nothing to their personal wealth or social standing, enslaved people could have conceived of acclimation differently than whites did, not as an asset but as a burden. Slaves were embodied capital, so acclimation enhanced the value and safety of that capital only for their white owners, while providing whites with a justification for relegating enslaved Black people to society's lowest social rung. John Wyeth, a traveler from Boston, recalled in 1833, "When a negro gets very sick" from yellow fever, "he loses all his spirits, and refuses all remedies. He wishes to die, and it is no wonder, if he believes that he shall go into a pleasant country where there are no white men or women."[113]

Gens de Couleur

New Orleans's large population of *gens de couleur libres*—who constituted about a quarter of the city's population at the high watermark in 1830—was not a homogeneous group. Highly atomized by class, ethnicity, religion, language, and profession, some free people of African descent could trace their Louisiana ancestry back multiple generations. Some had more recently arrived from Saint-Domingue or the eastern United States, with the city acting as a magnet for free Blacks from other jurisdictions. The richest owned slaves, whether solely for profit or to protect their families with a master's legal rights. Elite free Blacks worked in cotton warehouses and as commission merchants—and some socialized in white Creole circles. The majority occupied more menial positions, as professionals, managers, artists, and clerks.[114]

Like all Creoles, free people of color were assumed immune to yellow fever and malaria. And some appear to have leveraged their implied immunity or creolism in much the same way as whites did, to etch out lucrative positions in certain industries and demand social recognition. Georges-Alcès, a Louisiana-born free Black man, and his uncle Lucien Mansion ran a cigar factory in Tremé that employed two hundred people. Nicol Riquet, another cigar maker, who never left the city and died rich, developed a reputation as one of Louisiana's greatest songwriters, his most famous lyric being a tribute to the god Bacchus. Camille Thiery, born in New Orleans in 1814, ran the successful commission house Lafitte, Dufilho & Co. Pierre Casenave parlayed his earnings from undertaking into working in the commission business, and became the clerk of the wealthy Jewish philanthropist Judah Touro. Casenave amassed a fortune of over $100,000.[115] Bernard Soulié, a merchant and real estate broker, doubled his capital to $100,000 in the 1850s. Thomy Lafon amassed perhaps the greatest fortune of all—half a million dollars—through brokering and property speculation.[116]

Such wealth and success was exceptional—for any person. But lower-class free Black people also found footholds in certain industries where their alleged immunity to yellow fever gave them a leg up. Steamboat captains apparently preferred acclimated free Black men to white laborers, considering them less militant and longer-lived than Irishmen. Many free Blacks demanded large sums for grave digging and body-carting—as much as $5 per body during particularly bad epidemics.[117] Whether rich or poor, most of these *gens de couleur libres* had probably survived yellow fever in childhood; all sought to capitalize—directly or indirectly—on their creolism or acclimation. In doing so, they resisted the pernicious ideas and fragile excuses about the Black body that whites used to justify slavery and exclude Blacks from full membership in society.

Over time it became increasingly difficult for free Black people of any class to enjoy full freedom in New Orleans. Their social and legal status deteriorated dramatically during the 1850s, a decade during which the free Black condition was increasingly described by whites in the language of disease—a social abnormality that must be excised from a "healthy" and binary slave society. An 1852 act required all persons emancipating slaves to pay for their passage to Liberia, and all manumissions were banned in 1857. Free Blacks were also required to register their presence within the city or face fines. Within this increasingly hostile social and legal regime, many richer free Blacks left the city permanently, departing for France or Haiti. By 1860 the city's free Black population had dropped to just 6.3 percent. As the free Black population declined, the acclimation privileges accorded to *gens de couleur libres*—if they were ever material—dwindled. In essence, race trumped creolism in the rubric of immunocapital, with whites seeking to racially stigmatize this group, not enhance its power through immunity.[118]

A False Meritocracy

Depending on a person's race, class, and gender, acclimation could open or close doors. As one white New Orleanian said in congratulating a newly acclimated friend, he had "finally succeeded in getting out his *naturalization papers*. He is now in every respect a citizen of New Orleans, and long may he live to enjoy the glorious privilege."[119] As immunity for whites became a form of social capital, closely linked with the concepts of citizenship and legitimacy, slavery inverted the logic of immunity for Black people. Here, only white people could adopt disease risk—they claimed to own the risk of the people they enslaved—and therefore only white people could control immunocapital. This logic of risk and immunity justified a larger system of inequality, for the longer enslaved persons could survive to make wealth for their masters, the more it made sense to enslave them. The professed belief in enslaved Black people's natural immunity emphasized their statelessness, movability, and malleability—at once sub- and superhuman, incapable of living in freedom.

Those white elites at the top of New Orleans's economic and political life, all (allegedly) survivors, meanwhile, obtained a *de facto* moral legitimacy, a tropical (if ecumenical) twist on Max Weber's aristocracy of the elect. In their public willingness to roll the epidemiological dice and risk their lives, they classified themselves as victors in a harsh but essentially honest meritocracy. Equating survival with morality justified, in their view, the exploitation of unacclimated whites and all Black people. It also made New Orleans a miserable place to live for the majority of its inhabitants. Carl Kohn, an eighteen-year-old cotton clerk from Bohemia, in a letter to his uncle in Paris summed up the foul mood engulfing the city during the 1833 epidemic: "Is this the 'dear Orleans' of which you talked in your letters with such affection? Is that the place where you wish to lay now your mortal remains?" Kohn concluded, "Bye the bye that's a good idea, for it is only a place to die at but not to live."[120]

But Kohn did not leave. Instead he faced down yellow fever and survived to become one of New Orleans's most prominent businessmen, forming his own brokerage firm in 1842, serving as the president of the Union Bank, and marrying an acclimated woman named Clara, the daughter of sugar planter

Maunsel White. In September 1833 Kohn had expected yellow fever to "attack with as much certainty as a condemned criminal does expect the sentence of his execution"; by year's end, he cheerfully described his improving business prospects and plans for the future (much as his father-in-law had). Once a source of misery and anxiety, yellow fever now endowed Kohn with a future, transforming this onetime skeptic of New Orleans into a *bona fide* titan of it.[121]

4

Public Health, Private Acclimation

While journeying back from Oregon to Boston, adventurer John Wyeth found himself stuck in New Orleans at the height of the 1833 yellow fever epidemic. "It is an unexaggerated fact," Wyeth reminisced, "that I witnessed more misery" in nine weeks in New Orleans than "old men experience in a long life." Time itself seemed to ooze by. At a hazard rate of $2-a-day, Wyeth spent a month digging graves, eventually excavating a fifty-seven-foot trench in which he packed 300 people, nestling the corpses of small children into the gaps. Many people were tossed into the Mississippi River like "dead hogs." In one house, Wyeth recalled, twenty-five or thirty people had perished, discovered only when "a most pestiferous odor" reached the street outside. Rather than deal with the bloated corpses individually—some covered in worms, some partly eaten with entrails hanging out—the city ordered the house boarded up and incinerated.[1]

Wyeth found New Orleans's epidemic disorder, its lack of "good government," and its lawlessness disturbing, marveling at how unlike Boston—indeed how *un-American*—it all felt. All shops, taverns, and grocers shut up for want of customers. Half the city's population (25,000 people) left. Even the gambling houses went quiet. Potholes sprang into ripe cesspools "as green as grass," releasing a steam that could be detected half a mile away. No one seemed to be in charge. One day Wyeth witnessed an assault on an enslaved man returning from the carpenter. His attackers ran off with the rough-board coffin he had been carrying. When Wyeth fell sick with yellow fever, he spent all his money on medical care. His doctor dosed him with glass after glass of hot castor oil, so much he thought he "should have no insides left to go home with." Wyeth survived that season, though approximately 10,000 people—or one-fifth of the city's population—did not. Traumatized, he left New Orleans, feeling the city was "a dreadful place in the eyes of a New-England man."[2]

A century after Wyeth left New Orleans, Henry Dart, editor of *Louisiana Historical Quarterly,* challenged the glamour-saturated image of antebellum New Orleans in its ostensible golden age, a place immortalized and celebrated in movies, books, and memories. "There was no romance in the lives of average citizens or workers in New Orleans," wrote Hart. These "real people," living in the nation's deadliest major city amid extreme filth and terrifying annual fevers, "could scarcely have loved or respected the rulers (city and province) who permitted those conditions to exist."[3] Inversely, city officials—looking on as the hospitals and graveyards buckled under the immense pressure of dealing with the desperate living and increasing numbers of dead—could scarcely have felt much accountability to their constituents. Indeed, residents and visitors agreed that "city authorities" took essentially "no precautions against sickness," even though, as one reformer suggested, the death rate was "at *least double* what it ought to be." Another physician argued that one-half or even two-thirds of those who died could have been saved with some government action.[4]

The Weak and Sickly State

Why did politicians allow health to fall to such abysmal levels in New Orleans when even a little intervention—garbage removal, drainage, *cordon sanitaire,* hospitals, and quarantine—could have saved thousands of lives? Why did New Orleans reject the ameliorative systems employed to great effect in other nineteenth-century cities like Boston, Charleston, Philadelphia, Chicago, and New York? How was it that the same people who entered New Orleans politics with the conviction that "*yellow fever is an evil, remediable and extinguishable by human agency*" finish their terms deriding quarantine and eschewing sanitation?[5] Given the terrifying mortality, why was yellow fever not *the* primary political issue? How was it that the persistent waves of lethal disease did not undercut the stature, legitimacy, and reputation of government? Most of all, why did residents not revolt?[6]

New Orleans's political elite were neither crippled by mass sickness nor particularly concerned with fixing it. This was because few of the aldermen, mayors, and recorders running municipal government were professional politicians; they were, instead, merchants, planters, and enslavers—appointed and later elected on the basis of their commercial success. Enmeshed within a wider culture of Southern illiberalism and fixated on cotton, their policies were informed by their small-state fetishes, ardent support of racial slavery, and tax aversion.[7] And even though they lived in the deadliest city in America, immunocapitalists insisted that yellow fever was a problem with no solution; that all tax money spent on improving health was wasted; and that people would simply have to accept infectious disease as the status quo—just as they had. The worthy would survive and succeed commercially, and it was inappropriate for government to get involved in this process. Consequently, New Orleans's governing bodies "simplified" their mandate "to the utmost," officially limiting their focus to the legal "protection of [white] life and private property," greasing the wheels of commerce through deregulation, and ensuring the smooth movement of goods and people through the port. It was the "particular" job of city government to police "people of color." That many excessive deaths could be counted in New Orleans each summer might have been a personal tragedy, councilors conceded, but it was not the particular problem of government.[8]

New Orleans's indifference to the public's health was increasingly abnormal in the larger national context. During the nineteenth century, as historian William Novak has described, local governments gradually consolidated power in pursuit of the "well-regulated society," a large component of which was health reform. As early as 1800, municipalities from Boston to Savannah began reallocating certain responsibilities for education, policing, and especially public health away from budget- and reelection-conscious politicians. In such instances, the public health charge increasingly fell to independent and permanent health boards composed of trained experts, doctors, statisticians, and specialized clerks. Health authorities condemned buildings, collected vital data, cared for the sick, removed waste, initiated smallpox inoculation programs, and established hospitals. Some also implemented quarantines—the least popular and most draconian tool in a health officer's arsenal. The US Supreme Court upheld the state's authority in such matters. In the landmark 1824 case *Gibbons v. Ogden*, Chief Justice John Marshall recognized the "acknowledged power of a State to provide for the health of its citizens." This could encompass an "immense mass of legislation" and "health laws of every description"—laws that subordinated individual and commercial rights to the commonweal. By the 1830s many American cities (mostly in the North, but also in South Carolina and Georgia) had shown disease to be remediable, if not fixable; tasked a "health police" with drawing up and enforcing health codes; and proved that money spent on public health saved lives.[9]

New Orleans's politicians justified inaction and cheapness by adhering to a narrowly defined vision of what government could and should do. After 1816, Louisiana's state legislature ceded all control over health in New Orleans to its municipal government, giving its mayor and city council "full and entire power to make and pass all regulations or ordinances which they shall deem necessary to preserve the public cleanliness and salubrity." In 1827 Louisiana's Supreme Court affirmed the "extensive discretion" of New Orleans's city councilors over health legislation. Adopting a philosophy of health and government opposite to that outlined by Chief Justice Marshall in *Gibbons v. Ogden,* New Orleans politicians claimed that no laws could stop yellow fever; that health solutions might work in temperate cities but had no impact in subtropical New Orleans—and therefore it was folly to even try.[10] Moreover, they claimed, government should spend as little tax money as possible on comprehensive fixes like draining city streets, maintaining the Charity Hospital, and providing welfare to yellow fever orphans and widows. Quarantines were perennially a nonstarter. Clinging to the increasingly dubious theory of "anti-contagionism"—that yellow fever was neither contagious nor imported on ships—far longer than their counterparts in other cities, New Orleans's commercial-civic elite argued that quarantines were "inexpedient, vexatious and oppressive" rather than lifesaving.[11] To compensate for the problems left unaddressed by state minimalism, private and church-affiliated asylums and orphanages arose, but never at the scale required.

New Orleans's leaders continued to proffer two time-tested "solutions" to yellow fever: get acclimated or flee. The political answer to the great public health problem was thus not less yellow fever, but paradoxically *more:* drainage, sanitation, and quarantines only wasted money and delayed the inevitable process of acclimation. Elites repeated the line that while weak New Yorkers looked to their maternalistic government for health protection, independent white New Orleanians must rely on their hard-won acclimation, which would eventually propel them into the upper ranks of commodity capitalism. Viruses, however, do not respect state lines or city limits, and this non-approach to public health at New Orleans had terrible knock-on effects across the Mississippi Valley. In fact, New Orleans's health

policies became the *de facto* health reality of upriver towns, plantation hinterlands, and Gulf ports across the Yellow Fever South as every ship or barge
from the Crescent City propelled disease into their limits. Smaller cities like
Natchez, Galveston, and Vicksburg knew their commercial dependence on
New Orleans left them epidemiologically vulnerable. But they also knew
they could not force change in New Orleans. Dr. John McKowen—a critic
of New Orleans's "murderous" health philosophy—later recalled that with
all bayous and rivers leading there, "country Jakes were . . . compelled to
do what the merchants of New Orleans wished or they must do without a
Metropolis."[12]

This system of immunocapitalism, suspicious of any government action,
came to thrive and depend on epidemic disease because it perversely incentivized politicians to maintain not only a vast system of racial slavery
but also a broad and epidemiologically rendered white underclass. Many
American cities relied on property taxes and industry for funding by the
mid-nineteenth century; in contrast, New Orleans lined its coffers through
a system of fines, fees, and stealth taxes levied disproportionately on the
unestablished and unacclimated. Acclimated white elites considered this a
winning solution. Not only did it insulate the elites from paying essentially
any tax on valuable property—like real estate or slaves—but it also squeezed
a group of people who were mostly new to the region, had few connections, often could not speak French or English, and could not count on
steady employment. Crucially, only a narrow sliver of this group could vote.
About a quarter would be dead within three years; most of the remainder
would be so pummeled by arbitrary fines and fees that they could not ac-
crue any property. As for those lucky few who survived five years, became
naturalized US citizens, and gained the right to vote, the timing of elections, deliberately scheduled to coincide with the high-fever season, operated as a climate gerrymander—most unacclimated people were either
absent, too sick, or too scared of fever to vote. Should strangers run the
gauntlet to become both enfranchised and *acclimated* citizens, they would
surely come to vote with the interests of their epidemiological class, accepting or even relishing in the powerlessness of the unacclimated. The
system was exploitative, deadly, and self-perpetuating.[13]

At best, such an aversion to public health and reliance on individual acclimation corroded connections between state, citizen, and community. At
worst, perceptions of immunity gave the commercial-civic elite a scientific
excuse to disregard the lives of vulnerable constituents. They cynically col-

luded to enhance their own wealth—and preserve the value of their own immunocapital—through active negligence. The economic interests of a small minority took precedence, and welfare for the poor and vulnerable had no place.[14] The oligarchs of New Orleans actually came to celebrate disease: it saved them from a host of problems (infrastructure, welfare obligations, regulation) that would have otherwise required long-term political attention and serious expenditures. New Orleans's paltry health system—undergirded by an ideology of hyper-individualism, an acceptance of social asymmetry, and a religious-like reverence for private property—mirrored the wider violences of this slave society, which was predicated on devaluing reality in favor of convenience and prizing economic profit over human life.

A Diseased Political Culture

If we were to time-travel back to October 1833, when John Wyeth was digging mass graves, and sat in the Cabildo's public gallery to listen to the deliberations of New Orleans's city council, we might not realize that the city was in the grips of its worst yellow fever epidemic in a generation. We would hear detailed discussions concerning the oyster shells being used to pave a new road out to Lake Pontchartrain; debates about city attorney salaries; estimates for the amount of wood needed for a flying bridge; and fights about the cost of lantern oil for the cotton exchange. Across the road in the mayor's office, the conversation might center on city finances or the schedule of the city guard. There would be little to no discussion about the horrific situation at the Charity Hospital less than a mile away, where unclaimed corpses, baking under the sun outside, had recently exploded. Nothing either about the nearly 300 immigrants around the corner in Marigny, who had just died from yellow fever.[15]

The elite culture of apathetic fatalism ran deeper than silence. New Orleans's city fathers *actively* avoided discussing yellow fever even at the height of epidemics, instead preoccupying themselves with finances, zoning, and parochial matters like bread weights. Aldermen considered it a poor use of political capital to seek out means to solve or ameliorate disease. Some believed the fatal status quo was intractable and that there was nothing to be gained by raising controversial topics like quarantine, which did little but produce shouting matches and inflame the ire of businessmen. Others were weary of discussing disease, which inevitably morphed into conversations about other sensitive issues like taxes, regulation, or immigration. Mayors, the public face of the city, walked an especially fine line in their disease messaging. Mayors often campaigned on a health platform (a big issue for the mass of city inhabitants), and because eras of New Orleans's history bore mayors' names—the Roffignac administration or the Crossman period, for example—some worried that a bad epidemic could damage their reputation abroad and in history. But raising the disease question also had immediate consequences at home: it was a surefire way to anger aldermen and lose mayoral appropriations (which were subject to city council approval).[16] Some politicians, of course, surely felt overwhelmed by the scope of the problem. One physician-cum-alderman argued in the 1850s that the idea of solving the yellow fever problem was met by "every person" with "disbelief," and that nothing "short of draining, filling up, or reclaiming the whole of lower Louisiana" would make the city healthy and miasma-free, a project so expensive it would require "all the gold of California."[17]

Municipal officers may have been uninterested in discussing yellow fever, but they were not disinterested. Throughout the antebellum period, most politicians at the state and parish level (senators, representatives, judges, sheriffs) and the city level (mayors, aldermen, assistant aldermen, recorders, tax collectors) were also planters or merchants, had significant financial interests in sugar, banking, cotton, or slavery, or quite often drew wealth from many of those interests. Of the twenty-four aldermen who sat during the administration of merchant-mayor Nicholas Girod (a. YF ca. 1790s) between 1812 and 1815, for example, the majority were sugar planters or merchants. Many were doctors. All were slave owners. And almost all city and state politicians claimed to be Creole or to have faced yellow fever and lived to tell the tale. Their job, as they saw it, was thus not to prevent disease among newcomers but to help white survivors—like themselves—make money through commodities and slavery.

And make money they did, often by putting their personal commercial interests above their civic responsibilities. Many did not see these as conflicting interests. According to the credit-rating agency R. G. Dun & Co. (predecessor to Dun & Bradstreet), for example, Whig mayor Abdiel Crossman (a. YF ca. 1833) had come to New Orleans from Maine in the late 1820s with only $5 to his name. Standing just above four feet tall, Crossman had started off as a hatmaker but had insinuated himself among the merchant and banking classes, eventually serving as an alderman from the First Municipality. By the time he was elected mayor in 1846, Crossman had already "been a bank director many years" and accumulated bank stock.

He owned multiple lots and houses. For a public servant, he grew incredibly wealthy, even by nineteenth-century standards when the divide between public and private was often razor thin. Crossman was worth an estimated $100,000 in 1853.[18]

There were essentially no negative consequences for politicians who avoided discussing disease. Historian John Sacher estimated that in 1820, property requirements barred 57.8 percent of white men from voting in New Orleans. Though Louisiana's 1845 constitution established universal white manhood suffrage, in practice many people were still shut out. By 1850, 41.5 percent of white men in New Orleans were still disenfranchised. Excluding so many white males—while also excluding women, most free people of color, slaves, recent immigrants, the "floating" population, and children—meant that only a small proportion of city residents held politicians accountable. Luckily for politicians, those inhabitants who clamored for public health infrastructure quieted over time as they accepted the filthiness of the urban condition, gained immunity, fled, or died. This was no idle speculation. Statistician James Wynne calculated in 1857 that if one hundred immigrants settled in New York, nine people would die and ninety-one would become permanent residents within three years. In New Orleans, however, the number of dead shot up to twenty-four. And because naturalization required five years of residence, there was a strong overlap between the unacclimated, the nonpropertied, and the noncitizen. Figuring that a large percentage would die before becoming enfranchised citizens, politicians in New Orleans found the unacclimated an easy bloc to ignore. After all, dead men did not vote; acclimated men did.[19]

Absenteeism

Demonstrating how little concern they had for their constituents, most aldermen—even those who claimed immunity or creolism like William Kenner, James Carrick, and Félix Arnaud—fled to their country plantations when yellow fever appeared, joining the business and planting elite in playing "like truant children." Baron Joseph-Xavier Delfau de Pontalba (a. YF ca. 1793), a wealthy planter and landlord, related that when he fled the city in 1796, his party needed "the air of the country, the maladies in town having driven them all into a state of deep melancholy." In the country, "all news of that sort is taboo." Pontalba's party amused themselves with jokes, debauchery, and games in a scene reminiscent of Boccaccio's Ten fleeing the ravages of the Black Death. In one letter, Pontalba described a party so wild that he had to barricade his bedroom door with a table to keep the crowd from dragging him out. In another, he described how the women had stolen the breeches, shoes, and coats of the men, who were forced to return to the city in their night garments. Hung over and exhausted, they found it difficult to make it to their 11 a.m. meeting in town.[20]

The police, unwilling to venture into a diseased city, were not much better. Though police officers were legally required to increase their surveillance over Black people and white-owned property during epidemics, one night-watch report from September 17, 1840, noted that nine officers in the Second Municipality had failed to show up for work, Sargent Pincham was still sick with yellow fever, and three wards were left with no police whatsoever.[21] As one visitor joked, epidemics were a criminal's paradise, with "jolly bank-runners" carrying their loot "fearlessly under their arms," pickpockets working openly, and murderers roaming the streets and killing with impunity. Police officers were as vulnerable to yellow fever as anyone else, perhaps more so as their job often put them in contact with diseased people and spaces. In 1854, after some policemen died from yellow fever, many remaining officers determined that the risk was too high. Some abandoned their posts to flee town, forfeiting the bond the city had required them to pay to ensure their good behavior and physical presence.[22]

The elite of most any nineteenth-century American city had the privilege of spatial segregation from the "filthy" poor—they could retreat to their uptown mansions, seaside homes, or Europe—but this privilege took on a distinctly diseased flavor in Louisiana. Most acclimated merchants and planters saw no need to keep their families in town during the fever season, when business was slow and the mood was depressing. Having already demonstrated their immunity, the cotton and sugar elite could instead see to their country business—surveying their fields, checking accounts, trading slaves, and visiting creditors in New York and London—while delegating city tasks like bookkeeping and sales to their low-level clerks and agents, men who could not financially or socially afford to leave. Widespread absenteeism gave the city a "*hibernal*" feel during epidemics, but as landscape architect Benjamin Latrobe (d. YF. 1820) reasoned, why would a man endure the "*ennui*" of a New Orleans August if he could afford to enjoy a summer sojourn elsewhere?[23]

Political absenteeism during epidemics was the norm, and it crippled the government. In the autumn of 1804—a season when 1,000 to 1,500 people died—seven meetings of the city council were canceled for lack of a quorum, which required six aldermen in attendance. Of the twenty-seven meetings that did take place from July to December, there were six aldermen present less than half the time; future mayor Dr. John Watkins (d. YF 1812) appeared just once. In the deadly autumn of 1811, four meetings of the council were delayed due to disease.[24] Those politicians who were forced to remain in town during epidemics became skilled at putting disease out of their minds. By 1810, the city council banned the ringing of funeral bells between August and December, finding the constant noise too distracting. In many later years the council made it illegal for the city to communicate the death toll to the public. During some serious epidemics, the only prevention undertaken was to post "resolutions on strangers" in various languages along the levee, advising newcomers to leave immediately. Only occasionally did the mayor use his discretionary fund to ship "indigent foreigners" and "unfortunates" across Lake Pontchartrain, perhaps with a biscuit and some salt meat in hand.[25]

The dire consequences of political absenteeism reached their apex in 1853, the year of the city's worst epidemic. In June the council was under pressure to convene a board of health, but the decision was tabled. The council also discussed giving the Howard Association—a private benevolent group—$5,000 to care for yellow fever victims. Discussion reduced the sum to $2,500. This resolution was referred to the board of assistant aldermen (the body directly responsible for health after 1852), which further reduced the sum to $2,000. But because so many assistant aldermen had already fled—and multiple meetings had already been canceled—the requisite quorum of fourteen out of twenty-seven was not met and the meeting was adjourned.[26] Mayor Abdiel Crossman was so angered by the municipal councils' collective negligence that he called a special session of the assistant aldermen. Even then, only eight showed up, again insufficient for a quorum. Of the twenty-seven elected assistant aldermen and twelve elected aldermen, two-thirds had fled the city and would stay away for the entirety of the epidemic.[27] By mid-July—as the epidemic was claiming approximately one hundred lives a day—even the most pro-business paper in New Orleans, the *Commercial Bulletin,* implored the council to intervene. "The City Council meets to-night," the *Bulletin* announced: "Will they defer such trivial and ephemeral matters . . . to the great and all important consideration of Health? This, and this alone, at this time, if they are true and honest public servants, and faithful to their trusts, should occupy their attention."[28] The council and assistant council, however, did not discuss disease during their last meeting. Instead they bickered over "silly disputes"—including the accusation that one of their own, George Pandelly, was not a white person but a "man of color."[29]

At the meeting's close, the city council president, Dr. S. W. Dalton, avowed to the gallery of scared onlookers that although over 400 people had already died that week, he was "firmly convinced that the disease . . . is not by any means epidemic"—it was just "ship fever."[30] The city council adjourned until October, delegating its powers to a finance committee. For more than a month New Orleans was entirely without a government. J. D. B. De Bow (a. YF 1847), the planter and editor of *De Bow's Review,* wrote in December, "There is, perhaps, not another case on record of the authorities of a modern city" abandoning their constituents "to fly from a pestilence."[31] That year about 12,000 people died in New Orleans—as well as thousands more across the Lower Mississippi Valley—with countless more widowed, orphaned, impoverished, and starved. The government took no action to help them.[32]

Climate Gerrymandering

Such inaction might have been shocking to some, but it had little impact at the ballot box. This was because yellow fever factored heavily into election scheduling. In the decades following the Louisiana Purchase, New Orleans's main political divide was between the white *anciennes* and the new Americans (free people of color were barred from voting in local elections in March of 1805).[33] Wary of losing their influence, the white Creole majority in the newly formed state legislature lobbied in 1812 to set elections for July, precisely because Americans were more likely to be unacclimated and therefore flee the city. In another kind of climate gerrymander, the Creole majority on the city council changed the mayor's term from six months to one year, with elections mandated for the summer—when commerce was in the doldrums and Americans visited family up north. All of these measures were strategies to lessen the power of the American vote. Consequently, eight of the first ten mayors were white Creoles. American-born candidates left or died too frequently in the summer to build and maintain electoral viability.[34]

As time passed and more white Americans moved to Louisiana, New Orleans's political landscape shifted. In 1803 there were seven Creoles to every

American in New Orleans. By 1812 the ratio was three to one, and by 1830 it was two to one. Anglo-Americans had gained in population and power, but they remained frustrated at being subject to vestiges of French and Spanish law, they wanted to direct public funds to expanding the cotton port, and they were horrified by the city's racial fluidity. In 1836 the Creole-American rivalry reached a breaking point and New Orleans disintegrated into three semiautonomous municipalities, an arrangement that persisted for sixteen years. These municipalities—two francophone and one anglophone—shared one mayor but devolved to separate councils the powers for taxing residents and providing municipal services. These three sections corresponded roughly to the French Quarter (First Municipality), the American-dominated Central Business District or St. Mary's (Second), and Marigny (Third).[35]

New Orleans became a white-majority city for the first time in its history in the 1840s due to European immigration. As New Orleans's economy and population swelled, the ethnically driven political battles of the old days dissipated and new ethnically stratified political parties emerged. Broadly speaking, Louisiana Whigs became the party of "the classes": nativist planters, merchants, and bankers—many of them Creole—who felt President Andrew Jackson was using his powers to undermine sugar, an industry that required tariff protections, internal improvements, railroads, and a sound national banking system. Whigs vied against the Democrats, the party of smaller cotton farmers, Protestants, professionals, and naturalized immigrants. Many Democrats took staunch anti-tariff and anti-immigration stances. As immigration increased, so did the force of nativism. And in the 1850s, a major third party known for its intense xenophobia—the Know-Nothings—gained a foothold in Louisiana, especially in New Orleans.[36]

Partisans within this Second Party System took climate gerrymandering to the extreme. During the opening debates of Louisiana's 1845 constitutional convention, "Creole of Creoles" Bernard Marigny, a rare sugar-planting Democrat who would later migrate to the Know-Nothings, identified disease as a potential tool of disenfranchisement: "If you fix the elections in June or July, you place the result of the popular choice at the control of . . . the floating population—those birds of passage, who come to New Orleans for a limited season, and for some temporary purpose, and who are ready to quit at any moment, particularly at the period when yellow fever makes its appearance." Come September, the "birds" had "taken their flight," and the city was reduced to "the actual citizens—to those who have a real and permanent interest in . . . the preservation of our local interests." Marigny submitted that "no good citizen" was afraid of yellow fever: acclimation was "the baptism of citizenship," offering a "guarantee of devotion to the country." German-born Whig Christian Roselius, a lawyer who had come to Louisiana as an indentured worker in 1820, countered that the "political principle of suffrage . . . is inherent in every freeman, and I cannot see how it can be restricted and denied; because a citizen does not choose to incur the risk of contracting yellow fever." Virginia-born Charles Conrad agreed with Roselius and questioned Marigny's motives. Conrad stated that many of the "birds of passage," present in May, were still present in September because they were too poor to flee. Many of them were unacclimated noncitizens who could not vote anyway. Conrad suggested the real motivation behind Marigny's zeal for a September election was to eliminate the growing population of qualified Whig voters—"worthy citizens" who had made New Orleans their genuine "roosting place—who nonetheless lived in fear of yellow fever. Besides, noted Conrad, Marigny was native to Louisiana and had been "exempted by his birth from that baptism" of acclimation. He was, therefore "ignorant of its tortures and its suspenses." Had he known the tortures, Conrad concluded, "I am convinced . . . that he would be the last one to require so awful a proof of good citizenship."[37]

Though silent on how to solve the problem of disease, all parties sought to use epidemics to suppress the vote or somehow turn epidemics into electoral advantage. New Orleans–based Whigs implored "every true whig" in 1840 to "remain in his parish or district *until after the July elections*" to vote in state elections, and "return *before* November next" for the presidential election. Six years later, and shortly before he died from yellow fever, Irish immigrant and former Georgia congressman Richard Henry Wilde said that the scourge abetted "the Loco foco's [radical Democrats'] desire to run off all the Whigs . . . so that they can't be here to vote."[38] As the sun set on the national Whig Party in the summer of 1854, its members in Louisiana desperately tried to set state elections to fill two government vacancies for September—amid an epidemic that killed approximately 3,000 people—though the positions would not be taken up until January 1855. The Democrats, however, lobbied to move the election to October, November, or even December, months with "much pleasanter weather in which to go through the fatigues of a canvas." Additionally, the Democrats argued, the return of absent citizens would give the city a "much fuller voting population," resulting in a "truer reflection of the deliberate preferences of the constituency."[39]

Yellow fever electoral tactics went beyond scheduling, descending into all manner of chicanery. Some years the Democratic machine hired hearses to drive around the city loaded with empty coffins on the eve of an election, insinuating the arrival of an epidemic to scare off the Whigs. In other years Whigs hired men to don mourning bands and tell sad tales in taverns about their dead families to frighten the Democrats. There was also outright fraud. In the election of 1853, votes were cast for the Democrats by 4,000 Irishmen who had recently died from yellow fever, giving the "Demmys" a "tremendous majority" over the Whigs.[40] But when elections were over, "when not another timid vote can be scared away by this phantom of 'yellow jack,'" all political parties and their media instruments dropped the fever question. All returned to proclaiming the "uninterrupted health, and comfort, of our good city of New Orleans."[41]

The State of the City

Though politicians routinely manipulated yellow fever to their electoral advantage, there was bipartisan silence on the reality of sickness. Whigs, the party traditionally most comfortable with government involvement in railroad construction projects and protective tariffs, seldom pushed for public health infrastructure. Democrats, and later the Know-Nothings, actively discouraged it, instead celebrating the fact that yellow fever checked the increasing demographic and political power of the foreign-born.[42] This official silence, along with public health cheapness, was increasingly atypical for American cities. Even in the context of the larger South—a region traditionally less willing to levy taxes to support public services—New Orleans was especially parsimonious. While Charleston allocated 77 cents per person toward poor relief in the 1830s, New Orleans allocated only 22 cents for this purpose, less than half the national average. By the 1850s, New Orleans ranked last among major cities in poor relief (8 cents per person compared with $1.43 in Boston), and lagged seriously behind other cities in public health spending (about 4 cents per person compared with 69 cents in Boston, 23 cents in New York, and 19 cents in Charleston). Almost all funds earmarked for public health were spent cosmetically in the rich residential and commercial districts of the First and Second Municipalities.[43]

All nineteenth-century ports faced health problems due to overcrowding, poverty, and poor sanitation. Crowd diseases like tuberculosis, typhoid, and cholera ripped across Fishtown, Fell's Point, and the Five Points, striking down thousands crammed into water-logged basements and tenements. Reacting to widespread sickness and occasional devastating epidemics, many American cities mounted efforts to curb disease and refined their approaches guided by science. In fact, as historian Charles Rosenberg described, municipalities and states grew "in experience and power" while fighting off disease, and some had even temporarily attained "many of the functions of the twentieth-century government" by the 1830s.[44]

Following the deadly yellow fever epidemic of 1793 and a smaller one in 1797, Philadelphia augmented the power of health officers, installed a municipal waterworks, and greatly improved its quarantine system. During the 1797 yellow fever epidemic in New York, the health committee sanitized the city, erected two large temporary hospitals to care for poor patients, and hired three physicians to make home visits. The municipality cared for over 800 individuals in the Alms House and up to 2,000 each day at three relief centers, supplying the poor with soup, boiled meat, bread, and candles. Five hundred more families were given free food. As soon as yellow fever made its appearance in September 1805, New York's city council authorized the health board to spend $50,000 and gave it absolute authority to evacuate a large section of the city. These measures appear to have worked: aside from the greatly reduced death toll compared to previous epidemics, not one of the sixty physicians who attended the sick died. To promote health more generally, in 1811 New York health authorities filled in the Collect Pond; this once-tranquil water source that had become a cesspool, where the detritus of local slaughterhouses and tallow factories accumulated. And even though many physicians insisted that yellow fever was miasmatic, from 1800 until 1820 New York constantly operated two quarantine stations in New York Harbor for vessels arriving by sea (with spaces designated to isolate obviously sick passengers and for the "airing" of ships), as well as a floating hospital at Staten Island. In 1819, when rumors of fever again circulated, officials urged all ships to leave port and dissuaded New Yorkers from lingering around the docklands. Soon after, they evacuated and barricaded the docks. Only sixty-three cases and thirty-eight deaths from yellow fever were reported in 1819 out of a population of over 120,000— the same year that yellow fever killed between 2,190 and 6,000 people in New Orleans.[45]

Southern city governments also took steps to ameliorate disease, if more cautiously and cheaply than their Northern counterparts. Outbreaks of yellow fever in Baltimore in 1800 galvanized physicians and philanthropists to establish a free clinic for the needy. When yellow fever was rumored in Havana in the spring of 1799, the city council of Charleston (a major trading partner with Cuba) deferred to the separate medical society—not the merchant elite—on how to respond, funding street cleaning, quarantine, and sanitation. In 1802 David Ramsay, a prominent Charleston physician widely known for his two-volume *History of the American Revolution,* published a pamphlet in which he provided mortality statistics for the previous year, tracking who died from what and how often. Probably because of the application of information provided by these public health and data collection efforts, not one case of yellow fever was reported to Charleston's sexton's office between 1807 and 1817, even though the disease raged in the West Indies and in Louisiana.[46]

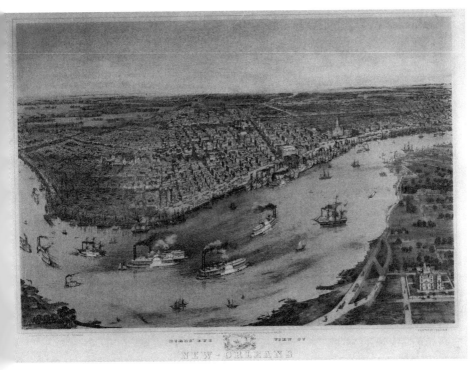

John Bachmann, *Bird's-Eye View of New-Orleans,* lithograph, 1851. The Historic New Orleans Collection, Bequest of Richard Koch.

Public health could scarcely have been worse in New Orleans. Unpaved streets stank with stagnant water, sewage, and rotting animals. Apart from the Ursuline nunnery, the Charity Hospital, and an array of benevolent societies funded through individual almsgiving or bequests (often ethnicity- or religion-specific), there were few resources in the city for poor victims of disease. The board of health seldom acted, making all disease—not just yellow fever—more lethal. Not until the devastating yellow fever epidemic of 1878, with over 20,000 deaths across the Deep South, and the following years of postwar economic depression and stagnant immigration, did "the cupidity of commercial men" wane and a new attitude that "Public Health is Public Wealth" take hold. Only then was government spurred to drain streets and implement quarantine more reliably.[47] But such progress was for a later generation. In the antebellum period, as one health reformer noted in 1844, medical authorities would "immolate hundreds and thousands of victims annually upon the altar of a blind incredulity."[48]

The "Incubus" of Quarantine

New Orleans veered most abruptly away from the national norm in its stubborn rejection of quarantines—installations that stopped and inspected ships, checked the health of sailors, investigated itineraries, and had the power to bar a brig from landing or leaving. Quarantines were a nonstarter in New Orleans, implemented only four brief times during the whole antebellum period. Science, insisted "anti-contagionists" and "miasmaticists" in New Orleans, was on their side. Repeating the claims made by French epidemiologist Nicolas Chervin in 1827—who surveyed 600 physicians about their views of yellow fever's "contagiousness," twenty-seven of them in New Orleans—yellow fever was not contagious and thus could not be imported. Ships carrying cotton and people briskly in and out of port could not carry the contagion, and therefore "lazarets and quarantines . . . neither serve to prevent, nor lessen the violence of the infection." Instead they were "onerous for governments and prejudicial to commerce." By this logic, quarantines only squandered money, hurt businesses, and became vehicles of patronage and corruption; they did not save lives.[49]

Merchants everywhere—from New York to Hamburg to Melbourne—grumbled about quarantines, blunt instruments that disrupted their commerce in the short term and only imperfectly defended against disease.

Whether merchants and planters in New Orleans earnestly believed yellow fever was not contagious is questionable, given that many planters quarantined their own plantations during epidemics, letting no one in but the doctor and nothing out but cotton. Dr. Stephen Duncan, for example, related in 1855 that he was shocked that a man he enslaved was attacked by yellow fever at his plantation in Homochitto and died with black vomit, insisting, "This man had not been off the place for years, and could have had no intercourse with any person or thing likely to communicate yellow fever." Whatever their personal beliefs, merchants and planters understood the expedience of invoking anti-contagionism as a matter of policy. Anti-contagionism allowed white elites to insist on an open port and to pose as the victims of quarantine—of despotic government overreach—when quarantines were implemented, instead of being the reason yellow fever spread needlessly. As physician William Chambers wryly noted in 1862, "Commercial interests are opposed to quarantines." Thus, most businessmen publicly maintained that yellow fever was noncontagious because people believed "what it [was] in their interest to believe."[50]

Many residents of New Orleans, probably a silent majority, believed anti-contagionism was quackery, finding ample evidence for yellow fever's communicability from infected ships, persons, and objects. After all, many residents of New Orleans had come from other places—Boston, Bordeaux, or London—where quarantines had proven at least partially effective against all manner of diseases, including yellow fever. And sometimes these contagionist voices shouted louder, if only for fleeting moments. Louisiana governor Jacques Villeré sent a message to New Orleans's city council in January 1818 as the city recovered from a devastating yellow fever epidemic, declaring that the evidence that yellow fever had been imported in 1817 was conclusive. Villeré recommended a quarantine law.[51] But the city council, endowed with exclusive control over all sanitation matters, ignored him. Conceding that his contagionist beliefs were controversial, Villeré again urged the council and state legislature to impose a quarantine in 1820, arguing that yellow fever must be contagious or it would not have otherwise ravaged those "persons heaped together" in the city prisons. Again he was rebuffed. In December of that year, Villeré's successor, Thomas B. Robertson, urged quarantine upon the council. So did 600 constituents of city councilor and soon-to-be New Orleans mayor Louis Roffignac, who wrote: "Shall we be deaf to their demands . . . and say their fears are ridiculous?"[52]

Not all anti-contagionists were necessarily anti-science or pro-business. Many doctors, for example, reached the conclusion that yellow fever was noncontagious through a rigorous analysis of their patient histories, unable to find legible patterns of disease transmission. But others did see clear evidence of communicability, and some Southern doctors of the contagionist persuasion agreed that any city that did not quarantine was "suicidal."[53] By the 1840s, works by three prominent Southern physicians—John Monette, Benjamin Strobel, and Wesley Carpenter—questioned the truism that yellow fever always originated organically in town. Carpenter alleged that the cost of even "the most expensive quarantine establishment in the world" would "be but trifling" compared with the aggregate costs of "physicians' bills, medicines, and funeral expenses, during an epidemic season."[54] In the *Picayune* in August 1853, a twenty-two-year veteran of New Orleans, writing under the pseudonym "H.," begged the health establishment to see plain facts rather than abstractions. He insisted quarantine had proved successful in New York in 1822 (giving the city "perfect immunity"). Quarantine had also worked in Vicksburg in 1847, allowing its residents to evade yellow fever even as the disease raged to the south along the Mississippi and in New Orleans. H. also noted that every epidemic of yellow fever in New Orleans could be traced to an infected ship from Havana or Rio de Janeiro. Should these facts, H. wrote, not matter?[55]

But New Orleans's authorities refused to speak of quarantine without dire references to an "incubus" or an "extravagant tax upon commerce."[56] The costs of *not* establishing quarantine after all—doctor's bills, medicines, life itself—were incurred by individuals, not industry, and therefore should not factor into any grand accounting. Commerce monopolized newspaper column inches to convince the public of the rightness of their side. One editorialist in 1843 derided New Yorkers, claiming they had "made themselves ridiculous in the eyes of the whole country" by "attempting to revive the long since exploded and obsolete doctrine, that yellow fever is contagious." "New York," the *Picayune* claimed, "persists in remaining a century behind the age." Another editorialist suggested in 1855 that if contagionists in New York could find "a single feeble crutch to support them, they must be more ingenious than the philosopher who extracted sunbeams from cucumbers."[57]

The degree to which even allegedly commercially disinterested professionals like doctors made objections to quarantine—often in highly emotional broadsides—is striking. Samuel Cartwright, one of New Orleans's most famous physicians, argued that it was "safer for the public health to let trade be free than to shackle it [with quarantine]." Dr. M. Morton Dowler went further and insisted that "our commercial interests" *and* "the cause of truth" required "every person whether physician or layman" to denounce contagionism, as "so monstrous a doctrine!" He also ramped up his attacks when it was suggested that a strict quarantine might actually enhance international capitalists' confidence in New Orleans: "There is not, in the whole dictionary, a word suggestive of more fearful associations than this word *confidence,*" Dowler roared. "Let the histories of rotten banks, broken hearts, dishonored virgins—nay, the history of the world bear witness."[58]

Many unacclimated people died because those empowered to implement public health reform clung to anti-contagionism. And not just in New Orleans. Without a quarantine at the mouth of the Mississippi, smaller up-river and Gulf Coast towns were sitting ducks, with every ship from New Orleans shuttling in potentially infected people and mosquitoes. These towns were dependent on New Orleans for trade, culture, and credit, so they had little leverage. The elite of Mobile, who reassured the public that they were "thorough non-contagionists" in 1829, nevertheless timidly asked, "Are our quarantine laws yet in force?" In later years the mayor of Mobile ordered health officers to inspect ships only from New Orleans. Health officials in Natchez even offered to help pay for a New Orleans quarantine after the 1853 epidemic. "As New Orleans exists, lives, and thrives by the Mississippi valley," Dr. Luke Pryor Blackburn stated, "the whole valley will indirectly contribute to the expense of a quarantine in New Orleans." Blackburn—who plotted during the Civil War to assassinate Abraham Lincoln with "infected" yellow fever clothing—insisted that such an expense, would be a "trifle compared with the lives of thousands, the happiness of tens of thousands."[59] Bigger cities farther afield could mount a more muscular response to New Orleans's ineptitude. In 1819, Boston imposed an expensive quarantine only on ships from New Orleans, as did New York, Philadelphia, and Liverpool in later years. Taking no chances, one Mediterranean port quarantined a Boston-based brig in 1834 for forty days because yellow fever was raging in New Orleans; Genoa, Italy, instituted a similar policy in August 1855.[60]

Some New Orleanians quietly worried that their city was squandering goodwill with its flagrant rejection of quarantine, diminishing its reputation and credit abroad. According to Dr. E. H. Barton, it was a fact that "capitalists . . . will not invest permanently where the mortality is double what it is elsewhere." Moreover, New Orleans's middle class of "mechanics, manufacturers, laborers, and others" would eventually give up on this death-trap and leave for more healthful locations—a trend that had already started by the 1850s. Then the dominoes would fall: the "tide of immigration" to Louisiana would be checked, the "confidence of capitalists abroad" would diminish, trade routes would shift away from the mouth of the Mississippi to Charleston or Memphis by railroads, property prices would plummet, and commerce would evaporate. All it would take was one devastating epidemic in another city, traceable to a New Orleans–based ship, to trigger the city's final demise.[61]

In time Barton's prediction would prove remarkably prescient. But for now, merchants and politicians in New Orleans remained resolute in their anti-contagionism. They did not have to change their minds or think about the health of other cities because they held the trump card: cotton. If the rest of the world wanted to finance, move, trade, or purchase it, they would have to deal with New Orleans, and accept its terms.[62] As Canadian visitor William Kingsford mused in 1858, New Orleans merchants' "feeling of geographic strength"—that their physical position on the Mississippi River dictated their future relevance and dominance—meant New Orleans would perpetually be the "great mart of the South West and of Texas." "And so it must remain," Kingsford concluded, warts, yellow fever, and all.[63]

Sanitation

Even though quarantines were too controversial to seriously consider, sanitation schemes like swamp drainage, street cleaning, and garbage removal could find bipartisan support. Such programs were cheaper than quarantine, and sanitarians also genuinely believed that suppressing miasmas and sweetening "foul airs" were crucial to disease prevention. Historian Melanie Kiechle has noted that according to nineteenth-century science, miasmas were the literal cause of illness. If a woman covered her nose while walking past a reeking abattoir or while descending into a dank cellar, this was not just a reflex—it was prophylactic. Visitors to New Orleans made a point of commenting on the city's uncommon filthiness and smelliness, noting that the swamps behind town emitted foul vapors; that the levee was trash-strewn; and that streets were indistinguishable from latrines after a light rainfall. The city's natural low-lying condition—combined with its heat and filth—created dangerous conditions.[64]

Early in the American Period, New Orleans's residents complained that the stench was unbearable—and the city council took steps, albeit small ones, to improve conditions. After several citizens protested in June 1804, for example, that the barges waiting in port were "injurious" to health because of "the putrid miasmes emanating" from "decomposing foodstuffs or . . . the filth of animals on board," the city council resolved that all barges carrying food and animals must unload above Poydras Street (uptown) or below the city's shipyard fronting the French Quarter. Violations would merit a $10 fine. The council also mandated that butchers remove all accumulated "blood, excrements, horns with bits of flesh, in fact all filth" from their shops and throw it into the Mississippi to prevent "very contagious diseases." Officials laced sausage with poison to kill rabid dogs and paid enslaved workmen to remove the canines' carcasses. It also barred soldiers from defecating on the river bank, which had offered "at once a spectacle of the most revolting indecency and nastiness" and also worsened "public health."[65]

But as the city's population swelled, so did the city's abounding filth. This became increasingly hard to ignore, even for those with the most ironclad stomachs.[66] Garbage and sewage were produced much faster than they could be removed. By 1851, Dr. E. H. Barton had estimated that New Orleans's 130,000 residents produced 5,633 tons of sewage and 43,000 tons of urine each year. Animals produced a further 50,000 tons of waste. And if the 3,000 dead bodies interred each year were added to the weight of "organic matter submitted to the putrefactive fermentation," this made for a whopping 150,000 tons of organic waste, within an area of 7.25 square miles. All this organic waste contaminated the purity of the air New Orleanians breathed, poisoned the water they drank, and caused epidemics. British sociologist Harriet Martineau described New Orleans as "peculiarly unhealthy" compared to all the other cities she had visited on her American tour in the 1830s. She was distressed to hear that parents would only let their children play outdoors if the wind was blowing in from Lake Pontchartrain. Otherwise, the air was too dangerous to breathe.[67]

The *Picayune* claimed in the 1850s that all townspeople agreed that "an efficient medical police system of internal sanitary measures" tasked with removing filth was necessary and important. But the arrival of such a system was overdue. New Orleans had no "judicious system of sanitary police"— making it the "only large city in Christendom" without one.[68] City officials, in fact, seldom saw the filth of their constituencies firsthand. On paper,

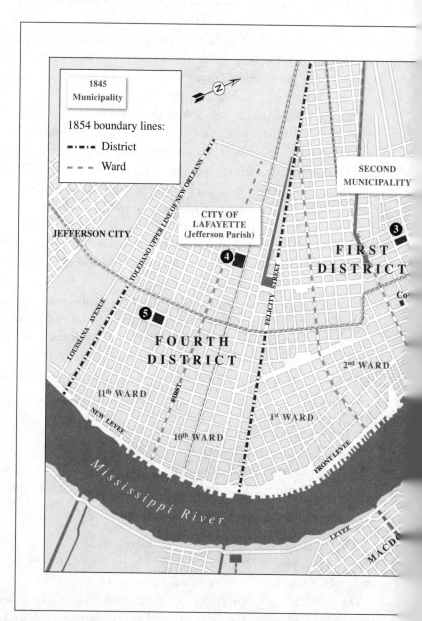

New Orleans, ca. 1855.

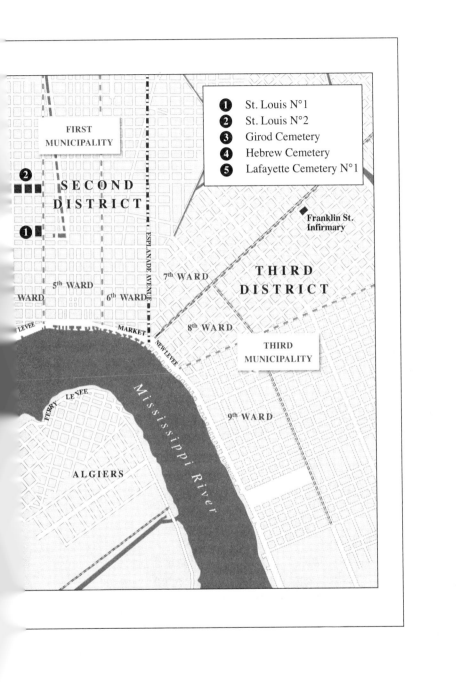

❶	St. Louis N°1
❷	St. Louis N°2
❸	Girod Cemetery
❹	Hebrew Cemetery
❺	Lafayette Cemetery N°1

FIRST
MUNICIPALITY

❷
SECOND
DISTRICT
❶

ESPLANADE AVENUE

5ᵗʰ WARD
6ᵗʰ WARD

WARD

7ᵗʰ WARD

Franklin St.
Infirmary

THIRD
DISTRICT

LEVEE
MARKET
8ᵗʰ WARD

NEW LEVEE

THIRD
MUNICIPALITY

FERRY LEVEE

Mississippi River

9ᵗʰ WARD

ALGIERS

aldermen and police officers were required to own property in the district they represented and walk around their wards twice a month. But most officials seemed to take any residency requirement as a suggestion rather than a mandate.[69] For most of the antebellum period, only about half of the city's aldermen lived in town full-time. Those who were technically permanent residents lived in wealthy neighborhoods in the First and Second Municipalities, even if they represented other city wards. As late as 1854 one physician implored aldermen to walk through their constituencies and see the filth for themselves: "Do not stop at Canal, or St. Charles, or Carondelet streets, where greedy contractors do make some *little* show of performance of duty," but leave the "atmosphere of newspaper politicians and truckling office seekers, and visit the 'back streets,' the abodes of the 'bone and sinew' of our city, on whom in reality depends its prosperity." If politicians took their duties seriously, they would be "fully convinced" that there was much more to be done.[70]

The perception of filth and its dangers correlated strongly with class, race, and geography. In 1849 the *Picayune* noted that "any resident of the First Municipality will tell you" the city "never was healthier." But in the "Third Municipality there is much sickness, and in one ward of the Second there is considerable; but these are notoriously the abodes of the poor upon whom the masses of emigrants are quartered." Indeed, it was well known that disease was always much worse in the "Dirty Third" because it was "most thickly populated by the unacclimated citizens."[71] Traditionally, affluent Creole and long-standing American areas had a much stronger political voice and were consistently cleaner and sweeter smelling.[72] The immigrant-heavy and most-populous Third had only seven aldermen—compared with eight aldermen in the more-affluent Second (Faubourg St. Mary) and twelve aldermen in the richest First (French Quarter)—so this district with more people had less power, before even factoring in the lack of representation provided by many Third Municipality aldermen. This meant the haunts of the elites were drier and smelled better than poor parts of the city. In the French Quarter, petitioners complained about a ditch full of smelly, stagnant water that was "very harmful to our health and very disgusting." This petition was immediately referred to the mayor, and the ditch was drained within a week. In the busy commercial districts populated by cotton and sugar merchants, the city council routinely authorized the mayor to pay to fill potholes, repave streets, expand sidewalks, and reinforce the levee. And in Faubourg St. Mary, the seat of richer American merchants, the council authorized city funds for the repair of cross-bridges at street corners.[73]

The city was conspicuously slow to answer petitions from the Third Municipality (Marigny) and Tremé, where many people were poor, recently immigrated, Black, and unable to vote. Though the mayor promised in 1817 that the ditches of Marigny would be excavated and cleaned by the men of the city workshop (prisoners and chain-gang slaves), the city council overruled him, decreeing that Marigny's inhabitants would have to do this work in front of their own respective properties, or suffer fines. Residents would also be held financially responsible for discarding their own trash and "feculent matter" in the Mississippi. In 1818 the council gave Léandre Lacoste the contract for cleaning Marigny and Tremé. The contract was for just $880 for the entire year, several factors less than the sum awarded to contractors in other parts of town.[74] One writer remarked that even by 1839, the majority of streets in the Third remained unpaved and unsewered, with "the filth and suds from the houses layering, or dragging a lazy course by the sides of the foot-paths." And yet "little or no effort is made to remedy this crying evil." If not the city, one reformer argued, then the "state of Louisiana, might, and ought," to install a proper drainage system, pave the streets, and clean the city, "if it value the lives and safety of its inhabitants."[75]

Frustrated citizens in poorer neighborhoods simply did for themselves whatever sanitation and draining they could manage. Tired of falling into stinking mud puddles, the recent Irish immigrant A. Philipps and his neighbors asked permission of the city council in 1829 to drain one roadway and build a stone crossing using their own labor. The mayor sold them the necessary stones at cost, but charged an importation fee.[76] One unacclimated resident sent "petition after petition" to Mayor Roffignac in 1833 about the condition of the city streets in the Third, promising him a "vote for every re-laid stone." Over the next two decades, over 80,000 feet of New Orleans streets were paved. But the poorest and unhealthiest districts—where the majority of inhabitants were renters, unacclimated, poor, and foreign-born—were last in line for critical upgrades.[77]

Healthy Filth

Some in the commercial-civic elite sought to turn the horrors of poor sanitation, perennial flooding, and government inaction into a positive, arguing that filth was not injurious but salubrious—a benefit to the poor and unacclimated. Making a case for filth, J. S. McFarlane—a North Carolina transplant, surgeon of the city's Marine Hospital, alderman from the First District, and vehement nativist—argued that "filth of every description, no matter how putrid and offensive, could neither create nor aggravate fever of any description"; instead "it was absolutely a retard, of yellow fever, rather than a creator of it." As evidence McFarlane provided statistics he had collected, purporting to indicate that the areas of greatest filth in the Third and Fourth Districts (District replaced Municipalities after the city reunified in 1852), comprising today's Irish Channel, Garden District, and Central City, experienced a relatively low yellow fever rate. Eventually, McFarlane argued, yellow fever would "wear itself out and disappear"— the government could do nothing to expedite its exit. And in the meantime, filth was actually beneficial for it hastened acclimation which *en masse* provided the best public health available. In a city where "acclimated" and "citizen" were inextricably linked, health and filth could also become synonymous.[78]

For some, the filth-is-health approach went beyond the already-stretched bounds of credulity. But as the *Commercial Bulletin* wrote in 1853, the "absurd" dirt-is-healthy theory "suited admirably the city authorities," enabling them in "their gross neglect of all those sanitary regulations and provisions which reason and common sense so clearly indicate." Concluding its chastisement, the *Bulletin* wrote, "The accumulation of filth and putrescent matter in our streets, we are told, is in no wise prejudicial to health; nay more, we are positively assured, that dirty streets are the most healthful localities." If the government could not or would not improve the city's condition, inhabitants would simply have to adapt.[79] It was citizens' job to accommodate the filth, and become healthier thereby, rather than for the authorities to take the sorts of obvious actions to clean the streets that were commonplace elsewhere. Of course, this approach had dire health consequences for new immigrants. The English-born architect Thomas Kelah Wharton noted in his diary in April 1854 that almost 2,000 immigrants had arrived in New Orleans over the previous two days. He worried about what would happen to them as the fever season approached, "with no Quarantine laws—no sanitary arrangements worth a straw—a feeble city government, and inefficient police, and an embarrassed city finance." He concluded, let "the Lord help the unacclimated stranger, and the citizen too—whom business ties here for the summer."[80]

Some reformers sought to reframe the issue in the only language the commercial-civic elite understood—money. Reform-minded physician J. C. Simonds wrote in 1851 that the economic "penalty" wrought by disease "is a costly one." He calculated that 37,785 people of all races died in New Orleans between 1846 and 1849—most of them preventable or excessive deaths. If each of these dead persons represented $400 in capital (he used the average slave price for reference, and perhaps to shock his white audience), Simonds estimated that the "positive loss" to the New Orleans economy amounted to over $15 million. To this, he added the lost interest on that capital; that is, what would have been the value of the dead's future labor. With a collective 4,347,750 days of lost labor, estimated as worth 50 cents per day (what the average unskilled white worker made in 1850), this amounted to a further $17 million loss.[81] When Simonds added the cost of sick care and death, he estimated that the city's total loss between 1846 and 1849 exceeded $45 million. Should New Orleans not, Simonds suggested, spend this money preventatively, on public health? Almost all aldermen and health officers scoffed at such a large sum. But given that many regular townspeople believed what was repeatedly told to them—that yellow fever was caused by miasmas—such official indifference to draining and sanitation was shocking. Some even believed, and not so conspiratorially, that political inaction on health was premeditated: their government was actively failing to prevent disease in some neighborhoods because it willed poor and unacclimated immigrants to die.[82]

Private Funding, Private Institutions

If the government would not prevent sickness, what would they do about sick people? No institution embodied the gross failures of public health in New Orleans more than the Charity Hospital, the place most poor New Orleanians—Black and white—ended up when they fell ill. Over half a million people passed through its doors between 1803 and the Civil War. During the 1830s and 1840s it admitted at least 122,317 patients, many of whom were undoubtedly yellow fever victims, given their nationalities, admission dates, and death rates. This made for an average of about 6,000 people per year.[83] In 1847 alone, 11,890 patients passed through the Charity Hospital, 4,959 of them very recent migrants. By the 1850s the annual admission rate topped 18,000 people. Perennially underfunded, overstretched, and decrepit, the Charity Hospital, one observer claimed, was merely a "nursery for the grave." Another declared it one of the "worst managed establishments of the kind in the world," believing that it "would be a greater charity" to let the poor "die in the streets" than for them to end up there.[84]

Perhaps this was correct.[85] In September 1809, after the hospital's director, J. B. C. Blanquet, refused to take the medical licensing examination, the hospital burned down. Three patients died. Twice the roof fell in, killing multiple "inmates."[86] On the eve of Louisiana statehood, hospital employees had to personally contribute to the endowment to keep patients alive, and Mayor James Mather appealed to Father Sedella, a Catholic priest, to collect money for the hospital during services. Even the new building erected by Henry Boneval Latrobe (d. YF 1817) had little to commend it. Reverend Benjamin Chase, a young Boston minister, said in 1819 that the hospital stood in a swamp, which for several months of the year made it "difficult to walk to it, except on bridges of logs or boards."[87] This "deep disgrace to any civilized or Christian country" was so understaffed that dead, contorted bodies stained in black vomit laid on the floor for days before removal. Dr. Charles Luzenberg, the house surgeon in the 1830s, was credibly accused of stringing up dead yellow fever victims and "shooting at them as marks with pistols." One visitor described the horrific conditions inside: "In one cot was a mother who had just died of the black vomit; in the next cot the daughter," near-dead from fever. Next to her was a woman "raving mad with the black vomit, and lashed down to her cot." Petrified of the hospital, many New Orleanians preferred to keep their deathly ill relatives at home, knowing that if they died there, at least they would not have had to face the horrors of that institution, even temporarily.[88]

No sector of government ever took responsibility for funding the Charity Hospital. In 1811 Mayor James Mather was begging Territorial Governor W. W. C. Claiborne for hospital funds, noting that hundreds of patients arriving at the gates were already in such a "wretched and desperate condition" that they died within hours of their admission. When Claiborne rebuffed him, wanting nothing to do with the hospital, Mather persisted. He asked if it was possible to apply to the US Congress, "or any other branch of the administration," for an annual subsidy, noting that the city covered less than 10 percent of the hospital's budget. Mather also asked the city council for more money but was refused. He then appealed to the governors of Tennessee, Kentucky, Ohio, Virginia, and Pennsylvania for help, on the grounds that "among the Patients admitted into the hospital gratis, the greater proportion were Inhabitants of the Western States and Territories who descend annually to New Orleans."[89] Pennsylvania was the only state to reply, enclosing a donation of $5,000 specifically earmarked for building a wing to the hospital and $500 "solely and exclusively" to fund the "relief of such persons employed in the trade from Pennsylvania, attacked by disease at New Orleans."[90]

Seeking to patch the hospital's budget, the state legislature enacted a law in 1818 stating that the proceeds from any ship illegally smuggling slaves into Louisiana would be split—one half for the commanding officer of the capturing vessel and one half for the treasurer of the Charity Hospital. But securing constant funding from a clandestine industry like slave smuggling proved too uneven. And even the "sales of effects and moneys found on deceased persons" in the hospital did not go far.[91] Thus, by the 1830s the hospital was mostly funded through a constitutionally murky head tax on passengers. A $1 "commutation tax" was levied on all foreigners entering the port of New Orleans in the 1830s and 1840s, raised to $2.50 on each passenger in August 1853.[92] By 1850, $42,342 of the hospital's annual budget of $84,711 came from the passenger tax, followed by state appropriations ($15,000), fees paid by patients ($5,501), fines on gambling establishments ($3,109), and ball licenses ($1,840).[93] Only certain "privileged" people—priests, nuns, and local notables—were allowed free admission to the hospital, and even the family members of patients had to pay 25 cents in "gate money" to gain entrance. Scrambling, the city council levied a tax on entertainment venues in 1856 to raise more necessary funds for the hospital. But theaters complained that the Charity Hospital tax levied on them—$500 per year—was unreasonable, especially considering that the New Orleans theater season was only five or six months compared with twelve in New York. Theaters, of course, were shuttered during the fever season.[94]

A Safety Net with Many Holes

When asked to do more for public health, city politicians always cried poverty; that they could not spend money they did not have. City finances were indeed a "gaping abyss" for large parts of the antebellum period, mostly because the municipality taxed its richest citizens—themselves—lightly. Most nineteenth-century cities raised funds through property taxes on both movable and immovable assets (generally real estate and slaves). But from

1803 until the Civil War, New Orleans had the lowest city property tax rate in the nation (20 cents per $100), far below the rates in Boston (82 cents per $100) and Baltimore (75 cents per $100). In 1820 the city raised only 9.6 percent of its revenue from property taxes (St. Louis, conversely, raised 85.3 percent of its revenue in this manner) and a scant $7,025 total in 1830.[95] By 1856 the state of Louisiana raised $2,223,869 in tax revenue through various avenues, but most of this money was earmarked for the sinking fund (funds periodically set aside to replace wasting assets) and federal debt repayment. Just 2 percent of state expenses—$46,500—was earmarked to fund drainage in New Orleans, port sanitation, tend to the sick, and care for all the state's orphans, widows, and foundlings. Only a small portion of this sum was given to the Charity Hospital.[96]

Tax-averse and without modern borrowing capabilities because they did not have sufficient creditworthiness, the city corporation took on loans from banks, private corporations, individuals, and sometimes Northern cities to fund municipal activities. Often they asked for "donations." When the Charity Hospital burned down in 1809, Julien Poydras donated $35,000 to rebuild it. Sugar planters and slave owners Étienne de Boré and R. Caune also gave large sums. The following year the city council asked Bernard Marigny, another powerful planter and enslaver, to provide the city with an interest-free loan of $2,226 to pay sanitation and levee-repair contractors in 1810.[97] But by 1822 the mayor begged the city council to stop spending money it did not have, noting that "at least one fifteenth of the promulgated revenues are annually set apart to assist about one-hundredth only of the population." Meanwhile, the city "remains forced to pay discounts and interest to her creditors—her treasury is empty; the obligations are pressing." The city struggled to find lenders, and the loans they did secure were expensive. In the 1820s, Vincent Nolte and Barings loaned New Orleans $300,000 for internal improvements at 7 percent interest per annum—borrowing at a higher interest rate than other cities. But New Orleans was riskier, and it desperately needed money to pave its roads in the busy commercial districts. Nolte was delighted to make $65,000 on this deal. Barings also did well, and made subsequent loans to New Orleans at high interest rates over the next decade. Though $300,000 was a lot of money, New Orleans was in such disarray that townspeople barely noticed the "improvements." As one Barings agent in New Orleans told the London office in 1830, "much yet remains to be done for the health and embellishment of the place."[98]

With politicians intent on avoiding (or exploiting) the yellow fever problem, private citizens stepped in to ameliorate the disease's worst social effects—though never at the level required. New Orleans was internationally famous for its charity, with its safety net—protections for the "deserving" unacclimated, sick, and widowed—constructed and financed almost entirely by private and professional associations, foreign consulates, and especially the Catholic Church. In 1841 the Howard Association, the Dames de Providence, the Samaritans, and the Firemen's Charitable Association collectively expended $15,151 to help "our distressed unacclimated brethren."[99] Recorder Baldwin noted that his office was overflowing with gifts from charitable citizens for orphan children, including "hams, flour, beans, corn, maccaroni, potatoes, bread . . . and in no small quantities." Thousands in the "Can't-Get-Away Club"—acclimated people compelled to stay in town—volunteered for the Howard Association and other caregiving charities in 1853.[100] A large number of Black-run benevolent societies arose to cater to the needs of Black sick, dying, and dead people barred from white charitable institutions. Two Black nuns in New Orleans, Henriette Dilille and Juliette Gaudin, opened a religious school to care for urban and indigent slaves suffering from yellow fever. They also went to neighboring plantations to care for sick slaves.[101]

Beyond small cash and in-kind donations, private citizens founded institutions across the Yellow Fever South that were designed to ameliorate mass mortality. Reacting to several documented cases of poor orphan girls being sexually assaulted when their mothers died of yellow fever, in 1816 seventy-four wealthy women of Natchez formed the Female Charity Society to "give instruction to the poor children." At the discretion of the subscribers, any surplus could be applied to poor widows in "extreme distress," but only to "those of reputable character." Women like Ann Seip (the wife of Dr. Frederic Seip, the first president of Natchez's board of health) and Catharine Minor (the daughter of Stephen Minor, one of the region's wealthiest planters) paid annual subscriptions of $10 to $20. Amassing an endowment of $670, the Natchez Academy opened in April with ten children, a teacher, and a matron for the orphans boarding with local families.[102]

The Catholic Church took particular charge of yellow fever orphans—as it traditionally did in Havana and Mexico City, and across the Spanish Americas. Between 1830 and 1850, it opened several asylums for Catholic youth. These children stayed for two to four years, were taught skills like sewing, and then were turned out to look for work.[103] Black Catholics endowed an alternate tapestry of institutions designed to aid needy Black people; many of these institutions were run by the Sisters of the Holy Family. These organizations included the Colored Female Benevolent Society of Louisiana, the Union Band Society, the Benevolent Association of the Veterans of 1815, Thomy Lafon's Asylum for Orphan Boys, and Armand Lanusse's La Société Catholique pour l'Instruction des Orphelins dans l'Indigence.[104]

Noblesse Oblige

Across the Cotton Kingdom, however, the largest and most ostentatious charitable contributions came from elite businessmen who used honorific displays of wealth to assert their social dominance. Upon his death in 1824, Julian Poydras, a Saint-Domingue native and pious Catholic, bequeathed over $100,000 to charity. This man who had been a sugar planter, slave owner, and former president of the Louisiana Senate directed $60,000 toward the "Marriage Portions" of poor orphan girls, an endowment for the Poydras Orphan Asylum (an institution filled with yellow fever orphans), and more property for the Charity Hospital (host to the majority of yellow fever patients). Nationwide, Americans lauded his generosity: "Like the Pyramids of Egypt," one New Yorker opined, Poydras's donations "stand as lasting monuments of his renown." Saved from a life of squalor, immorality, and death, "thousands of female orphans, as yet unborn, will bless the name of POYDRAS!"[105]

Philanthropy gave certain elites incredible power and privilege. Public education in New Orleans was funded almost entirely through one private donor, a devout Protestant named John McDonogh. McDonogh was a real estate speculator notorious for his miserly and litigious manner. He was obsessed with his land holdings and bored all those around him with endless chatter about his 1,600 properties in New Orleans. McDonogh was effectively a slumlord: he rented to the poor, seldom improved his buildings, and was known for renting houses to prostitutes in wealthy neighborhoods to drive down property prices—only to buy up surrounding property at a reduced price. In true Croesus form, as novelist Baron Ludwig von Reizenstein put it, this "philanthropist" McDonogh also paid very little tax on his vast property empire, working out a deal with the Democrats on the city council—he had been a city councilor himself—that allowed him to pay only half of his tax burden in the 1840s. And from his position of power, McDonogh successfully fought against city and state ordinances intended to raise funds for railroads, which he believed would depress the value of his land and increase his tax burden. Instead, he agreed to purchase 116 municipal bonds in the late 1830s, worth $1,000 each.[106]

Upon his death in 1851, McDonogh was rumored to be the largest private landowner in the country, his wealth estimated at 0.07 percent of the entire US gross national product. Vincent Nolte even speculated that McDonogh owned four-fifths of all uncultivated land in Louisiana.[107] McDonogh did not quite possess riches at this mythological scale, but he was incredibly wealthy, and he left the bulk of his cash fortune—about $2 million—to the cities of Baltimore and New Orleans for the purpose of constructing about thirty public schools for poor children. This was both unprecedented and controversial, and more complicated because he died without heirs—the only relation he had was a brother, a steamboat pilot, who had died from yellow fever years before. The executors contested the will, and the case went all the way to the US Supreme Court. It took eight years for New Orleans to receive the $700,000 McDonogh had bequeathed to the city. There was a catch, however: if New Orleans accepted this windfall, "an immense expenditure, which would otherways have come out of its coffers," McDonogh demanded in his will that all of his donated property in New Orleans remain "exempted forever by Law, from all Taxation."[108] Such was the power of the richest capitalists. They could control the function of government even after death.

Private philanthropy, altruistic though it could be, was not a sufficient replacement for government support. And it made individuals like Poydras, McDonogh, Beverly Chew, Nicholas Girod, and Judah Touro—those with their names on schools, orphanages, asylums, and hospitals—into gatekeepers, the ultimate authorities on who was deserving, who could access welfare, and on what terms: mostly young girls, and decidedly not their "filthy" immigrant parents. The *Picayune* lamented in 1860, "Is it not the duty [of the citizenry] to aid in the benefaction demanded by the fatherless, the orphan, and the sick stranger found in our commercial capital?" The potent combination of rampant disease and government inaction compounded society's asymmetrical status quo. Acclimated elites gained extra social capital through honorific displays of charity, often while deriding the efficacy of quarantines, refusing to pay tax, or actively lying about the region's salubrity in anonymous editorials. Meanwhile, the unacclimated poor came to rely on this privatized patchwork system of charity for their survival. Most people quickly accepted New Orleans's harsh reality: public health was private acclimation.[109]

Lopsided and arbitrary philanthropy had other social costs. White and Black people who fell outside the categories that private philanthropists delineated were forced to undergo the humiliating process of begging the city council for assistance. After waiting in the council's anteroom for hours, dole-seekers were obliged to present a petition declaring their state of poverty certified by at least three trustworthy persons and have their names appear in the official record. The vast majority of "city charity" recipients were women. One typical city charity roll read: "a sum of twenty-five dollars in one payment is granted . . . [to] Widow Baquet, Widow Dumonbrin and Widow Pierre Gonzales" and "a sum of fifteen dollars in a lump sum is likewise granted . . . [to] Widow Astin and Widow Ste. Ménière."[110] Another widow appealed to the council on behalf of herself and her four young children. Four witnesses testified that she earned what she could "by her needle" but circumstances often forced her to accept charity. The council granted her $10, with no promise of continuance. In 1815 Widow Bayon asked the city council to "ameliorate her sad and miserable situation as well as that of her large family." The council gave her one lump sum of $50, mindful not to set a "precedent for the future." Widow Crussol begged for financial assistance from the council to allow her, considering her "penniless condition," to continue to care for a white foundling child who had been left on her doorstep.[111] In 1857 the city council maintained that any help to orphans and foundlings should be supported "at the lowest possible price" to the city. This simply codified long-standing practice, as most grants from the government to the poor appear to have been one-time only. Given the feeble subsidies available and the absence of good job opportunities for women, it is not surprising that prostitution in the city was rife, with many women and girls "notoriously abandoned to lewdness."[112]

Keeping the City Afloat

Health reformers understood that official cheapness on public health came at a social cost. Dr. J. C. Simonds argued in the 1850s, "The cost of the Charity Hospital alone, during eight years (1842–'49) has amounted to nearly half a million of dollars. The cost of your Orphan Asylums I do not know—but it must be enormous." Not only was the cost of the police system also high, Simonds added, but "who can tell how much of the crime has been due to the poverty caused by sickness and death, widowhood and orphanage, and the want of parental control and education." Moreover, the "number of beggars upon your streets has, of late, increased to such a degree as to have become a public nuisance." But many politicians, looking at their cash-strapped coffers, with no sales or income tax to rely on, did not see this social chaos as a problem that needed fixing. This was because New Orleans effectively had one asset that no other city had, or at least that no other city was willing to exploit quite as ruthlessly: a large population of politically impotent, predominantly immigrant, disproportionately poor, *unacclimated* people. Through a complex system of professional licensing fees, head taxes on arriving passengers, arbitrary fines, and stealth taxes, this population came to be the source of much of the city's revenue in one way or another.[113]

In this system, what funding the city did enjoy—specifically "auxiliary" expenses like the Charity Hospital and city cleaning—came disproportionately from those least able to afford it and those most vulnerable to disease. Until the Civil War, residents of the immigrant-heavy Third District paid substantially more in tax, on average, than residents of the First and Second paid.[114] Politicians aided and abetted this system, even bragging about it on the campaign trail, calling the unacclimated "worthless," "dissipated," and "vile." Politicians knew this epidemiological shakedown would cost them nothing politically: many of those "worthless" residents would shortly be dead and quickly replaced. And while those residents were still alive, the commercial-civic elite sought to fully capitalize on the nonimmune who were politically impotent or too distracted by everyday difficulties to protest.[115]

The ever-shifting tax code suggests just how much the burden of financing the city and port fell on the lower classes. Complaining at the state constitutional convention in 1845 about the "partiality" of Louisiana's system of taxation, slave owners successfully lobbied for a simplified tax code with "uniformity clauses." Thereafter, real estate was taxed at an *ad valorem* rate—that is, "according to value" at the time of transaction, like a stamp duty or value-added tax—and it became illegal to tax chattel more than other kinds of assets.[116] In 1856 the *ad valorem* rate was set at $1.67 per $1,000 on the "full cash value" of real estate (land, lots, buildings, improvements, and machinery), slaves (valued at low, flat rates), animals, carriages, ships, corporate stock, and capital invested in "any kind of commerce."

With the general rate set so low, this effectively reduced the tax burden of large property owners and slaveholders in Louisiana relative to other states where tax rates increased in proportion to wealth. A typical Louisiana planter who owned a townhouse in the First District and a plantation worked by twenty slaves, for example, paid only about $20 in taxes per annum. In contrast, a New Yorker of similar wealth and social class to that Louisiana planter paid nearly ten times as much in taxes, or $15.05 per $1,000 on property.[117] Slaveholders—who were skilled tax evaders in any case—claimed the flat tax rate system was fairer and more practical than scaled rates based on wealth, as flat rates were easier to assess and collect. But the uniformity clauses did not create a uniform burden on all residents. In effect, the average person in the Third District paid much higher "consolidated" rates than the average person in the richer First—up to 33 percent more. After 1856 the comptroller stopped disaggregating tax data by district, perhaps because the gap was so glaring.[118]

New Orleans routinely introduced new licensing fees specifically targeted at working-class laborers and professionals, and at occupations predominantly held by recent immigrants. By the 1850s a peddler on horseback paid a $25 licensing fee, plus a tax on his horse and inventory (capital invested in commerce). Coffeehouse operators paid $100 for a license, plus a tax on urban real estate. Insurance agents paid a $500 fee; out-of-state agents paid $1,000; liquor retailers and wine houses paid $100; money brokers, pawnbrokers, and racetrack managers paid $100; brewers paid $20; lawyers, notaries, doctors, dentists, and druggists paid $10.[119] Anyone who could not produce his or her license immediately to a tax assessor or police officer was fined $2 to $5 per offense. Certain industries were hit harder than others. Coffeehouse proprietors, for example, were collectively charged $362,000 in licensing fees between 1836 and 1851, whereas merchants contributed less than $23,000 to the city coffers in the same period.[120] Licensing fees, mostly levied on the working classes, amounted to $965,519 in 1853 and $1,192,328 in 1854. In comparison, the city raised only one-fourth as much in property tax.[121]

Though other American cities also used licenses to raise revenue, New Orleans took this system to the extreme, licensing just about everything it could outside of cotton and banking. With just over $41,000 in the city treasury in 1858–1859, the city council passed a resolution to "appoint an assistant whose especial duty it shall be to ferret out all persons who sell goods by sample in this city" and exact fees. Commissioners were incentivized to seek out as many people as possible by being paid 10 percent of all sums collected instead of a regular salary. Most licensing fees were shifted onto consumers, making the costs of goods, services, and rents reportedly more expensive in New Orleans than in any other American city. Indeed, workers experienced a 100 percent increase in their rents during the 1850s.[122]

Peccadillos

New Orleans also criminalized a whole host of activities associated with destitution. Laws were drawn up to entrench a system whereby extracting money or labor from the replaceable unacclimated became self-reproducing, perpetual, and ostensibly blameless. Though J. Livingston, the city attorney, stated in 1854 that "it never was contemplated that the city should make money out of fines and penalties," by the 1850s the city's laws appear to have been *explicitly* designed for this purpose. New Orleans had one of the highest crime rates in the United States during the antebellum period. But it also had a much higher rate of arrest.[123] Police arrested 25,417 people in New Orleans in 1858 (population ca. 160,000). That same year, the police arrested 21,537 in Philadelphia, a much larger city (population ca. 500,000).[124] Crimes were liberally defined. Most fines were levied for non-violent, even trivial offenses popularly referred to by locals as "peccadillos." For example, any person entering a theater without a ticket was fined between $5 and $15. Any person who kept his hat on after the rise of the curtain was fined $50. Any Black person sitting in a white person's seat was fined. Anyone selling underweight bread was fined $25 to $100. In 1852 recent immigrant Thomas Clark was arrested and fined in the Third for "having no place of abode," after being discovered sleeping under the platform of the Pontchartrain Railroad depot.[125] N. J. Hackney was fined for "using obscene language on St. Charles street, and behaving in a disreputable manner." New Orleanians paid hefty fines for small offenses like "disturbing the peace," trespassing, pickpocketing, resisting arrest, public drunkenness, gambling, and petty theft. Drunks, particularly in the fever season, were municipal windfalls. For example, Martin Connolly was fined $10 in 1858 for "disturbing parties sick of yellow fever" by singing loudly while intoxicated.[126] Daniel Sotteland and Jacob Jacobs were both fined $10 for "trying the speed of their nags while under a superabundance of whiskey." Persons who could not pay the fines, or post a $100 bond to guarantee good behavior, ended up in the workhouse—or if they were enslaved, they were whipped.[127]

Recorders elected from each municipality were tasked with keeping legal records as well as raising city revenue. In the 1840s and 1850s Summers, Long, Seuzeneau, Ramos, Adams, and Wiltz raised thousands of dollars per month for the municipality, sometimes hundreds of dollars each in a single day, from small fines. Acknowledging the recorders' (and the city's) dependence on fines, the *Picayune* joked during the 1841 epidemic that "the city police magistrates have quite a sinecure of it now. Yellow Jack has driven off blacklegs and burglars, ropers-in and rowdies, pickpockets and their 'pals.'" Recorders competed to bring in the most revenue. It was noted in December 1858 that First District recorder Henry Summers—the future mayor—added to the city treasury, "as the result of fines for small peccadillos, the snug little sum of $1810.65." This was "nearly equal to that collected from all the other districts." Recorders were incentivized to collect revenue through fines rather than imprison offenders. They therefore tended to set fines in the range of $10 or $20, high enough to raise real money for the city, but low enough that a person could actually pay.[128]

Regulations changed so frequently and arbitrarily that it became nearly impossible to follow the law. In 1816 a new tax was levied on two- and four-wheel carts "for the profit of the city." Those who did not immediately take out a license were fined $10 on the spot.[129] In 1817 it became illegal to put human waste on street-cleaning carts. Thus, women had to carry detritus from their houses to the Mississippi River to dump it, which for some was a precarious journey of more than a mile. If anything spilled on this journey, they were fined. Another ordinance dictated that toilet trenches had to be emptied when they reached to a foot below the brim. But this operation could only take place in darkness, starting one hour after curfew—between the hours of 11 p.m. and 3 a.m. Offenders were fined $10 per offense, though many were unsure exactly which aspect of the law they were guilty of, since they could not abide by one rule without violating the other. New ordinances were posted on a weekly basis outside the Cabildo, but only in French and English. A series of recently immigrated German women were fined between $1 and $3 on one day in 1855 when they failed to comply with a new law stating that all sidewalks abutting property were to be swept daily before 10 a.m., and all galleries "watered" before 6 p.m. When they protested that they were unaware of the new law, they were fined a further dollar a piece for disturbing the peace.[130]

Prostituted women—a sizable portion of them yellow fever widows—were hit hard by ever-changing laws and arbitrary fines. At times prostitution was legal under the "Lorette Law"; at others, it was illegal. And this could change in an instant, block by block. Small-scale bordellos (places policemen and politicians regularly patronized themselves) were routinely targeted by raids and were forced to pay an annual $250 license. Recorder Seuzeneau commented in a campaign speech that such action against small brothels generated revenue for the Charity Hospital, and that licensing fees from "dance halls"—rented out by larger brothels—made even more money for the city.[131]

In 1853 two "vagrant white women" were fined $3 for "being caught coming out of a drinking shop in Phillippa street," an area notorious for prostitution. In 1856 Lucy Schaffer, Emeline Sheppard, Mary Wilson, Annetti Martinas, Margaret Hanaw, Bridget Malony, and Jane Boyle—all women who had been in the city for less than two years—paid a fine of $10 each for "leading disreputable lives on Dryades and Perdido streets." In February 1857, twenty-four women were arrested on Gravier Street for "leading lives of lewdness." The "poor things," representing "all degrees of female degradation," were fined $20 each or required to spend "thrice twenty days in the Workhouse." Even when prostitution was technically legal—a city decree in March 1857 allowed prostitution in some areas—prostitutes were still vulnerable to arrest and fines, only their crimes were rebranded. In August 1857, Jane Boyle, an Irishwoman charged in 1856, was rearrested on Perdido Street along with Mary Williams, Mary Johnson, Kate Lyons, and Mike Golden (their pimp or *maquerelle*) for "creating a general disturbance of the peace and for being vagrants in the worst sense of that term." Each paid a fine of $10.[132]

These fines were often unpayable. Consequently, prostitutes were "sent down" to the workhouse, where they made rope for use in the port, or otherwise generated revenue destined for city coffers. On a single day during the epidemic of 1858, Elizabeth McCarty and Margaret Dailey, unable to afford the fine for prostitution, were sent to the workhouse—kicking and screaming—for six months for "being drunk and disturbing the peace" on Dryades Street; Elizabeth Henderson of Perdido, a "habitually drunken vagrant and street walker," was also sent to the workhouse for six months; Mary Summers, another "drunken vagrant" from Basin Street, was sent down for three months. Susan Wilkes, a "drunken brawler" was also sent down for a month, with Recorder Summers noting that her residence on St. Paul Street was known for its "misery, filth, and degradation." Her living conditions might have been "disgusting in the extreme," but the workhouse was worse.[133] It was a dangerous, disease-ridden space where prisoners were chained together, heads shaven, and dressed in red caps and trousers. Many investigations found that prisoners were confined, naked, in damp cold cells. In 1829 multiple convicts in the workhouse fell sick and died, and during epidemic years, between 20 and 50 percent of inmates could die from yellow fever, evidence that this population was largely new to the region and unacclimated. Violence was common—and many women doubtlessly faced sexual violence behind bars. Making matters worse, once arrested for prostitution, a woman was permanently barred from receiving public charity, trapping her in an endless cycle of poverty and crime.[134]

State and Citizen

In 1850 commissioners for the sanitary survey of Massachusetts articulated a modern, holistic approach to welfare: either a city paid now or it paid more later. "Debility, sickness, and premature death, are expensive matters," the commissioners wrote, "inseparably connected with pauperism." These problems must be paid for "directly or indirectly," and a "town in which life is precarious pays more taxes than its neighbors of a different sanitary character."[135] In New Orleans, city wisdom held precisely the opposite: that poverty brought on disease, not that disease brought on poverty. The white poor would have to accept their filthy living circumstances, get acclimated, and join the economic climb with no help from government, which appeared determined through inaction to let as few immigrants as possible break through the immunity threshold. Making matters worse, during their period of unacclimated limbo the immigrant and poor were considered fair game for police officers and judges, who sought to squeeze as much money out of them as possible before they either died or experienced a New Orleans rebirth as acclimated citizens with a political voice. And despite overwhelming evidence that public health measures were effective against yellow fever in other cities, New Orleans's leaders righteously insisted that those examples did not apply. Immunocapitalism, after all, worked for those whites who survived.

5

Denial, Delusion, and Disunion

With astounding hubris, the editors of the *New Orleans Medical and Surgical Journal* declared in November 1852 that yellow fever could soon be "numbered among the diseases that have passed and gone." Five officially epidemic-free years had elapsed, seeming to prove that the city's negligible public health interventions—a partial draining of the swamps behind town and some street paving—had staved off terrible outbreaks, which in turn justified not doing more. Now, the editors concluded, Louisiana could rejoice in a "corresponding augmentation in our wealth, character and standing as a community," confident that "the time is not remote, if it be not already at hand, when the existence" of yellow fever "will be known only in the recollection of the older inhabitants." It was true that by the spring of 1853, many of New Orleans's 120,000 residents knew of epidemic yellow fever only by reputation. About 57 percent of the population was foreign-born, and a midcentury spike in European and enslaved migration meant that at least a third of the city's inhabitants were unacclimated. A majority of these people had been in New Orleans for fewer than five years and had seen only summers with sporadic cases. But others remembered epidemic times and doubted the rosy talk of the city's breathless boosters, even if that was impolitic to express publicly. Gagging at the garbage-laden streets, hopscotching around pools of green stagnant water, and watching dilapidated shacks pop up across the Third and Fourth Districts, residents had good reason to worry that yellow fever would return.[1]

Enter patient zero. On May 6, 1853, a twenty-seven-year-old German man named Johanes Kein hobbled into the private practice of Dr. Bennet Dowler. Four days later he was dead after spewing black vomit. Kein's wife died five days after that. Dowler remembered little about the Keins—he lost his memorandum book that summer—beyond that they were poor and lived in a "*very filthy*" quarter of the city with many soap factories, and that yellow fever had killed them. This was two full months earlier than yellow fever normally appeared, however, so on the official death certificates Dowler ascribed their deaths to "bilious malignant fever." He did not wish to "create alarm" so uncommonly early in the summer.[2]

Two weeks later, a German sailor unloading the ship *Augusta* from Bremen fell to his knees on the levee, complaining of severe body aches and fever. Dr. Martin Schuppert noted only that the patient recovered, and that the *Augusta* had been on the same tow up the Mississippi as *Camboden Castle*, recently of Jamaica. On May 26, nuns at the Charity Hospital found a burning-hot twenty-six-year-old Irishman named James McGuigan outside the gates. He collapsed in the arms of his friends, his shirt soaked with rainwater and black vomit. McGuigan died two days later. Then Dr. Schuppert was once again summoned to the *Augusta* to tend to the delirious John Haar, a ship cook. Haar died bright yellow on May 30. That same day, another hallucinating sailor on the *Augusta,* twenty-five-year-old Gerhardt Woetle from Oldenburg, appeared at the Charity Hospital. A postmortem autopsy revealed that Woetle had "two ounces of the black vomit" in his stomach.[3]

By early June, yellow fever had struck every corner of the city, especially the "crowded and filthy tenements" and the docklands fronting the Mississippi. A laborer got it here; a butcher died from it there; a stevedore was buried, and then his wife and children soon after; one clerk at Circus Street Infirmary shook with delirium, then a whole factorage fell sick; every tenant in a boardinghouse was carted off to the Charity Hospital. Exodus ensued. Enslaved porters readied their masters' carriages to spirit them away. Feverish foot passengers, children and baggage in hand, bribed steamboat captains to let them aboard any outbound ship.[4] Then the usual rumors of opportunistic slave revolt arose with unusual force. From local papers, New Orleanians learned that a white, Jamaican-born schoolteacher named James Dyson was organizing enslaved men and disgruntled whites to rise up in every quarter of the city. Billowing smoke, apparently, would be a signal to the 2,500 slaves on surrounding plantations, along with free Black and

Cuban compatriots, to attack. Dyson was arrested, and Mayor Abdiel Crossman asked army units to stand at the ready to quell civil unrest. Police ramped up surveillance, and slave patrols were told to arrest all Black people and white strangers found on the streets at "unseasonable hours."[5]

By mid-June, hundreds of weak and feverish people were arriving at the Charity Hospital each day, crowding the wards and corridors past capacity. And yet newspapers remained silent, wary of printing reports that would give the "wrong impression" of New Orleans both "here and abroad" and "entail severe loss on merchants and shop-keepers."[6] On June 22 (a day with twenty-four confirmed yellow fever deaths), the *Crescent* crowed that "yellow fever has become an obselete [*sic*] idea in New Orleans" and encouraged all absentees to return immediately; on June 23 (a day with twenty-six confirmed yellow fever deaths), the *Picayune* proclaimed that the danger "does not exist," brushing aside all epidemic talk as "Madam Rumor" raising false alarm. The press remained quiet even after two editors at the *Picayune,* one editor at the *Delta,* and one editor at the *Crescent,* died.[7] Doctors also conspired to downplay the epidemic, saying it was "*too early in the season*" for yellow fever, that patients with textbook cases were "*too yellow*" or that their yellowness was "*not exactly of the right hue.*" Others said that what was "pronounced *black vomit*" was too red, or too dark, or "*too black.*" Only when a twenty-two-year-old Irish servant named Margaret Russell turned bright yellow and threw up a considerable amount of "*unmistakable, old fashioned, coffee-grounds black vomit*" did doctors admit the obvious—yellow fever was back with a vengeance.[8]

The problem was now too big to control and too widespread to cover up. As usual, the city government adjourned for the summer in late July without appropriating any funds for health care or constituting a board of health—an abdication of duty one critic called a "burlesque on municipal government."[9] Mayor Abdiel Crossman, a Whig who had campaigned on a promise of sanitation, failed to summon the aldermen back. The sick, dying, and widowed still in town were left to the care of private charities—particularly the Howard Association, which spent over $150,000 in three months on medicines for the poor, nurses' fees, and doctor reimbursements. The Howards also established three orphan asylums for the 241 children and ninety-one nursing infants "left totally destitute" by the deaths of both parents from yellow fever. Cemeteries could not handle the influx of so many dead bodies. Corpses, bloating and stinking, piled up outside graveyard gates until workmen—paid an extraordinary $5 an hour—shoveled them onto carts and threw them into trenches, covering the dead with lime to hasten decomposition.[10]

News spread across the country about the calamity unfolding in New Orleans. Obituaries for victims of the "prevailing epidemic" dotted every domestic newspaper; vivid hospital scenes were rendered for European readers; the Glasgow papers called New Orleans "the most vicious and reckless city in America," lamenting those "poor wretches" who died amid "bacchanalian orgies" of disease.[11] Charity concerts, fundraisers, and food drives were staged in New York and Boston to aid Louisiana's "distressed unacclimated." New Yorkers sent more than $20,000 to New Orleans; Philadelphians more than $11,000. Irish immigrants in San Francisco—many of whom had passed through New Orleans on their journeys to California's gold fields—raised $12,000. Mayor Crossman even received a check for $1,000 from the citizens of Wheeling, Virginia, population 12,000. The Howard-backed "due-bills" or *bons*—tickets exchangeable for ice or beef—circulated as currency around the city.[12]

By August, 1,000 people were dying each week from yellow fever. As one volunteer for the Howards described it, "The whole city was a hospital," the streets deserted except for "the hasty pedestrian on an errand of mercy" and the body carters yelling "Bring out your dead!" Religious leaders preached that the epidemic was divine punishment. After Sunday, August 21—the so-called "black day" when over 300 people died—the bishop of the Episcopal Diocese of Louisiana, Leonidas Polk, declared a fast day. He prepared a special prayer asking God to "turn from us the ravage of the pestilence, wherewith for our iniquities, thou art now visiting us." Unitarian minister Theodore Clapp suggested that the unusual virulence of the epidemic was a clear "display of God's anger." But Clapp insisted God would look kindly upon New Orleans again; that in spite of the pestilence, "there is as much of God's love in New Orleans to-day as there ever was *before,* or ever will be *hereafter.*"[13]

Though old-timers said that "the fever will fail for want of food" by September, the epidemic had still not abated. City authorities still considered it too dangerous to reopen schools. With no customers, most businesses remained shuttered. "Nothing can be had here for love or money" wrote Mary Copes, the wife of a cotton merchant and insurance agent, in mid-September. With "nothing in market to eat and nothing brought from the country," she was anxious about the epidemic's long-term economic consequences. "This fearful epidemic will be so disastrous to the prosperity of

N. Orleans," worried Copes, "that it will take several years for her to recover from it, even if it should be healthy for several successive years."[14]

The Aftermath

Unseasonably early frosts in mid-October finally brought the epidemic to
a close. In five months, approximately 30,000 people had sickened with
yellow fever and 12,000—about 10 percent of the city's population—had
died. As always, the epidemic took a staggering toll on particular groups: at
least 3,500 people from Ireland (one-fifth of the city's Irish-born population) perished. As Dr. Dowler, a longtime fever watcher, put it, "The blood-
iest battle-fields of modern times scarcely can compare with the New Orleans epidemic of 1853, which destroyed five times more than the British
Army lost on the field of Waterloo." Though observers focused on the
devastation felt by white people in New Orleans (once again, no reliable
mortality estimates for Black people were committed to record), tragedy
rippled outward. Sick refugees imported yellow fever to Natchez and
Galveston, and by Christmas, thousands across Alabama, Mississippi,
Florida, and Texas had died. Even landlocked towns far from the epidemic's
epicenter were devastated. On September 2, 1853, a note on a mail bill
from the small village of Thibodeaux, sixty miles west of New Orleans, read:
"Stores closed—town abandoned—151 cases of yellow fever—22 deaths—
postmaster absent—clerks all down with the fever."[15]

Even for a disaster-steeled people like Louisianans, the "Great Epidemic"
of 1853 was too serious a catastrophe to be written off as an act of God about
which nothing could be done. And while many white survivors wanted to
get back to making money as quickly as possible, returning politicians
struggled to revert to business as usual. Much to their chagrin, outsiders
blamed them, the slavery-based system of cotton capitalism they governed,
and the public-health-as-private-acclimation system they endorsed for
the magnitude of the epidemic. Upon reconvening in late October, the
city council established multiple *ad hoc* committees, tasked with investigating why the epidemic had been so lethal. Hearings ensued, with performative outrage on full display. Written reports followed. Channeling the
anger of committee member J. C. Simonds (who had warned in 1851 that
such a disaster was nigh), the chair of the newly formed Sanitary Commission, Dr. Edward Hall Barton, directly attacked the see-no-evil attitude of city authorities, writing in his 542-page report: "It required a great

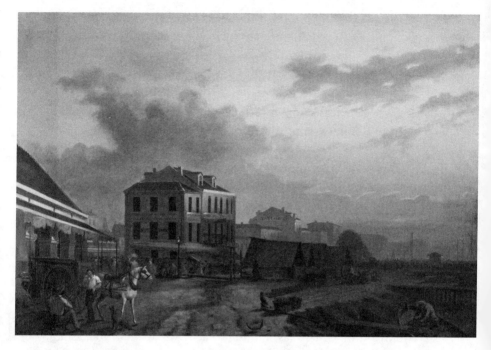

Louis Dominique Grandjean Develle, *French Market and Red Store,* ca. 1841–1844.
The Historic New Orleans Collection, The L. Kemper and Leila Moore Williams
Founders Collection.

calamity, like that of 1853, to open our eyes to the actual truth" that "ignorance is not bliss." Barton estimated that the epidemic had cost the city millions in future earnings, damaged its prosperity and reputation, devalued
its real estate, and swelled the ranks of orphans and widows. "Shall we say
then," Barton asked, "that all this *could have been prevented?*"[16]

But the Sanitary Commission resurrected the same minimalist nonsolu-
tions always proffered in the aftermath of epidemics. It concluded that
yellow fever was not contagious, that it differed from other fevers only in
degree, and that it resulted from a combination of local meteorological and
geographical conditions. It made seventeen lackluster recommendations—
other American ports might have considered them self-evident—for improved health: it called for a sewage and privy system; city-wide drainage;
more paved roads; extending the water works; building an "extensive shed"
across "the entire front of the business part of the city"; filling in defunct
canals; moving slaughterhouses out of the city center; and banning burials
within city limits. The biggest and most expensive recommendation was

to establish a Health Department and a quarantine station, both under the control of the city council. All of these reforms would cost about $1.43 million, Barton estimated. Anticipating the sticker shock, he recommended the city council sell swamp lands, secure $35,000 on credit and $400,000 in a loan from John McDonogh's estate, levy a tonnage duty on arriving vessels, tax the property of absentees, and raise the remaining revenue through a lottery.[17]

Immediately, the vultures swooped. Dr. Bennet Dowler—author of a competing report—bitterly attacked Barton for dilettantish posturing, calling his report "really a tedious book, abounding in absurdities, extravagances, and self-glorification." To the Commission's claim that yellow fever would be ameliorated by more rigorous public health infrastructure, Dowler scoffed:

> Think of that, ye who live! Hear it, ye angry ghosts of the dead! Let "the filthiest city in the civilized world" open wide the door of its treasury to the inspired Commission, and yellow fever shall henceforth be "an impossibility." Allah is great! but the Commission are the true yellow fever killers.[18]

The pile-on continued. In his thirteen-page introduction to the mortality lists from 1853, Dr. J. S. McFarlane—famous for his filth-is-health theory—bizarrely dedicated about half of his text to deriding quarantines, adding a plea that the city not put its health destiny into the hands of "hygienic visionaries." Instead, he insisted that authorities should "do nothing in a hurry."[19]

The city and state governments, hiding behind their commission pageantry, took McFarlane's advice. No health board or department was established. No future plans for quarantine were drawn up. That would take more epidemics and many more deaths. By December 1853 the council had returned to its more pressing business: preparing for the new business season and redrawing election wards. As the very conservative *Bee* put it in a brief moment of chastisement, the "languid sympathies" and "drowsy consciences" of New Orleans's city authorities have "evinced ignorance, apathy and neglect." Indeed, the dreadful mortality "seemed to bewilder and stupefy without adequately arousing them." Any other city, the *Bee* continued, would have actively sought to "discover [yellow fever's] cause and to prevent its recurrence."[20]

Denying the problem, of course, did not fix it. Another epidemic struck in 1854, killing over 3,000 people. Once again the newspapers remained silent (the *Picayune* never acknowledged that yellow fever was epidemic); politicians fled to the country without appropriating money for health care; no quarantine was installed; no board of health was established. Clearly frustrated, Barton wrote another account for the Sanitary Commission, copying whole sections and recommendations from the previous year's report. But this time he took sharper aim at the apathy of those with the power to affect change: "When pinned to the wall to account for this frightful mortality occurring year after year, the impudent and ungrateful reply is—'it only consists of immigrants!' immigrants who have made this city what it is, and consists now of no less than two-thirds of the white population." The filthy condition of the city and its astronomical mortality "is not, at this day *a matter of opinion,*" Barton insisted, "it has, unfortunately for us, passed from opinion *to fact,* about which there is no room for dispute by any honest inquirer."[21]

The Paranoid Style

Barton's call to action would have been equally potent if he had written it in invisible ink. The state legislature—recently moved to Baton Rouge—recognized that New Orleans's city council, if left to its own devices, would never impose quarantine, collect comprehensive data, or otherwise intervene to ensure the health of the region, and so the legislature constituted a State Board of Health. The landmark "Act to Establish Quarantine for the Protection of the State," passed in March 1855, empowered a nine-member panel to institute quarantine—with three members appointed by the New Orleans city council to represent commercial interests. All members were required to possess "known zeal" for quarantine.[22] But predictably, New Orleans businessmen styled the law "an act to harass, impede, shackle and injure the commerce and navigation of New-Orleans." They mounted such an opposition that the quarantine imposed in 1855 was quickly dismantled. That summer another epidemic killed over 2,000 people, but that too was absorbed by New Orleans's elite without serious concern. Instead, in its official report on internal resources, the city council celebrated that for the past ten years "New Orleans has advanced steadily and healthfully in the chief elements of a commercial greatness." Epidemics went unmentioned, and the fact that 12,000 had died in 1853 and 3,000 in 1854 was smoothed over by extolling the record exports of cotton and sugar.[23] In short, New Orleans's economic system of intensive commodity production and export worked well for those at the top *in spite* of disease. Why spend money fixing a system that was not broken? As novelist George Washington Cable put it, elite minds "turned only to commerce; and the commercial value of a well-authenticated low death-rate he totally overlooked. Every summer might bring plague—granted; but winter brought trade, wealth. It thundered and tumbled through the streets like a surf."[24]

Immunocapitalism certainly worked, in its way. But it was fragile. If slavery were to be abolished, if New Orleans were to lose its apex position in the cotton export trade, or if white immigration were to be rerouted even more extensively to other locations like Chicago or California—a trend that was already beginning by the 1850s—the system could collapse. The white elites of New Orleans, knowing that their fortunes and way of life depended upon *replacing* people, not keeping them alive, got to work on more intensely framing the yellow fever question as being, not a matter of science and mortality, but instead one of politics and sectional loyalty. Much like slavery, health and death became highly charged political issues, lightning rods in the antebellum culture wars that increasingly divided the slave South from the free North. What a white person in Louisiana said (and did not say) about disease became a litmus test for their positions on other pressing political questions: the proper role of government, states' rights, territorial expansion, and—most of all—slavery.

In the increasingly paranoid social and ideological context of the 1850s, anonymous boosters penned numerous glowing articles about New Orleans, professing that its sanitary condition was first in the nation, that yellow fever was barely a problem, that acclimation was a mild process easily undertaken, and that the city's reputation as a "necropolis" was just a jealous Northern fiction. Their public essays, speeches, and "anti-panic salvos" followed a strikingly similar pattern we might call "disease denialism." This had six steps. First, deny the validity of empirical data and adamantly discredit any accounts of sickness as outliers, propaganda, or wild exaggeration. Second, cast survival as a choice and blame victims of yellow fever for bringing the disease on themselves. Third, emphasize that acclimation was an easy, even blissful, process. Fourth, claim Northern attention to yellow fever was actually a proxy for antislavery hysteria, which was hypocritical because Northern cities also had their share of disease and labor-based suffering. Fifth, assert that any monetary penalties incurred by Southerners

for yellow fever—especially the "climate premiums" levied on white Southerners seeking life insurance—were unfair. And sixth, cast all criticism—
whether internal or external—as Northern in origin, the grumblings of a
region that was conspiring to malign the South as sickly, even though
Northern wealth depended upon it.[25]

Viewing plain facts like death rates with skepticism and discounting eye-
witness accounts of grave digging as anecdotal, some extremists cast doubt
not only on the scope of a given epidemic, but also on whether yellow fever
was a problem *at all*. Such views may have been illogical and unbelievable,
but their righteous repetition successfully shifted the terms of the debate.
In time, it became acceptable even for those who conceded yellow fever
was an occasional danger to claim it was a social panacea, screening out
alcoholics, filthy immigrants, and lesser men only. And by the late 1850s all
disease denialists came to espouse the crucial points of their argument: that
Black people were intellectually inferior but immunologically superior to
whites; that only abolitionists—the ultimate outsiders—died of yellow
fever; that *freedom,* not disease, was what killed Black people; and that Black
slavery was key to white public health, as "without the productive power
of the negro whom an all-wise Creator has perfectly adapted to the labor
needs of the South its lands would have remained a howling wilderness."[26]
At its apogee, disease denialism asserted that Black people were biologically
adapted to work *specifically* in the American South. Why else would Black
people possess the "gift" of yellow fever immunity, denialists demanded, if
God did not intend them to be enslaved in Louisiana?

Not one of the claims made by disease denialists was true. Indeed, to
subscribe to this logic in its entirety required a special kind of delusion,
with the argument collapsing under the weight of its own inconsistency.
But truth and good faith were never the point. The goal of disease denialism was to construct a worldview of aggressive aggrievement in defense
of the South and racial slavery through the rhetoric of annihilation and
resentment. Such thinking was, by definition, not rigorous. Boosters—
vacillating between cynicism, deflection, and hysteria—persisted in denying
obvious facts, elevating anecdotal evidence, and undermining or eliding
inconvenient truths.

Disease denialism was a paranoid ruling-class ideology, prone to, in the
words of Richard Hofstadter, "heated exaggeration, suspiciousness, and conspiratorial fantasy."[27] But New Orleans's elites worked hard to generate
this worldview so wholly at odds with reality. And by the 1850s, they had

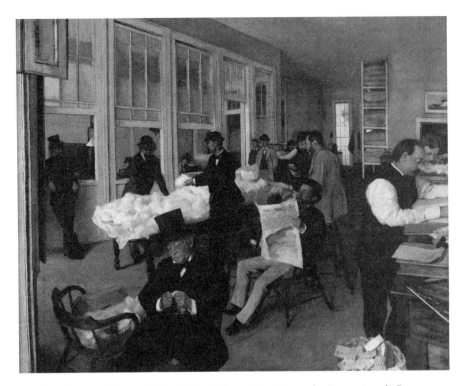

Edgar Degas, *A Cotton Office in New Orleans,* 1873. Musée des Beaux-Arts de Pau, France.

convinced or manipulated the vast majority of white townspeople into accepting disease denialism as the status quo—even those subordinates, especially recent immigrants and the unacclimated, for whom denying yellow fever was decidedly against their interests. Propaganda does not simply disseminate and magically delude people into "false consciousness"; cultural hegemony is not achieved by fiat. Rather, disease denialism resonated with whites across every social class because it reinforced the racial and economic order they wanted. Its logic tracked the logic of proslavery ideology, the South's "dominant fundamental" worldview, which was similarly fact-allergic and rooted in denial. Surviving yellow fever was considered a test of an individual's worth. Whether they then stuck to the disease denialists' script was considered a test of loyalty—to New Orleans, to racial slavery, and to cotton. We should think of proslavery thinking and disease denialism as two parallel, occasionally intersecting ideologies. Both cloaked anti-Black racism in the language of natural science. Both heaped opprobrium on an outside enemy—malicious Northerners—whom Southerners were already primed to mistrust. And both foreclosed alternate ways of thinking about the city's future: New Orleans was what it was, and it could be no other way.[28]

There were internal critics of this system. Drs. J. C. Simonds and E. H. Barton were two thorns in the side of merchants and capitalists in New Orleans, mostly because they criticized the health establishment and came by their view that the region's yellow fever problem was both acute and ameliorative honestly. In 1851, upon returning to New Orleans after attending a meeting in Boston, where he heard many negative comments about the Crescent City's health, Simmonds sought to demonstrate that New Orleans was just as healthy as any other American city. But upon study, he found the opposite. He scathed, "If New Orleans can only be sustained by a concealment of the truth, and a criminal immolation of unsuspecting victims on the altar of Mammon, the sooner it falls the better." He concluded, "Do not any longer say that the deaths occur in the Charity Hospital—that they are of poor immigrants, who are unaccustomed to the climate—that they are due to the want or imprudence of strangers and the unacclimated, and consider this a sufficient apology for a high rate of mortality." Barton echoed Simonds's sentiments in 1855: "It has become a kind of moral treason to admit that people die here at all! and all who attempt to stem this torrent of lies and toadyism, are held up as enemies of this city—as attempting to 'write down' New Orleans." The "facts—the painful, stubborn facts" were that the mortality hovered between 6 and 9 percent per year with 77,338 people dead between 1847 and 1855 alone. "Is it not time," Barton concluded, "that this veil of concealment and falsehood should be withdrawn—and that we should look the facts steadily in the face?"

Barton was right: thousands of people died from yellow fever whether elites admitted it or not. The power of disease denialism, however, was that—like a black hole—it sucked naysayers into its rhetoric of grievance. Even those who did not believe it rallied to it because to defend the diseased status quo was to defend the white wealth and power New Orleans generated. Even Barton came around eventually, as we will see, as did thousands of others.[29]

To ask why skeptics capitulated to disease denialism runs parallel to a fundamental question about Southern culture: Why did non-slaveholding whites fight for the Confederacy?[30] Yellow fever is not the answer. But it can provide a clue. In how unacclimated whites came to reflexively deny disease, in how quickly recent German immigrants attributed any critique of the massive death rate to meddling abolitionists, and in how immunocapitalists gladly conflated criticisms of their scant public health measures with wholesale attacks on slavery, we can see just how besieged many members of this society felt. And with their false equivalency and whataboutism masquerading as a legitimate counterargument, health boosters successfully convinced most white Deep Southerners by the mid-1850s that they were "*an injured people!!,*" the victims of wicked Northerners who were focused on destroying them through falsehoods about slavery *and* yellow fever. As the *Picayune* wrote at the outset of one epidemic, channeling the hostility many New Orleanians felt: "The Northern prints are trying their best to make it out that we have the yellow fever in this city. Go ahead gentlemen. You cant [*sic*] kill any of us by your mere 'say so.'"[31]

Health Boosterism and Sectional Tension

As yellow fever cut a path across New Orleans in May 1853, the city's press focused on what it perceived as a larger threat: abolitionist Harriet Beecher Stowe had recently landed in Europe and was promoting her new book, the *Key* to the best-selling *Uncle Tom's Cabin.* The *Picayune,* like the rest of the Southern press, was staunchly anti-Tom. In repeated editorials, it derided Stowe as an ignorant fantasist who had invented the horrors of Southern slavery out of whole cloth. One editor hoped that Stowe would be exposed to true slavery—that is, the "wage slavery" experienced by white mill workers—in Glasgow. These poor Scots lived in such "sin, misery, drunkenness, ignorance and depravity," the writer mused, that they would be pitied even by "the hardest worked, poorest fed and worst clothed negro on the most miserable plantation south of Mason & Dixon's line."[32]

Stowe did not have to travel to Europe to see urban poverty. There was plenty of it in her native Connecticut, as there was around the corner from the *Picayune* offices in New Orleans—though the editors seldom mentioned that. But a hyperfocus on abolitionists like Stowe and the alleged sins of industrial capitalism was increasingly common by the mid-1850s, when longsimmering tensions between North and South were threatening to boil over. Northerners spoke of the "slave power conspiracy" in which Southern oligarchs plotted to spread slavery into every nook and cranny of the nation, to Kansas then to all the western lands taken from Mexico in the Treaty of Guadeloupe Hidalgo, and perhaps even farther afield. The evidence of

Southern grasping seemed to grow clearer by the year: first it was the Fugitive Slave Act of 1850, then the Kansas-Nebraska Act, then the filibusters departing New Orleans seeking to annex Cuba as a US slave state, and then the potential reopening of the African slave trade. Southern slaveholders feared the South was "shrinking"—that limiting slavery's extension anywhere would reduce the South's political power and would inevitably lead to general emancipation. Soon, white Southerners feared, they would be relegated to permanent minority status. They hated the degenerate appellations they believed Northerners had appended to them: that every enslaver was a Simon Legree; that racial slavery was backward; that malaria made them lazy and lethargic, hookworm emaciated them, and yellow fever killed them.[33]

By the 1850s Southern health boosters fought back against the idea that the South had special public health problems in much the same style as they defended slavery—through deflection, denial, and whataboutism. They deployed selective evidence about death rates, smeared critics as jealous, and insisted on their unique authority to speak about local disease. This script was decades in the making. As early as 1806, for example, one Louisiana booster calling himself "An American" proclaimed in a Washington-based newspaper that "many erroneous ideas are entertained in the distant parts of the United States, respecting the salubrity of this country." To prove Louisiana was healthy, the writer analyzed the mortality data from select plantations and parish churches for the year ending August 1, 1806, within a 150-square-mile region around New Orleans known to be the "most unhealthy" for its "unusual number of fevers." The writer calculated 699 total deaths out of a permanent population of 32,038, thus deriving a death rate of one in every forty-seven white people or one in every forty-five Black people. This showed, he insisted, an "extreme degree of health and small degree of mortality."[34]

Yes, the writer conceded, *some* people died. But the "lamentable" truth was that nine in ten migrants died not from disease but from intemperance. As if anticipating pushback to this bold claim of near-universal alcoholism, he pivoted: "Should an enemy of Louisiana here raise the hue and cry against us of *yellow fever,*" he asserted, "I would reply to him by asking whether Massachusetts, Rhode Island, New-York or Pennsylvania have been looked on as the certain grave yards of strangers, because their capitals have been sometimes afflicted with this scourge." Yellow fever appeared in Louisiana "seldomer" than in most of the ports of the United States, and long-term residents remained "perfectly free and secure from its ravages."

Moreover, cautious newcomers who moved "ever so little a distance into the country" were certain to escape it. The author closed by promising that Louisiana's rewards far exceeded the risks, detailing the Caribbean-like fortunes of Louisiana's biggest planters.[35]

As epidemics in New Orleans increased—and news of epidemics traveled faster on steamboats—boosters honed their critique. Now they claimed the problem was not yellow fever misinformation *per se,* but instead a lack of context and precision in discussing epidemics. "Medicus," a fixture columnist in many Deep Southern newspapers, wrote in the *Natchez Gazette* in April 1826 that the practice of publishing the sexton's reports of deaths in the summer months—common in most major American cities by the 1820s—was immoral and misleading to potential settlers. For eight months of the year, there were few deaths to report, Medicus wrote, news which would be "gratifying to those interested in the welfare of the City" and would redeem it from "the imputation of being more sickly in the *annual aggregate* than towns similarly situated in the Northern and Eastern States." Medicus was clear about his intentions: he wanted to keep up the "emigration of moneyed capitalists and others" who were otherwise "prevented from settling here from imaginary danger." He ended with a jab at the North, declaring there "can be no doubt that, taking a whole year together," the amount of sickness and death was proportionally smaller in New Orleans than in New York, "with possibly one or two epidemics excepted."[36]

By the 1840s, boosters were more likely to sign their essays, publish in Southern journals, and insist that only they—men who had directly experienced yellow fever and understood its local logic—were qualified to discuss it. Positioning themselves as righteous Davids, this generation erected strawmen Goliaths to attack, normally characterized as effeminate, puny New Yorkers with poison pens but no sense. These prejudiced outsiders, J. D. B. De Bow asserted, were hell-bent on portraying New Orleans "as a perfect charnel-house—a Golgotha—a 'whited sepulcher' . . . 'filled with dead men's bones.'"[37] Even Barton, who generally pushed for health reform, canted that "so much has been said about this 'horrible' climate . . . that it is like opening Pandora's box, or visiting Botany Bay to come here." But, he said, a "scrutinizing analysis" of "*actual facts*" would compel "our northern brethren, who sit quietly in their libraries" to reach a different, more accurate conclusion. Dr. Josiah Nott of Mobile, Alabama, agreed that sober inquiry was necessary, and—like Barton—blamed the Deep South's sickly reputation on Northern ignorance. Nearly all writings about Southern health stemmed from pens "north of the Potomac" and Europe, Nott claimed, and therefore many had been led to "grave errors" about the actual state of health in Louisiana. He charged Northerners to come south, view the data he had personally collected, and see for themselves that the "native or acclimated inhabitants" of New Orleans "are, perhaps, the healthiest in the United States."[38]

In September 1855 the *New-York Tribune*—a Republican Party paper owned by Horace Greeley—printed two columns entitled "New-Orleans and Its Unwholesomeness," nestled between articles about the ongoing violence in Kansas, Texas elections, and the temperance movement. Asserting that New Orleans took "chief rank of any city in the Union" in the lists of "unqualifiedly sickly places" and was "never designed by Nature for a city," the *Tribune* cautioned against immigration. Why should men become "willing martyrs" by moving to New Orleans? Louisianans were scandalized. One writer at the *Picayune* expressed shock that the *Tribune* would engage in such a "flagrant demonstration" of yellow journalism. The editorialist chided the "persistent fanaticism" of "conceited speculators" spewing false information about New Orleans "at a distance," when only those people "who, from long residence, close observation and experience, have a right to give an opinion" on health in the city. Rather, the *Picayune* argued, even with yellow fever New Orleans was "as healthy" as any other large commercial city, referring to "the years 1844, '45 and '46, and the years of 1848, '49, '50, 51 and '52." Conveniently omitting the lethal epidemics of 1847, 1853, and 1854, as well as the one still unfolding in 1855, the article concluded: "We hardly know whether most to smile over" the *Tribune's* arguments "for the ignorance they display, or to despise them in consideration of the motives in which they originated."[39]

Trickle-Down Denial

New Orleans newspapers infamously suppressed the truth about yellow fever and systematically spread misinformation. John McGinnis, owner of the Democratic-leaning *True Delta*, later recalled that "the first and last step to success in any undertaking in New Orleans was persistent falsehoods about yellow fever." McGinnis adhered to this maxim so stringently, in fact, that he would not even warn friends in private correspondence or telegrams about cases of fever in town, lest the news be traced back to him.[40] Suppression was so widespread that during some serious epidemics, New Orleans's papers, like the *Bee* or *Picayune,* would report nothing on the subject, even while it was front-page news in Philadelphia or New York City. Media reserve—combined with the customary official silence—meant that the average person could not accurately gauge the scope of a given epidemic outside of their own idiosyncratic experience. This led many New Orleanians to express a feeling that *their* lethal experience did not align with reality. As a result, many townspeople, both acclimated and unacclimated, found it easier to lean into disease denialism. Novelist George Washington Cable, in fact, wrote that "it was the confident conviction and constant assertion of the average New Orleans citizen, Creole or American, on his levee, in the St. Charles rotunda, at his counting-room desk, in the columns of his newspaper, and in his family circle, that his town was one of the healthiest in the world."[41]

The moment many people transitioned from living in mortal fear of yellow fever to denying its seriousness was acclimation. And just as the "Unacclimated Stranger" was a recognized figure, so too was the man he transformed into if he survived—the "Acclimated Man." He was the fellow who said he had survived yellow fever back in 1847 and "therefore knows all about it." Even at the height of epidemics, this man "strongly affirms" that his city is "one of the healthiest and most delightful cities in the world," deploying a "long string" of "admirably arranged" statistics to support his claim. "Figures never lie," he says confidently. And when this man was confronted with data showing a fast-mounting death rate, "he has the most facile way of . . . shifting the responsibility of the disease from the shoulders of New Orleans to the back of Emigration." Acclimation was not just about surviving and gaining immunity; the next step in a man's acclimation journey was an expression of fidelity to the core tenets of disease denialism.[42]

It was difficult to get newcomers and outsiders to buy into this image of New Orleans as a health spa, but boosters considered this imperative in order to encourage continued immigration. New Yorkers and Londoners might be unconvinced by glowing and anonymous paeans to New Orleans's health. But they were more likely to believe what their sons, husbands, and nieces told them. The real trick, therefore, was to get newcomers to buy into the boosters' worldview or at least become emissaries of this ideology. Upon arriving on the levee—or perhaps later at their consulate or boardinghouse—foreigners were inundated with travelogues and self-help pamphlets, many of them explicitly providing stock phrases and talking points for what they should tell health-skeptical family and friends abroad.

Gibson's Guide from 1838—published by John Gibson, editor of the vehemently nativist *True American*—fed new arrivals various lines: "No country in the world has suffered more unmerited obloquy than New Orleans, in relation to health." "Probably there is no portion of America where the mortality is less than with our native and acclimated population." "The process of acclimation is not difficult to those who take the proper steps." Though the annual mortality of New Orleans "averages in ordinary years, about 3,800," *Gibson's Guide* assured readers that Louisianans were a long-lived people, with far more centenarians than Boston or New York. Moreover, there were multitudes of charities, municipal councils, banks, and chartered companies dedicated to helping strangers through the acclimating process. The laudatory picture of charitable benevolence *Gibson's* described admitted something deeper to anyone reading between the lines—that New Orleans had no government concerned with protecting the public's health. But this was spun into a positive. "Almost all of our charities are bestowed upon strangers," the guide insisted, "for there are but few, very few, of the ancient or permanent population, that need assistance."[43]

By the late 1840s many sources show just how quickly recent white immigrants adopted these talking points, first in daily conversations and then in letters home. They said that yellow fever was mild, its dangers overstated; that it attacked only drunks; that any suggestion that New Orleans was especially fatal was preposterous; and that any disease risk was worthwhile, because the city's commercial opportunities were unparalleled. For example, James McMartin told his brother Peter back in New Jersey in 1849, "I am delighted with New Orleans and think it is one of the best places I ever saw . . . if I had now about $500 by me I could double it every month." He wanted his brother—the former mayor of Jersey City—to join him, telling Peter he "could make enough here in 5 years" to buy "Jersey City out and out." As if copying the boosters' boilerplate, James continued, "Your objection to New Orleans seems to be that it is sickly, but there is a great mistake that we have in the North about the sickness here. Except in seasons when the epidemic rages this is the healthiest city in the Union." Though James expressed some trepidation about the looming summer, he concluded New Orleans was generally salubrious. "To see the healthy look of persons that I know who have been here for ten years and more" James wrote, "is the best evidence to me of the fact."[44]

Isaac Charles, who had recently immigrated from Philadelphia, was similarly sunny in a letter to a cousin in 1847, reassuring him that he had just survived an attack of fever "sufficient to answer all purposes of Acclimation" and now felt as "strong as ever." Charles chastised his cousin's ignorance regarding Southern health: "As for our Fevers Ned, I must beg of you to speak of them in a more respectful manner. You seem to place your 'City of Brotherly love,' against or rather before, our beloved 'Crescent,' as regards health—But there I think you are wrong." Charles then embarked on the usual pattern of argument: Between 1842 and 1847, he claimed, New Orleans had experienced only one yellow fever epidemic and New Orleans's total mortality within that period was the same or less than Philadelphia's. "And besides," Charles wrote, "the Yellow Fever is not so terrible a disease after all"—it was dangerous only to lower-class drunks with "by far the greater part of the victims . . . Irish & the Dutch." If his cousin could smell the "*stench*" and "see the miserable, filthy, loathsome manner in which the lower orders live," said Charles, he would understand why yellow fever "should spread & become as malignant as it does" among them.[45] In an era of intense nativism, many newcomers found attacking poor people—especially Irish poor people—to be a winning argument across sections. One saddler, for example, told his business partners in Hartford, Connecticut, "Nine tenths of the funerals that have been seen by the writer within a fortnight were *Irish*. These die as a matter of course."[46]

The mental gymnastics required by health boosterism were clearly taxing for some. Edward Henry Durell—son of a congressman, future alderman and mayor of New Orleans, future District Court judge, and pseudonymous fiction writer—sought to convince his sisters in New Hampshire that New Orleans was the picture of health at the height of the 1853 epidemic, when the hospitals were overflowing and panic was everywhere. "Poor New Orleans is and ever has been very much misrepresented abroad," Durell lamented in July, adding, "Cousin John, it seems, gets news at a distance of 2000 miles, which I have not been able to pick up here." Rest assured, he continued, "we have no more of yellow fever, or of Cholera, among us than is usual at this season of the year. . . . The city at this time enjoys its usual health, and there is, therefore, no cause for the alarm." This was a lie and Durell knew it. By August, approximately 1,000 people were dying each week—death he saw firsthand as a volunteer for the Howard Association. In fact, he fell sick and almost died from yellow fever that summer. But he lied to his sisters about this, too. And two years later Durell was still lying about health in New Orleans, offering that "N. York, Boston, Philadelphia, Baltimore and Charleston, our commercial rivals, seize upon every occasion to belittle and to injure us." But Durell remained sure that "our grand geographical position will bring us out in the end."[47]

How could boosters deny disease in good conscience, when the evidence clearly showed that the Deep South was a death trap for immigrants? When they surely knew many people—in their own households and neighborhoods—killed by yellow fever? When a stroll by the Charity Hospital in August would be punctuated by the shrieks of yellow fever victims dying inside? For acclimated merchants and bankers, the motivation was clearly to promote immigration and expand the economy. But why would regular, unacclimated people like McMartin, Charles, and Durell echo these talking points? Why did it become one of the city's "fashions" to lie about disease, and the "part of a good citizen," as George Washington Cable observed, to "debate with loud assertions" New Orleans's superior health?[48]

In the absence of solid statistical information, some "timid minds" surely believed the boosters' propaganda; that their city was not "The Wet Grave-Yard" at all, but instead "a fair and healthy city, a beautiful spot on the face of nature."[49] More likely, ordinary townspeople knew that New Orleans was incredibly unhealthy, but preferred the myth of immunological reward to the fatal reality. Many figured that worried mothers and brothers abroad would prefer lies about New Orleans's healthiness to the truth—or perhaps lies were all they could muster. Most of all, the mercenary attitude—that the economic health and reputation of the Cotton Kingdom must be protected at all costs—subsumed reason. Yellow fever denial metastasized into the culture because it tied into the city's other foundational beliefs: that New Orleans's condition was natural and unchangeable; that the city would remain important in perpetuity due to its geographic position; that external critics were just covetous of the city's cotton and commercial supremacy; and that racial slavery was climatically necessary. Questioning one aspect of this belief structure forced uncomfortable questions on the margins. Whatever the motive, denying disease was certainly cheaper than fixing health, and less stressful than obsessing about it.[50]

Life Insurance the "Southern Way"

Boosters' primary aim was to convince immigrants that everything they knew, saw, and heard about yellow fever was false, but they found their arts had no effect on one particular group: life insurers. To disease denialists' repeated displeasure, actuaries rejected their pugilistic style, rosy talking points, selective data, and, most of all, vexed definitions of acclimation. Instead, actuaries proved through data and tables that dying in the South was likelier than in the North, and that dying in and around New Orleans was, in fact, much likelier.

Before the Civil War, the American life insurance industry—worth approximately $100 million—was overwhelmingly white and Northern. (Policies on enslaved Southern lives accounted for a very small percentage of the overall market.) By 1860, policies on white Southern lives accounted for less than 7 percent of all life insurance in force—just under $6 million.[51] This North–South popularity gap has generally been explained as the product of protectionist state laws and uneven regulation. Louisiana, for example, levied a $1,000 licensing fee for out-of-state insurance agents, twice the fee imposed on locally chartered operations, in addition to a tax of 1 percent on the gross amount of the premiums earned each year. This was much more than the $100 licensing fee out-of-state agents paid to do business in Pennsylvania. Historians have also argued that white Southerners were less likely to insure themselves because they already had a large investment in the lives of their Black slaves that could be marshaled in case of emergency.[52]

But slaveholders were never considered the primary customers for life insurance in the South. Instead, Joseph Copes, a Louisiana agent for New York Life & Trust (NYL&T) in the 1850s, targeted non-slaveholding professionals in their twenties with dependents, those individuals willing to spend about $10 a year for peace of mind—clerks, bookkeepers, and accountants.[53] Copes was not alone in his thinking. Louisiana newspapers featured almost 5,000 advertisements for life insurance alone between 1840 and 1861, running alongside job postings, consumer reports, and death notices, all aimed toward white middle-class professionals. And here, as Dr. Josiah Nott, a sometimes insurance examiner, put it, where "the calculations of the merchant—the harvest of the planter—the fate of a ship at sea—the very existence of the world for another day, are all but probabilities," the market for white Southern life insurance was potentially massive.[54]

Southern coolness toward life insurance boiled down to the touchy subject of climate premiums, a surcharge levied on white Southerners and especially those in "Class VI"—the area immediately surrounding New Orleans along the Mississippi River and below the 32nd north parallel.[55] Most mutuals knew they had to surcharge Southerners if they wanted to stay profitable, but where this premium should be fixed was a matter of (educated) guesswork, and also of politics. Not only did the Deep South produce little accurate vital data, but existing life tables like the English Carlisle and Northampton tables did not apply to subtropical climates. Region-specific rate hikes always provoked the ire of new customers and agents alike. But incautious inclusivity could anger existing policyholders: adding new policyholders on standard terms from an unhealthy area like the Deep South could be seen as a tax on those in temperate places. If healthy regions were forced to, effectively, subsidize the less healthy, this would be "a violation of equity"—a violation of the entire basis of mutual life insurance.[56]

Without accurate vital data upon which to base their actuarial tables, how would mutuals determine their rates for such a notoriously unhealthy region? When NYL&T began selling insurance in the South in the 1830s, it simply guessed. It surcharged policyholders residing around New Orleans an extra $5 for every $100 of insurance contracted. Adding the Southern supplement to the standard rate meant Southerners were charged a little under $7 per year for every $100 of insurance they took out, effectively triple the amount a healthy twenty-year-old Bostonian paid. NYL&T also assessed any policyholder wishing to travel south at any season a 10 percent ($10 per $100) supplement.[57] Southern agents claimed these policies were just too expensive to sell. Competition, in the form of the Mutual Life Insurance Company of New-York (MONY), answered the agents' call. MONY offered a cheaper product, adding a much smaller supplement of 25 cents on every $100 of insurance for applicants living between the southern border of Virginia and the 32nd north parallel, and 50 cents on every $100 to those living farther south. The cheaper rates allowed MONY to attract about 10 percent of its total business from policy-seekers south of Virginia.[58]

But deaths from this region astounded underwriters. MONY complained that 16 percent of their policyholders who died in 1849 had perished in the New Orleans area, even though *all* of their Southerner policyholders constituted only 10 percent of their business.[59] William Bard, president of NYL&T, also complained that the largest portion of his company's death claims came from people living in or traveling to New Orleans, though they were only a small portion of those insured. As Bard explained, "There can be no doubt that Life is not so good in the Southern States as it is in those North of Virginia." Bard determined, "Compared with New York or Baltimore, the risk of life in New Orleans is more than 2 for 1 . . . Taking well-known facts into view, our Life Insurance Companies will feel bound, in duty to their own customers, to enhance their rates on lives South of Richmond, Virginia."[60]

Southerners would have to pay more. But how much more was still not settled by the 1850s.[61] Company directors and officers turned to internal statisticians and analysts, hoping data could inform policy decisions and make premiums more palatable to a Southern clientele. MONY hired statistician Charles Gill in 1851 to analyze the company's historical experience. In his 1854 report, Gill affirmed the necessity of climate supplements generally, concluding that all Southern policyholders should pay substantially more. Gill may have based his conclusions on solid data (he stressed, however, that the decade of data he worked with ended in February 1853, prior to "the fatal epidemic so destructive to life in the South Western States"), but he justified his recommendations in moral, anti-Southern terms. He told the board: "In some States the parties insured live simply and frugally and labor steadily and long, while in other States more bountifully favored in some respects, they toil less, live fast and soon accomplish their aim and end." In 1854 MONY's board raised rates for people in Texas, Louisiana, Mississippi, and Alabama, using Gill's findings for political cover.[62]

Regional premiums were not enough to generate profit. In 1859 NYL&T reported that the Southern mortality rate was much higher than average: death claims from Southern policyholders consumed more than half of total premium payments, although they constituted only one-quarter of its policies. Penn Mutual's internal data showed that for every 10,000 lives exposed to the chances of mortality for one year, about 186 died in the Deep South, making mortality in that section 98.5 percent greater than the Northeast. Thus "to render the risks among the two classes of Members equal," Deep Southerners should pay an "extra premium of $2^{26}/_{100}$ per cent. on the amount assured," and agree to travel restrictions. Travel restrictions became common in all policies on the logic that if it was easy to fake immunity to yellow fever, it was harder to move a dead body. New Orleans, in fact, was so dangerous that Maryland Life and Knickerbocker Life each declared that any policyholder who traveled to the Deep South when yellow fever was epidemic voided their life policy altogether. Prudential also banned policyholders from traveling to New Orleans or the West Indies between May and November, whether or not an epidemic had been declared.[63]

Acclimated Risks

Some mutuals felt the best, most politic approach was to differentiate *between* Southern risks. Medically verified "acclimated" persons would pay a smaller premium; "unacclimated" persons were denied coverage unless they paid much more and agreed to travel restrictions. South of Virginia, NYL&T initially surcharged those medically verified as "acclimated" by 0.5 to 1 percentage point; "unacclimated" policyholders paid a premium supplement of 5 percent and were not allowed to live in or travel to the South between June and November. Soon NYL&T president Bard decided that even these modifications were insufficient. He increased the surcharge to 2 percentage points for acclimated persons and from 2 to 6 percentage points for unacclimated persons, while "declining altogether Insurances for the whole year in New Orleans or in other Southern or particularly unhealthy places."[64] Other mutuals followed suit. By the late 1850s the Knickerbocker Life and the Mutual Benefit Life and Fire Insurance Company of New Orleans both required Southern policy-seekers to prove they had resided for more than two years in a city where yellow fever had prevailed or their application was denied entirely.[65] Mutual of Baltimore forbade policyholders from going south of 34° north latitude (roughly Columbia, South Carolina) and required "those residing in the States of North Carolina, Tennessee, South Carolina, Mississippi, and Arkansas . . . to keep 50 miles distant from the Mississippi river, and from the Atlantic Ocean"—essentially, to avoid New Orleans.[66]

Acclimation screening was part of a medical exam in which policy-seekers answered an array of questions about their profession, medical history, mental health, and alcohol consumption. Answering "Is the party acclimated?"—a standard question on many insurance forms—fell to the examiner's discretion. Most medical examiners were physicians who made a bit of extra money certifying insurance applications. Southern doctors, however, were socialized to treat acclimation as a biological *and* cultural marker and had to rely on the often hazy, and at times aspirational, memories of the insurance-seekers, who had to remember the specific year and month of their brush with yellow fever (often decades later), recount all of their symptoms, note if they had fallen sick with any other kinds of fever, and produce witnesses—preferably an attending physician. Thereafter, it fell to the medical examiners' prudence and expertise.[67]

Josiah Nott developed specific criteria for determining whether a party was acclimated, which he published:

> If the subject lives in one of our southern seaports, where yellow fever prevails, and has been born and reared there, or has had an attack of yellow fever, I answer, *"Yes."* If, on the other hand, he lives in the country, I answer *"No;"* because there *is no acclimation against intermittent and bilious fever, and other marsh diseases* . . . An attack of yellow fever does not protect against marsh fevers, nor *vice versâ.*"[68]

Nott's schema was somewhat accurate. But his and other models translated only haphazardly to real, idiosyncratic people with scant knowledge of their own medical histories. For example, forty-four-year-old cotton broker Robert Purvis applied to New England Mutual for a $4,000 whole life policy in 1845. He wrote on his application, "Born in Scotland, Resides in Mobile. Came to this Country in 1821. Have lived ever since in the Southern country—and I consider myself as an acclimated Southerner."[69] Was Purvis acclimated? Purvis noted that his brother had died of yellow fever in Guadeloupe while in the British military, but insisted he had a superior constitution and had only ever had one small attack of "country fever" many years before. Purvis's insurance agent and three business acquaintances provided affidavits that he was healthy, lived in a place "safe from yellow fever," and was therefore a good risk. On this basis, Purvis was extended a policy. This turned out to be a good bet: Purvis died in 1871, aged seventy-one. John M. Gould, a twenty-eight-year-old Massachusetts-born shoe merchant in New Orleans, was also a good risk. He bought a whole life policy in 1846 for $1,000, declaring on his application that the only time he had ever seen a doctor was in 1839 when sick with yellow fever and was therefore "guaranteed" acclimated. He died in 1887.[70]

But the disproportionate death claims from the South showed that plenty of bad risks passed their medical exams, only to be mowed down when epidemics struck. Surely some people willfully lied about their acclimation status to secure a cheaper rate, while others were genuinely unsure if what they had suffered with in the past was yellow fever. The result was that "acclimation" became a word with many meanings—and therefore none at all—for actuarial purposes. In fact, life companies sent explicit definitions of acclimation to their agents and medical examiners in 1856, hoping to establish an ironclad system, stripped of local meanings and privileges, for assessing who was a good risk. MONY's circular decreed: "Acclimation against Yellow Fever is not considered complete unless the party has had it, and has continued since to reside in places where it is epidemic." Seeking to quell dissent among agents operating in the Deep South, it added that if this definition was meticulously followed, climate premiums on acclimated lives could potentially be reduced across the board, meaning they could sell more policies.[71] But even with acclimation screening, insured people in New Orleans still died at disproportionate rates. One underwriter lamented in 1858 that the Deep South "has been a source of loss to the Company. The extra rate charged for the first ten years was found, on examination in 1854, to be entirely inadequate, and was advanced on acclimated risks from ½ to two per cent., and on unacclimated risks from 2 to 5 per cent. *extra*. Judging from experience, the present rates are not too heavy."[72]

White New Orleanians hated climate premiums. They hated them for quantifying a risk that contradicted the myths they had constructed about their region—its healthiness, their virtue, and the value of whiteness. The idea of Northern actuaries reaching their own definition of acclimation and determining that Deep Southern whites were riskier and sicklier—and therefore must pay substantially more for the privilege of insuring their own lives—was understood as a prejudicial slight against their entire system: against whiteness, slavery, and the commodities the system generated. Balking against the idea of levying any climate premium, at least eighteen *Southern* life insurance companies that expressly did not charge such premiums opened during the late antebellum period. One Richmond-based agent declared that "the Philadelphia & New York offices . . . have a greater dread of the Southern risks than we."[73] The short-lived Ocean Insurance (1835–1841) of New Orleans advertised: "The absence of any institution in this city for insuring lives and the extravagant rates of premium demanded by the Northern and European companies for granting life policies to persons residing in Louisiana" opened a market gap. The company reiterated that "no addition whatever" would be "made for difference of climate." Such rhetoric might have played well among white New Orleanian men, those who staked much of their identity on their acclimation. But it did not make them live longer. In fact, all climate-premium-flouting insurers failed.[74]

In the decade before the Civil War, many frustrated life insurers from the North began to pull away from the Southern market. MONY reported in 1858 that Class VI had been a source of loss to the Company and that "we do but little new business in this Class."[75] Right before the Civil War, the company quadrupled the rates previously charged on all new Southern policies. But even these rates were not fully remunerative and worked only to excite extreme "dissatisfaction among applicants."[76] By 1860 New England Mutual had only two agents working in South Carolina, one agent in Alabama, and no agents in the rest of the Deep South; it had seventeen agents in Maine. And after the Civil War, companies turned their sights westward rather than returning to the South, preferring the vast, less-diseased space that was starting to fill up with white people who would never encounter yellow fever, or perhaps even malaria. As one company declared in its 1866 annual report, "the loss of the South has been more than compensated for by the gain of the great West."[77]

To Deep Southerners, actuarial truth did not matter. Instead, climate premiums were derided as an unjustified punishment concocted by Northerners to undercut the South and discourage immigration. Insurance broker Nelson Sayler of Ohio reported, "The Southern people"—especially residents of New Orleans—"do not look upon life insurance as we Northern people do." Though Southern risks were not as good as Northern risks, "the almost universal belief *there* is that [they are]." Sayler added that to "tell an Alabama or Mississippi planter that he is shorter-lived than an Ohio farmer, would be considered the height of absurdity."[78] Adhering to the dominant ideology that white people's health was personally established, not publicly protected, the medical and political establishment of the Deep South responded to the insult of higher premiums by claiming that white inhabitants had no need for life policies anyway. Their longevity was a personal choice; they could "self-insure" by getting acclimated. Collapsing the rhetoric upon itself, acclimation was not the pathway to securing life insurance; it literally *was* the insurance. All those Northern actuaries, with their notions of acclimation risk and climate premiums, were not welcome. And if risk taking was essential—and indeed celebrated—in the South, there was no explaining this to Northerners, who had an entirely different understanding of what constituted prudent and reasonable behavior. One editorialist summed up New Orleanians' feelings about Northern insurers: "Laissez Nous Faire, Let Us Alone."[79]

Slavery for the Health of the South

White New Orleanians were capable of denying reality when it came to the epidemiological fact of disease and the actuarial fact of high mortality. But denial did not end there. By the 1850s, enslavers had developed an elaborate "science-based" script to legitimate racial slavery which was rife with anecdotes and reflexively paranoid. Whitewashing the cruelties of slavery and disease denialism were not the same. But these ideologies became increasingly entangled in style and substance during the high antebellum period as end goals aligned: to project a sunnier, more rational vision of the Cotton Kingdom than actually existed. Both hierarchies—racial and epidemiological—legitimated massive disparities of power and wealth, concealed violence and risk behind a facade of meritocracy, and naturalized slavery and immunocapitalism as scientific necessities. In this way, white New Orleanians came to interpret an attack on the city's response to yellow fever as an attack on slavery, and vice versa.

The notion that only Black people could physically do the labor of sugar and cotton production had persisted across the Atlantic world since the early seventeenth century. Dozens of writers—many of them physicians—insisted the torrid zone was too hot, humid, tiring, and deadly for whites to labor in. Bryan Edwards, the self-styled Jamaican gentleman who chronicled the Haitian Revolution, attributed superpower health to slaves. He observed that "the Negroes enjoy higher health and vigour than at any other period of the year" during the high summer, when they "are employed in the mill and boiling-houses," often working "very late, frequently all night."[80] During the era of the "second slavery" in the United States—when the domestic slave trade was powering the physical expansion of slavery further and further west—yellow fever (and malaria) took an increasingly central role in the proslavery argument, especially the claim that Black people of any origin were uniquely immune to this disease. Philip Tidyman, the Charleston-based physician-planter, wrote in 1826, "Nature has, with a special regard to the safety of blacks, rendered them almost proof against the insidious attacks of this terrible disease." Even when a slave was "assailed" by yellow fever, Tidyman claimed, they were "buoyed up by hope, from a consciousness that few of his colour are destroyed by it." In the Southern states, Tidyman saw enslaved people "working with cheerfulness and alacrity," even as white laborers would become "languid and sink from the effects of a torrid sun." Black people's unique health characteristics were thus "of great importance to the agricultural prosperity of the United States, and closely connected with the general welfare of the nation."[81]

By the 1850s, propagandists for slavery in and around New Orleans fully bought into Tidyman's assertions and took them even further. Now whites were likely to cite Black people's immunity to yellow fever as a God-given gift, while holding Black people responsible for creating this dreadful disease in the first place. Dr. William Holcombe put it: "From its color, its black vomit, and its special ravage of slave-holding countries, we might have known long ago that the negro was at the bottom of it." Reinforcing racist cultural cues were everywhere equating yellow fever with Black people. Newspapers described serious cases of yellow fever as "African fever," and steamboat pilots warned strangers against heading into town when the "African plague," "African poison," or "Congo fever" was at its peak. "Yellow Jack" was a favorite, though not exactly beloved, character in operas and plays—a sneaky mulatto who preyed upon the unacclimated Irish at the docks, waiting to trick or kill them. Factors and agents mused in their offices that yellow fever was a perfect crime against whites, as the "native African has no such fever. The African brought to the West Indies never has yellow fever. The West Indian negro brought to the United States is not liable to it." Some Deep Southerners, especially clergy, might have even quietly agreed with the abolitionist reading of the situation, that yellow fever's special focus on New Orleans—the hub of the nation's slave trade—was God's punishment on whites for the sin of bondage.[82]

White Deep Southerners, however, were more likely to cleave to the claim of Virginia-based proslavery theorist George Fitzhugh: that a free society was "afflicted with disease" whereas a slave society was always "healthy."[83] Late in the antebellum period, few white New Orleanians publicly challenged the Black immunity orthodoxy, nor did they question the authority of self-described fever and "black disease" specialists like Josiah Nott and Samuel Cartwright (a. YF 1823), even when these physicians' theories about yellow fever and Black people became increasingly tortuous and at odds with reality. In medicalizing race, Cartwright and Nott ultimately sought to defend slavery, a system that conferred outsized benefits on white people. Science, they said, made differentiating between races—physiologically and psychologically—intellectually respectable. They also held up epidemiology as proof that God had relegated Black people to permanent enslavement. Nott and Cartwright were progenitors of the American school of ethnology, a field that built on the work of European scientists and tapped into transnational networks of anatomists, phrenologists, and skull collectors like Samuel Morton. By the ends of their careers, both men went against the prevailing Christian orthodoxy of monogenism—the belief that all humans descended from Adam and Eve. As polygenists, they argued that Black and white people were of different descent. Yellow fever was a key piece of evidence they twisted into their theories about racial difference, white supremacy, and Black inferiority.[84]

Josiah Nott was born in South Carolina and completed his medical training at the University of Pennsylvania. Following a residency in Paris, he moved to Mobile in the 1830s to open a surgical practice. In Alabama he became fascinated by yellow fever etiology. During the 1840s and 1850s he worked as an insurance examiner and wrote prolifically on yellow fever's differential racial impact, stressing that Black immunity was near-total. If the "population of New England, Germany, France, England, or other northern climates, come to Mobile, or to New Orleans," Nott wrote in *Types of Mankind,* about half would die shortly of yellow fever, but "negroes, under all circumstances, enjoy an almost perfect exemption from this disease."[85] Nott honed his ideas further during his tenure as an anatomy professor at the University of Louisiana, in 1857 publishing *Indigenous Races of the Earth,* a 650-page meditation proposing a supposed natural hierarchy of the races, with his sometimes-research partner Egyptologist George Gliddon. Nott and Gliddon described six ways Africans were different from and inferior to other races—and the most distanced, intellectually and physiologically, from "Caucasians" or white people of European heritage. They argued that Black people, "native of the hottest region on the globe" go "naked in the scorching rays of the sun, and can lie down and sleep on the ground in a temperature of at least 150° of Fahrenheit"—an exposure that would kill whites (and, in reality, would kill anyone). One of the major differences between the races, Nott said once again, was that Black people "are exempt in a surprising degree from yellow fever."[86]

Nott was no yellow fever neophyte. By the mid-1850s he claimed to have cared for more yellow fever patients than any other American doctor, and he theorized the mosquito connection forty years before this transmission hypothesis was widely accepted. He also lost four children to yellow fever in 1853. But Nott's yellow fever analysis was political in nature, ultimately geared toward establishing the righteousness of Black enslavement and proving white intellectual superiority. As he worked to elevate prejudice to the level of science, his etiological explanations for yellow fever and racial difference became increasingly convoluted. He charged that "negro blood is an antidote against yellow fever, for the smallest admixture of it with the white will protect against this disease." His proof was the "curious" fact that he had "seen many hundred deaths from yellow fever, but never more than three or four mulattoes, although hundreds are exposed to this epidemic in Mobile." Rather than follow this argument to its next logical step—that interracial mixing potentially saved lives—Nott doubled down on the utility of strict racial purity. Though "negro blood" was a prophylactic against yellow fever (as good as a "vaccine against small-pox"), Nott also argued that the decreased intelligence whites would experience through miscegenation was not worth the immunological protection. Yellow fever, he said, was created by "excitements" of the brain and nervous system; Black people's smaller brains and less-extensive nervous systems kept these excitements to a minimum and thus reduced the impact of yellow fever on them. Black immunity was thus a natural by-product of their anatomical and psychological inferiority. Citing no statistics, Nott claimed that slavery was a kindness to Black people, who lived long lives in the South when treated according to their "particular" physiology. Conversely, Black people died in large numbers when free. Again citing no evidence of his own, Nott wrote that "Negroes die out and would become extinct in New England, if cut off from immigration, as is clearly shown by published statistics."[87]

Samuel Cartwright of New Orleans spent his career seeking to reconcile yellow fever, Blackness, and the American body politic. Most famous for his "diagnosis" of Black-only diseases like *drapetomania* (the "disease" that causes slaves to run away) and *dysaesthesia aethiopica* (rascality), he also had strong opinions about the virtues Blackness conveniently conferred upon those who were required to labor in the Deep South. In the 1840s Cartwright traveled around the southern bayous by canoe and determined that the *Jussiaea grandiflora,* a plant common in the swamps, was a prophylactic against miasmatic and bilious fevers—especially for Black people. In the sugar regions surrounding New Orleans, Cartwright declared that the Black population was "considerable" and "remarkably healthy and long-lived," containing "more negroes over one hundred years of age, than five New England states put together." Cartwright transformed these claims about Black health into a vision of how society should be structured. Later Cartwright would insist that the Deep South's climate was too torrid for the "master's race of men"; that it "scorns . . . the aristocracy of the white skin." Nature "has issued her fiat, that here at least," whites "shall not be hewers of wood or drawers of water . . . under the pain of three-fourths of their number being cut off."[88]

This was not only a massive overestimation of white morality; it was also a scandalous underestimation of Black death. But Cartwright's selective mix of science, race theory, economics, and religion, he said, explained not just why Black people should be enslaved, but why slavery was a healthy *system*. "If the prognathous race were expelled [from] the land," Cartwright argued, "and their place supplied with double their number of white men," Southern agriculture would be crippled and the sugar and cotton industries would cease to exist. Only Black "muscles" could "endure exercise in the smothering heat of a cane or cotton field," he said. As evidence, Cartwright pointed to Illinois, where half of white laborers were "prostrated with fevers from a few days' work in stripping blades in a Northern cornfield." Cartwright conflated malaria with yellow fever, and he wildly overstated the unhealthiness of Illinois. But this, Cartwright believed, still proved that Black emancipation would lead to white extinction. According to nature's laws—as he defined them—it was impossible to overwork a Black person in Louisiana: "A white man, like a blooded horse, can be worked to death. Not so the negro."[89]

Yellow fever featured with increasing regularity in Cartwright's work in the 1850s, and provided a popular line of proslavery argument for laypeople. On the second page of his 1857 treatise "Ethnology of the Negro or Prognathous Race," he argued that Black people never died from yellow fever "when treated with regard to [their] ethnical peculiarities." In fact, "so strong are they in this favor that, even under mal-practice, death is the exception—and recovery, the rule." He conceded that a number of Black people had died in 1853, but argued that their deaths had been "more from panic" than from yellow fever, as "panic is very apt to kill a negro." Cartwright then raised the specter of Benjamin Rush in 1793, who, he claimed, regarded "the negroes as black angels, sent by a kind Providence to nurse the sick during the terrible yellow fever which ravaged our Northern cities." Cartwright claimed to have studied under Rush, which was untrue. And Rush had famously recanted his original bullish opinion about Black immunity after many Black people died in Philadelphia while nursing the sick at his behest. Cartwright most certainly knew this and denied it. Instead, he declared, "the great Rush," and "many other good and distinguished men" had been mistaken about yellow fever and Black people for too long, and that they should correct their assumptions "in the light of ethnological science."[90]

Cartwright's and Nott's theories about Black people, yellow fever, and the overall healthiness of the slave system proved contagious. Matthew Estes, a lesser-known proslavery theorist from Mississippi, similarly argued that "the Negro was made for the south—is always found there, and cannot exist and flourish in a northern climate." Stating that Black people could labor in diseased spaces "without the slightest injury to his constitution," Estes maintained that "the African is naturally inferior to the Caucasian," endowed by God and nature "with certain qualities which fit him for the condition of slavery, as it exists in the Southern parts of the United States." Estes, like all proslavery theorists, masked economic and social arguments with soliloquies about slavery's mutuality, altruism, and inevitability; that, in his rendering, immunity was a God-given gift to Black people and thus slavery was a social kindness.[91]

But even if Black people were naturally immune, why would *slavery* be medically or ethnologically necessary? Proslavery physicians concocted an answer for this: paradoxically, slaves lost their immunity in freedom. And if it was already established that emancipation would lead to white extinction (as whites died too quickly from yellow fever), they said that any wide-scale manumission would lead to Black extinction, too, because they would be newly vulnerable to yellow fever. Emancipation would also create a host of social problems, they said, as Black people could not independently care for their own health and well-being and required white oversight. Philip Tidyman claimed freedom weakened Black people constitutionally and claimed that the death rate among free Blacks was at least three times higher than among slaves. His evidence was one Baltimore bill of mortality from 1825 showing that over the previous year, 368 free Blacks had died in comparison with only 48 slaves.[92] Cartwright held that Black freedom was particularly pernicious for Black women because their "husbands hold them in abject slavery; they dare not kill them, as in Africa, but they beat and maltreat them in the cellars of New York, and other places in the Northern States, which they dare not do in the South." He even proclaimed that Black people's immunity was "due to a special Providence," giving them a "special opportunity"—longevity—"to display their gratitude" to their civilizing and Christianizing white masters, whom they looked upon as "akin to Gods," meeting them with a "ready bow and grin."[93]

John Van Evrie, an intensely racist New Yorker with strong Southern sympathies, would take the supposed dangers of Black freedom to their furthest extent. He claimed in 1861 that "free negroism, as shown elsewhere, is a social abnormalism, a diseased condition, that necessarily ends in extinction." Van Evrie argued that "those ignorant and terribly mistaken" abolitionists who "seduced" free Black men to go to "the bleak and forbidden North" were leading them to their death and thus "unconsciously commit[ing] a crime that would appall [sic] them if they could truly comprehend it." He concluded that "crime, disease, and death mark the career of Free Negroism."[94]

Such thinking about the magical loss of immunity and Black extinction was nothing short of alchemy. But it stuck. By midcentury many whites took it as an unassailable fact that they could not gather firewood in swamps, plant sugar cane in August, or repair levees by themselves. If whites took the place of slaves in the cane fields, the *Weekly Delta* opined, "mortality among the laborers on the plantations . . . would nearly extinguish the sugar culture in Louisiana." It argued that as divine punishment for seeking freedom, enslaved people would lose their natural resistance to yellow fever. The evidence was that of the few Black victims in the epidemic of 1853—almost all of them had been free, and therefore "slavery is the condition best suited" to Black people, saving a bondsman "from a destructive disease, to which [he] would render himself liable by the exercise of his freedom."[95] Another article maintained that three-quarters of all deaths from yellow fever were among abolitionists. "Slaves and masters rarely die," the article posited; those who did die backed "abolition theory." Some people even reversed the logic: If a person died from yellow fever, then they must have been an abolitionist all along. The *Delta* argued that yellow fever was actually generated not by miasmas but by the practice of "rank poison abolitionism," which forced whites to make "negroes of themselves by doing the work in a hot noonday summer sun that negroes ought to do." Slavery, as society's best prophylactic against yellow fever, was thus a "blessing in our Southern States to both races."[96]

"No One Provokes Me with Impunity"

Disease denialists repeatedly lied to potential white settlers about the healthiness of the Deep South, doubtless luring many to their premature deaths. They lied to immigrants in telling them that yellow fever was a

mild ailment and that acclimation was easily attained. They lied to insurers, claiming the South was as healthy or healthier than other regions,
and cast Northern dissenters from this orthodoxy as liars. They also lied
about Black people's perfect safety from yellow fever. Even though disease denialism was internally inconsistent—and obviously incompatible
with reality—it became a fundamental worldview among whites in New
Orleans. To concede that the Cotton Kingdom was diseased would have
undercut a series of powerful, interconnected myths about bodies, commodities, and whiteness on which their slave society was founded, at a
time when sectional tension was at a breaking point. To disease denialists, it did not matter if Black immunity was fiction. Deploying the
language of objective "science," of reason and epidemiological certainty,
was a fantastic trump card—a way to bend a lethal environment into
a state; a way to establish that on Black people, as South Carolina planter
and politician William Harper put it, "nature has indelibly written—
slave."[97]

Nevertheless, professing total confidence in something so clearly untrue
required a fantastic capacity for cognitive dissonance, compartmentalization,
and ability to dismiss contrary evidence as false or malevolently inspired.
Even those who doubted whether New Orleans really was healthy for white
people concluded that boosterism was proper. The ends—redemption of
the South's reputation and its economic progress—justified the means.
Dr. E. H. Barton, once a lonely voice in the wilderness arguing for health
reform, illustrated how the need to adhere to and bolster the dominant ideology could produce striking mental about-faces. In an 1856 speech before
the Academy of Sciences at New Orleans—excerpted in newspapers across
the country and reprinted in full in *De Bow's Review*—Barton now sought
to redeem the reputation of the "much slandered southern States" by ex-
amining the respective climate, health, and commodity output of North
and South. Barton found the South superior in all respects, noting that
Southern diseases—from fevers to intestinal ailments—were mainly of a
"*preventable* nature." And while some ill-health could be avoided through
public projects like improved drainage, most important of all was "private
hygiene."[98] Barton tied this complete reversal of his earlier position into a
meditation on "our *peculiar domestic* institution," a benevolent and recip-
rocal arrangement in which Black people were improved and whites lived
longer. Barton concluded, "The south is accused of weakness, indolence,
and effeminacy" but it need not "shrink in comparison with the northern

portion of this Union," as "*Here,* in fact, resides the goose which lays the golden eggs." Not only did Southerners make all Americans rich, but also, Barton said, the South was "comparatively free from sectarian disagreements, no bigotry, no ridiculous humbugs about women's rights, false philanthropy or pseudo religion, each attends to his own business." The South, then, should be proud of its leviathan-like successes, especially as so many obstacles—disease, Northern ingratitude, and abolitionist meddling—had been thrown up to prevent it.[99]

Barton had tossed aside his earlier calls for health reform, falling in line with his Southern brethren. "The Scotch motto, 'nemo me impune lacessit'"—no one provokes me with impunity—"is the instant impulse of every true southron," he said, "when he sees his country assailed" by graceless and ungrateful Northerners. This "little quarrel" about health, value, and resources between North and South, Barton continued, should be "decided by the proverbial good common sense of our people, by a proper array of facts, not prejudices." Barton, of course, was not actually interested in facts by this point, at least not too many facts and certainly not facts harmful to his case. Thus, he ended with a rallying cry that would soon become common across the South: "The value of the Union to us is above all price; but that of liberty, which, we are determined, shall not be endangered."[100]

6

Incumbent Arrogance

When Louisiana seceded from the United States in January 1861, the now six-state-strong Confederate States of America was relieved. Louisiana's secession secured for the South the port city of New Orleans, along with the Deep South's millions of pounds of slave-grown cotton and sugar. This gave the South leverage. American cotton—the majority of which flowed through New Orleans—by the late 1850s accounted for 77 percent of the 800 million pounds bought by British mills, 90 percent of the 192 million pounds purchased by France, and 92 percent of the 102 million pounds milled by Russia. In 1860—a banner year—the combined value of all cotton and sugar receipts at New Orleans amounted to more than $500 million, making it the United States' second largest export city, behind New York. Cotton meant power, perhaps enough power even to coax Europeans to recognize the South as an independent, sovereign nation. As South Carolina senator and planter James Henry Hammond put it, "No power on earth dares to make war upon it. Cotton *is* King."[1] But because New Orleans was an economic and military lynchpin for the Confederacy, recapturing it was a chief Union goal—key to General Winfield Scott's Anaconda Plan to strangle the Confederacy through a naval blockade. It did not take long for the United States to re-seize "the elephant." In April 1862, New Orleans fell.[2]

New Orleanians did not take well to Union occupation. Many harbored hopes that "his Saffron Majesty" would deliver them from the military governorship of Union major-general Benjamin F. Butler; that, come summer, yellow fever would kill off so many Yankee soldiers that the North would abandon the city. That spring, prayers were put up in church for plague and Jefferson Davis to save New Orleans from its suffering, in full earshot of worshipping US officers. Schoolchildren taunted privates with songs, including "Yellow Jack will grab them up and take them all away." Newsboys set up next to patrols and whispered loudly, "Jimmy, have yer heard the news? . . . They have got the 'yeller' fever down in Frenchtown prime . . . The Yanks will catch it awful." One citizen approached Union soldiers with a tape measure, telling the boys in blue that he had a contract from headquarters for making ten thousand coffins—he needed a rough idea of their height so he could get a head start.[3]

Most of the 5,000 Union soldiers stationed in and around New Orleans in the late spring of 1862—boys who had come of age to horror stories about the Great Epidemic of 1853—felt their days in this "death-giving region" were numbered. Most had never traveled this far south before, and, making Union leadership nervous, nearly all Northern soldiers were "full-blooded, fresh-lipped men, as entirely unacclimated" to yellow fever "as could possibly be found."[4] Like a century of visitors, Union soldiers were utterly appalled by New Orleans's "perfect nastiness." They gasped at open sewers flowing "to and fro with the tide in the blazing sun," groaned at the fetid green puddles, and gagged at the ghastly smells emanating not just off the levee but around all government buildings. In fact, New Orleans was so obnoxious that some soldiers believed civilians were conspiring to worsen the city's sanitary condition so that Yellow Jack could lay claim to his "hereditary rights."[5] Battle-hardened officers became so agitated at the prospect of an epidemic that they presented General Butler with "every excuse"—headaches, backaches, toothaches—to be discharged from duty in New Orleans. Butler grew so exasperated that he threatened to publish their requests for leave, alongside his denial, in his new official newspaper.[6]

Butler—already famous for establishing the first field policies concerning "contrabands of war" at Fort Monroe in Virginia—was an intensely pragmatic (if egotistical) man. He too was concerned about yellow fever and the vast numbers of unacclimated men in his army, especially as none of his surgeons had seen the "hideous foe" before. Seeking to avoid an epidemic catastrophe, he consulted with local doctors hoping to tap into their vast reserves of knowledge about tropical disease. But he was shocked by how little even veteran physicians—those with decades of experience practicing medicine in New Orleans—knew or cared about yellow fever. He was likewise disturbed by the commercial elite's seeming indifference to epidemics. Merchants shrugged off Butler's inquires with "Why, what is the matter? It is always so." It was the attitude of public officials that troubled him most. The superintendent of streets and canals insisted that there was nothing unusual about the city's filthy condition, telling Butler "he didn't know of anything that could be done or why anything should be done, and he had been there a great many years." Simply, acclimation was, and had always been, New Orleans's sole public health strategy. Just ignore the animal carcasses bobbing in the canal and the unbearable stench, public officials said—and hope for the best.[7]

Not one for sitting and waiting, Butler issued a string of General Orders that flew in the face of all New Orleans's public health precedents. First, he established a strict quarantine station below the city and doubled the salary of the quarantine officer. Merchants protested as usual. They clamored that quarantine would only constrict their already throttled business; exports had dropped from $500 million in 1860 to just $52 million in 1862 because of the Union embargo. But Butler remained firm. Next he ordered heads of household to sanitize their homes, to the satisfaction of a military inspector. Butler also wrote to Mayor John T. Monroe, a vehemently proslavery Know-Nothing, instructing him that civilian health was a municipal, not a military, matter. Noting the many vulnerable women and children trapped in town—as well as the swelling numbers of now-idle cotton clerks and bookkeepers—Butler insisted that Monroe appropriate funds to hire 2,000 laborers at a rate of 50 cents per day to clean the city, protect its health, and give jobs to the unemployed. Monroe delayed, eventually responding that the city could afford to employ just 300 men. Eventually, the city council refused to hire anyone.[8]

Bristling, Butler issued Order No. 25. This chastised wealthy politicians as disloyal obstructionists indifferent to the welfare of the poor. It also levied new taxes on elites and distributed supplies of seized Confederate beef and sugar to the unemployed. Louisiana's scandalized governor, Thomas Overton Moore, eighty miles away in Baton Rouge, sought to rally the dissatisfied poor whites of New Orleans back to the Confederacy's cause, stating that Butler "comes from a section of the country that has done more than any other to degrade and cheapen labor and reduce the laboring man to the condition of the slave . . . He wishes to prejudice you against those in authority by falsehood and slanderous misrepresentations."[9] Butler reacted to Moore's remonstrance by moving faster: he mobilized teams of men to scrub and sanitize the city; censored the pro-Confederate press; investigated foreign diplomats for specie-hoarding; raised three regiments of Black infantry; and arrested seditious whites. In May, Butler threw Mayor Monroe and various city councilors in jail.[10]

Butler's reforms worked. Only two cases of yellow fever appeared in the summer of 1862, demonstrating, as Butler said in his farewell address, "that the pestilence can be kept from your borders." In ensuing war years, only sporadic cases appeared. Under the command of Union general Nathaniel P. Banks, two yellow fever deaths were reported in 1863, six in 1864, and one in 1865—a great triumph considering that over 100,000 mostly unacclimated soldiers passed through the port each war year.[11] Probably more died from it than the official record reflected. As one Union soldier wrote in an "objectionable" (censored) letter in 1863, yellow fever was spreading among Union troops though "it is considered a crime to mention it." Most soldiers were likely surprised to agree with New York corporal Ambert O. Remington, who wrote to his worried parents, "We are very pleasantly situated here . . . as New-Orleans has entirely recovered from the *plague* of twelve years ago." "Not *one* (U.S.) has died of yellow fever, this season," a healthy reality, said Remington, that was nothing short of a miracle.[12]

Congress approved the Militia Act in July 1862, allowing—"for the purpose of constructing intrenchments, or performing camp service or any other labor, or any military or naval service for which they may be found competent"—the enlistment of "persons of African descent" in the Union army. Following this and the 1863 Emancipation Proclamation, over 200,000 Black men—80 percent formerly enslaved—enrolled in the US military, mostly from the border states.[13] But the War Department was especially glad to see surging enlistments in the Lower Mississippi Valley; Black men, as Navy Secretary Gideon Welles put it, could provide ample "acclimated labor" for ships' crews.[14] Still others in the military considered the deployment of acclimated Black men essential around Natchez and Vicksburg, where more than half of the nonacclimated soldiers ordered to construct a canal had died of fevers in 1862.[15] If these Black men were furnished "with white officers of skill and accustomed to the climate, who shall drill and discipline them," as the pro-Union *Natchez Daily Courier* put it, there was no good argument against the *"enrollment and arming"* of Black men. "They have been employed in the ranks of the Confederates themselves; they make good and tractable soldiers," and moreover, the *Courier* continued, "we can safely reckon not only on their fidelity, but on their immunity from climatic diseases."[16]

Many white Northern military leaders, including Ulysses S. Grant, uncritically accepted that all Black recruits from the Deep South were "acclimated"—that all could survive a stint on the "fever breeding coast of Secessia."[17] But eerily echoing the logic of Southern slaveholders, the military brass saw whites as the chief beneficiaries of Black immunity. In this logic, Black acclimation was primarily useful not as a personal protective asset for the Black soldiers who possessed it, but as a means to protect *white* soldiers' lives and increase their glory. In May 1862, for example, Benjamin Butler justified mustering Black men on the grounds that his white soldiers could not "stand the climate" of lower Louisiana, "therefore the negroes must be freed and armed as an acclimated force." Nathaniel Banks authorized raising eighteen Black regiments of the *Corps d'Afrique,* though he did not intend to use these men in battle. "The Government makes use of mules, horses, uneducated and educated white men, in the defense of its institutions," he argued. "Why should not the negro contribute whatever is in his power for the cause in which he is as deeply interested as other men?"[18]

Acclimation, General Henry Halleck told Grant in 1863, meant Black soldiers could safely do the drudgery work of war while allowing white men to fight. If Black soldiers could hold key posts along "the Mississippi during the sickly season," and work as "laborers, teamsters, cooks, &c." said Halleck, it would "afford much relief to our armies." Colonel Thomas Ewing of Kansas described how Black acclimation could be marshalled for white benefit in the starkest terms: "The trenches will be dug by black men, and not by whites . . . hereafter, when the [white] soldier dies, he will die from wounds received in the glorious shock of arms, and not from fever and fatigue in the foul swamps. He will fall beneath the folds of his Country's flag, and not toiling under the fierce sun where the acclimated negro can labor without injury."[19]

Black soldiers resented that white officers used their alleged immunity to demote them from brave freedom fighters to a blue-clad support crew for white soldiers.[20] Grave- and trench-digging were tasks of drudgery akin to their work while enslaved; they were not the jobs, they imagined, assigned to valued soldier-citizens. Such a racial caste system within the army was insulting, especially as Black soldiers earned significantly less than white soldiers, and, because of disease and battle, suffered a higher overall death rate. And, despite what white military leaders said, not all Black soldiers or sailors were acclimated. Yellow fever, along with smallpox and typhus, killed many of them, as well as their family members who were still trapped in contraband camps or on plantations (75 percent of the enslaved were still in slavery by the Battle of Appomattox). As Olivier Blanchard, who had been enslaved in Louisiana as a young boy, remembered, "The yellow fever came durin' that war and kill lots. All the big plantation have the grave-yard for the cullud people. That fever so bad they get the coffin ready before they dead."[21] This war might have ultimately destroyed slavery. But it did not destroy yellow fever, nor did it stamp out the practice of manipu-lating disease for racially expedient ends.

Too Little, Too Late

Over the four years of Civil War, about 752,000 people had died.[22] Not only were approximately a quarter of the Confederacy's white men of mili-tary age dead by 1865, two-thirds of assessed southern wealth had vanished. Large parts of the South were ill prepared for recovery. Two-fifths of southern livestock had been destroyed or confiscated and half its farm machinery had been destroyed, thousands of miles of railroad had been torn up, and thou-sands of farms were in disrepair. Many plantations were strewn with de-caying bodies and corroding bullets, and had been overtaken by weeds. When one white planter eyed the destroyed cane fields west of New Orleans, he la-mented: "I felt as if in a funeral procession . . . This vast country, once the Eden of America, is a desert over which the weeds of mourning flourish and the clouds of sorrow weep." In 1860 New Orleans had been the foremost transshipment point for the nation's cotton, sugar, and tobacco from the Mis-sissippi Valley. But after four years of war and the boom in industry to the north and west, New Orleans's once dominant position was in jeopardy. Its banks, which had prospered from providing capital to the plantation South, now held worthless notes. As the Confederate dollar collapsed, cotton factor-ages on the levee faced ruin; many shut their doors. The steamboat trade had been seriously disrupted by military campaigns along the Mississippi. What white Louisianans lamented most of all, however, was that this war had de-stroyed the institution that had underwritten southern prosperity for two centuries. Following the ratification of the Thirteenth Amendment, in De-cember 1865, more than four million people were permanently freed from slavery across the nation—more than 331,000 in Louisiana.[23]

White planters had never needed slavery—they had just wanted it.[24] And to unionists, Republicans, freedmen, and carpetbaggers, Reconstruction offered an unprecedented opportunity for southern states and cities to rebuild modern industrial economies *without* enslaved labor. In time, radicals imagined, northern capital would return to the South, railways would be extended, port cities would be dredged to accommodate larger ships, infrastructure would be modernized, and the landscape would slowly recover. The political landscape would also be repaired and modernized as freedpeople went to school and participated in a contract-based economy, and as Black men began to vote and take up political office. To Democrats and their affiliates, however, Reconstruction was an abomination. Once again, New Orleans's white political elite looked to yellow fever as justification for blocking changes to society and citizenship in the post-emancipation order. While Radical Reconstruction, at least for a time, sought to establish a new kind of American citizenship, immunocapitalists fought furiously to keep alive the old way of doing things: worshipping King Cotton while accommodating Yellow Jack, subjugating Black people and the unacclimated, and always aiming for maximum personal benefit.

To mobilize the old system of immunocapitalism within this new political economy, postwar elites found they needed different tools to dominate, but they were determined to try. Now they massaged the logics of racial immunity to meet the needs of the post-emancipation order. Louisiana planters had long insisted that without Black *slavery,* the Lower Mississippi would revert to a wilderness. But looking back to the glory days of the Confederacy, apologists now claimed that Blackness had not been the key to yellow fever resistance; instead, *enslavement* had been. They invoked the high postbellum mortality rate of freedpeople to "prove" that Black people were incapable of full citizenship or capitalist participation. Just as they had misrepresented science to justify slavery before the war, the white elite now manipulated acclimation and its mysteries to attack their Reconstruction enemies and undercut them politically. They systematically distorted how yellow fever worked and spread misinformation about epidemics. They once again climate-gerrymandered to effectively disenfranchise Black people, carpetbaggers, and Republicans. Thus, yellow fever was re-weaponized to entrench white, neo-confederate power, taking its place alongside harsher methods of postbellum oppression such as obstructionist lawsuits, Black Codes, and terroristic violence.

Postwar elites maintained the arrogance of the incumbent: that New Orleans's past advantage dictated its future prosperity. They were sure the Crescent City would always dominate St. Louis or Atlanta, just as other nations would always prefer American cotton to Egyptian or Indian. The city's position at the mouth of the Mississippi was their trump card against disruptive market shifts, they maintained—even against modernity itself. Geographic determinism had always been at the foundation of the elite worldview, the belief that New Orleans's position—and therefore commercial future—was fixed. But what if geography, an advantage in the steamboat era, became a disadvantage in the railroad age? As it became increasingly clear to immigrants and capitalists abroad that yellow fever risk was a drag on Louisiana's progress, the state's commercial-civic elite remained remarkably blind to the sea changes in transportation, health, and commerce taking place around them, transformations that in fact had already been happening by the 1850s.

First, the postwar Yellow Fever South no longer had a fixed and enslaved labor force. The city experienced an upsurge in its Black population, as people from the countryside flocked to southern cities where opportunities were more abundant.[25] But with freedom to move, tens of thousands of "Exodusters" also fled Louisiana's political repression and white supremacist violence for the farmlands and cities of Illinois and Kansas. Second, New Orleans's attractiveness to immigrants was declining. By the 1870s, European immigration had dropped off precipitously as people increasingly bypassed the sickly South for other places of opportunity like the Middle West—where the land was plentiful and yellow fever was absent.[26] Third, by the 1870s, Chicago, St. Louis, and Atlanta could compete with New Orleans in the cotton trade, their multiple railroad lines transporting product faster and more reliably than New Orleans–bound steamships. By the 1870s much of the product and people that had once fueled the Crescent City's growth had moved elsewhere. Staring the unsustainability of their racially stratified, immigration-dependent system in the face, some whites tried to tie Black people to the land as sharecroppers. Others imported "coolie" laborers from China. Even still, the labor force shrank. As Edward Henry Durell, a Republican wartime mayor of New Orleans, had prophesied: "What is this miserable city to the growing giant of the West?"[27]

The death knell for immunocapitalism came after the 1878 epidemic, which killed 5,000 in New Orleans and 20,000 across the Mississippi delta. New Orleans' elites tried to absorb these deaths as tragic but unavoidable, just as they always had. But they were shocked to find that merchants in Memphis, planters around Galveston, and shopkeepers in Natchez held *them* responsible for the scope and deadliness of this region-wide epidemic. And now these smaller cities in the Yellow Fever South could take their business elsewhere; they no longer had to swallow New Orleans's health backwardness as their status quo or take unnecessary mortality in stride. Without slavery, sufficient immigration to replace the dead, and with New Orleans's cotton-market dominance waning, immunocapitalism could no longer be justified or sustained. Staring irrelevancy in the face, city leaders finally, reluctantly adopted the sanitarian's mantra: that "Public Health is Public Wealth."[28] But these changes were much too little, much too late. New Orleans, once the great southern metropolis, was fading into a necropolitan backwater.

Same Disease, Old Tricks

If the white elites of New Orleans had honestly reflected on the city's Civil War experience, they would have seen that many of their fundamental truths about disease were baseless. The war had proved that Black people were not entirely immune to yellow fever; that the city's health could be improved; that quarantines were effective; and that northern critics of their system were not ignorant quacks but actually had some good ideas. To shake its image as a backward, sickly city and to position itself for future prosperity, New Orleans and its hinterlands required a number of things to happen quickly. New Orleans needed a reliable laboring population to pick and process cotton; a speedy inflow of capital from the North and Europe to modernize its infrastructure and diversify its economy; and a return of river-based steamboat traffic to prewar levels. Perhaps above all, New Orleans would need new rail connections, and to repair the Jackson and Opelousas lines that had been damaged and degraded by the war.[29]

In fact, New Orleans was in as good a position as any southern city— better, even—to bounce back from the war. Having been occupied early, it suffered little structural damage. No other major southern city escaped so intact. Large portions of Atlanta, Charleston, Vicksburg, and Richmond had been razed by shellfire. By many metrics, in fact—health, infrastructure, and population—New Orleans had actually *improved* during the war. Indeed, the city had never been so clean or healthy as in 1865. Perhaps *because* New Orleans had suffered so little damage in the war, and because its leading citizens associated its current cleaner condition with the "Beast"

Butler and Northern despotism, they did not take the South's defeat as a prompt to rethink the city's purpose and prospects. Instead, the postwar merchant elite—essentially indistinguishable from its prewar counterpart—were hyperfocused on resurrecting the river-dependent cotton economy and reinstituting slavery in all but name, even if that meant a return of yellow fever.

Under wartime occupation, Louisiana's board of health had been converted into a military bureau with the Department of the Gulf's medical director serving as its president. After New Orleans was returned to civilian control in March 1866, the state's health board reverted to its prewar form, with six members appointed by the governor and three by the New Orleans city council. This reconstituted board of health was "not a Reconstruction body" concerned with progressive health improvement. Instead it focused on protecting the health of the reemerging cotton industry and thus "delayed and protracted their actions" on all health questions, especially quarantine. The hotheaded wartime mayor John T. Monroe, once jailed and exiled by Butler but reelected to the mayoralty in 1866, supported a policy of public health cheapness. He also stacked the police force with specially pardoned former Confederates, men who showed little interest in promoting the public's health and much interest in harassing freedpeople.[30]

Predictably, filth returned. The *Picayune* reported that the city lacked a "health police" and nobody was enforcing any sanitation rules. By August 1866 one doctor commented that "the city is now filthy in the extreme."[31] Provost-Marshall James Bowen, who had served for two years in the Union army in New Orleans, predicted that "with the usual lax administration of such laws by civil authority, the city will once again be subject to [yellow fever's] visitation." Dr. Edward Fenner agreed, writing that the city's recent cleanup represented a "Herculean task," though a futile one for New Orleans in the long term, as only the "military despotism" of General Butler "would have accomplished it."[32]

These prophecies proved correct. Cholera and yellow fever killed hundreds in 1866, coinciding with a brutal massacre in which ex-Confederates killed dozens of Black people at Louisiana's Constitutional Convention. And in 1867 New Orleans suffered through its worst yellow fever epidemic since 1858. In late August of that year, General Philip S. Sheridan—commanding officer of the federal forces in Louisiana—telegraphed Washington that yellow fever was again epidemic in New Orleans, though local health authorities and the city's press remained unconcerned. The *Pic-ayune* prodded the city to repeal the quarantine, called it a "folly," and re-minded readers that "seventy-seven deaths in a week"—seven-eighths of them unacclimated Europeans and northerners—"does not create much alarm in a community that has suffered in the same space of time to the number of twelve hundred." And besides, this iteration of the disease, unlike that of 1853, was "mild" and "easily managed."[33]

The press was characteristically unfazed, but many townspeople were scared, especially the many freedpeople who had flocked into New Orleans from its plantation hinterlands. Many of these unacclimated people were destitute and, when sick, forced to depend on feeble institutions within this city's already second-class health care system. Though they could go to the frightful Charity Hospital, most Black people received their care at the newly established Freedmen's Hospital on the east side of town, adminis-tered by the radical—though overstretched and underfunded—Freedmen's Bureau. Established by the War Department by an act of March 3, 1865, and its charter extended twice by acts in 1866 and 1868, the Freedmen's Bu-reau was the South's primary welfare institution for the emancipated mil-lions who had no land, education, or money. It was tasked with serving the needs of the destitute, establishing schools, negotiating labor contracts, helping Black soldiers and sailors collect pensions and back pay, and re-uniting families torn apart by war and the domestic slave trade. Health was a major concern of the Bureau, especially in the immediate aftermath of the war as massive smallpox epidemics ripped through contraband camps and communities of unvaccinated freedpeople, killing thousands.[34]

While medical facilities were thin on the ground for Black people across the rural South, larger cities like Richmond and New Orleans did have Black hospitals with professional staffs and dispensaries that provided med-ical care for a nominal charge. Patient records from the Freedmen's Hos-pital in New Orleans display a wide array of sicknesses, many of them crowd diseases or ailments exacerbated by malnutrition and poverty. Each year, cholera, syphilis, pneumonia, hepatitis, and tuberculosis killed hundreds. Each August, fevers of all description—ship, scarlet, intermittent, and remittent—filled the wards. In October 1867 the hospital's chief surgeon described the abject filthiness of the establishment. "For the last three Sunday nights," Dr. David MacKay wrote, "the scavengers employed to clean the sinks attached to this Hospital have, instead of removing the filth, emptied a part of it into the canal . . . a proceeding very detrimental to health of patients in our Hospital and persons living in the neighborhood." Other administrators commented that hospital conditions mirrored those that freedpeople were forced to live in all the time. After inspecting a home on Julia Street filled with feverish Black patients, the surgeon-in-chief noted the "wretched sanitary condition" of the premises, complete with "an unsightly heap of decomposing and putrescent vegetable & animal matter, which cannot but breed disease." Moreover, he wrote, "the sink or privy is filled, and the stench from it is unendurable."[35]

Over 3,300 people died in New Orleans from yellow fever in 1867 (including 200 occupying Union soldiers), one hundred times more than had died in the battle to recapture New Orleans in 1862. Most of the dead were white northerners and Europeans. Approximately 150 Black victims of yellow fever entered the Freedmen's Hospital and dozens died from it there. If this information was known, bureaucrats noted the dead's names, age, nativity, marital status, the name of their former owner, and their cause of death. But so much was unknown. Theodore (age thirty) and Williams (age twenty)—no last names mentioned—died of yellow fever in September 1867. Probably they, like many Black victims that year, had only just arrived in the city, perhaps to reunite with family or to find a job in an economy in turmoil. Matilda Taylor, a twenty-three-year-old woman from Kentucky, died of yellow fever in mid-October 1867, as did Leander Claire, a twenty-four-year-old man from Georgia.[36] Their bodies were carted to the lonely and secluded Freedmen's Cemetery, just downriver at Chalmette, the site where Andrew Jackson won his victory over the British in 1815.

The official reaction to the epidemic of 1867 was a facsimile of the past. Most politicians fled town when the epidemic ramped up in August, and most health officers still clung to anti-contagionism. Willfully forgetting just how well quarantine had worked during the war, some health officers insisted *during* the 1867 epidemic that there was no evidence that yellow fever was imported, and therefore quarantine was useless. Besides, the *Picayune* reasoned, "why shut the door of the sheep pen, now that the wolf has come in!" Even Stanford Chaillé—a professor at Tulane Medical School, later head of the 1879 US Havana Yellow Fever Commission, and one of the most respected voices on yellow fever in postbellum New Orleans—concluded that quarantines had historically "proved worse than useless."[37]

Much of the bill for this epidemic was footed by philanthropic northerners and firms, who sent funds to the Howard Association to alleviate townspeople's suffering. The ultraconservative *Bee* thanked "our friends of the North," adding the tongue-in-cheek rejoinder that northern "Charity"— not northerners' physical presence—"is the noblest and most effectual means for our reconstruction." Once more, the dead mattered less than the cotton crop. By 1867 the cotton economy was showing renewed vigor, even though a hurricane hurt many farmers' crops and the larger South was gripped by a postwar depression. New Orleans exported just under 200,000 bales in 1864–1865 but 867,316 in 1866–1867. The city's press continued to downplay disease—obsessing instead about the politics of Radical Reconstruction—and extolled New Orleans's commercial prospects glowingly: the city was rapidly restoring its "lost prosperity," said the *Picayune,* and New Orleans would once again "become, one of the most important shipping and commercial points in the country."[38]

Cracks

The response to the epidemic of 1867 was predictable. The leaders of New Orleans used their old playbook and thought it would work. But they did not catch on that southern trading and immigration patterns were reorienting. Atlanta, Georgia, for example, had been reduced to rubble during the war. But the municipality had invested in railroads, courted northern investment, modernized and diversified its economy, and constructed new commercial facilities. All five of Georgia's railroads—largely destroyed during Sherman's March to the Sea in 1864—were functional again by 1866, pumping cotton in and out at a fiery pace. Atlanta's rapid postwar growth, in fact, was a bellwether of national trends. In 1855 the railroads had carried only 7,661 bales of cotton from the Mississippi Valley to the East; by 1860 that number exceeded 108,000 bales.[39] Railroads were set to displace steamboats as the cheapest and most efficient way to transport bulky commodities. Mississippi had just three railroad lines in 1853, but within twenty-five years, 1,127 miles of track crisscrossed the state. These railroads largely bypassed New Orleans and drained trade away from it.[40]

New Orleans's merchants were also too slow to notice the telegraph wires following these tracks, providing connections that gave new relevance to inland market towns—New Iberia, Grenada, Shreveport, and Memphis. The multiple country stores, warehouses, and taverns popping up around rural rail stations also signified a localization of cotton marketing.[41] For the first time, inland merchants could trade directly with the North and bypass the trading firms in coastal cities that had traditionally monopolized southern commerce. No longer were country planters as reliant on their onetime metropolis, New Orleans, for information and financial services; now they could access almost instantaneous information about the price of goods in Chicago and New York, as well as news of disease outbreaks along the Gulf Coast. Within a decade of the war, Louisiana had built only 200 new miles of track, bringing its grand total to 539 miles. New Orleans found itself unable to compete with St. Louis for access to the expanding cotton trade of East Texas. The *Picayune* issued this warning in 1869: "Texas can do without the railroad to New Orleans, but New Orleans cannot do without the railroad to Texas." The railroad must be "completed quickly to save the Crescent City."[42]

New Orleans probably could have retained more of its prewar market share—and attracted more northern capital for investment—had it dredged its port earlier. The Mississippi River might have been the great American artery, but silt deposits near its mouth had made it inaccessible for larger oceangoing ships. New English steamships, with screw propellers, four-cylinder engines, and massive hulls, had taken over most transatlantic traffic, but they could not safely enter the South's shallower ports, including Richmond, Charleston, and New Orleans. Increasingly, products from the Upper Mississippi Valley diverted via rail to deep-water ports like Baltimore and Norfolk, rendering many merchants in the shallower ports obsolete.[43]

As product flowed away from New Orleans, so did streams of people. The postwar drop in in-migration was a major problem for a society built on replacing the dead with newcomers rather than keeping people alive. Many New Orleans elites grumbled that the "best class of her citizens"—enterprising white yeomen, capitalists, and skilled clerks from Europe—had died during the war and only "the indolent masters remained; the slaves remained; those free whites who were too poor and helpless and ignorant either to desire or to be able to remove, remained." Wary of what stalling immigration would mean for a state based on agriculture, Louisiana's House of Representatives passed Act 105 in 1866, establishing a Bureau of Immigration "for the purpose of encouraging immigration to the State of Louisiana, by diffusing information abroad and protecting and assisting such immigrants as may settle therein." Most of the $15,000 appropriated to the bureau went to salaries, however—the rest was spent on printing promotional literature in English, French, and German. All sponsored materials fell back on familiar denialist canards, stressing the unparalleled commercial advantages of Louisiana and the healthiness of New Orleans. Materials also insisted that Creoles were long-lived, acclimation was easy, and all "gradually adapted to the climate."[44]

In 1869, a correspondent for *Harper's Weekly* attended a meeting of the immigration bureau, reporting that the commissioners passed "rather lightly over the yellow-fever" and resurrected talking points ripped right from the antebellum script. "Louisiana, contrary to the general impression," insisted one commissioner "is shown by the statistics to be one of the most healthy States in the Union." And if New Orleans's "mean of three years unaffected by yellow-fever" was used and compared against the mortality rates of other cities, said another commissioner, immigrants would understand that New Orleans was far healthier—and more prosperous—than New York or Boston. By 1870, the immigration bureau had little to show for its efforts. It was out of money, employed only two agents in Europe, and had succeeded in attracting few newcomers to New Orleans.[45]

Growing increasingly desperate for immigrants by the early 1870s, several boosters more forcefully insisted tradition had wronged New Orleans. One editorialist for the *New-Orleans Times* told outsiders that the "Queen City of the Southwest" had been "terribly victimized" by "ghastly exaggerations" about yellow fever. The writer traced the germ of these falsehoods to antebellum capitalists in New Orleans who, "conscious that they were possessed of special commercial and financial advantages," had "looked upon new-comers with distrust." Not wanting "too many participants" in the "good thing they enjoyed," New Orleans's elites had "encouraged the circulation of romantic tales of the doings of 'Bronze John and his saffron steed,' and of the hair-breadth escapes which all acclimated citizens were supposed to be the heroes of." But now, the *Times* wrote, these "old traditional fancies" could not stand up to census data and statistics which, the writer claimed, showed New Orleans to be the picture of health, "undoubtedly the best landing place for immigrants, bound south or west, to be found in this entire country." With the census showing a "constantly diminishing" death rate, another writer argued, "New Orleans is becoming more and more healthy with every successive lustrum."[46]

These glowing portrayals no longer seemed to have the same attractive effect, at least on white immigrants—especially after the Panic of 1873 reduced the economy even further. In the past, ambitious men had risked their lives for a shot in New Orleans. But now, as travel writer Edward King described in 1875, the "lines of emigrant wagons filled with hard-featured men and women" bypassed the Crescent City, and were instead headed for

Texas and Arkansas.[47] As with all southern ports after the Civil War, immigration to New Orleans diminished to such a degree that, as historian Richard White put it, "the borders of the old Confederacy might as well have been a dam." Indeed, the percentage of foreign-born people in the South—the majority of New Orleans's population in some prewar years—fell sharply between 1860 and the beginning of the twentieth century, with the foreign-born amounting to just 5.3 percent of the population by 1920.[48]

As white immigration tapered off, the city's Black population nearly doubled, with about 23,000 African Americans migrating into New Orleans between 1865 and 1878, seeking new opportunities and safety from terrorism, nightriders, and Ku Klux Klan violence. Economic prospects were better in New Orleans than they were in the countryside, where the no-exit sharecropping system dominated. Between 1860 and 1870, the number of Black sailors and steamboat-men working on the levee grew from 84 to 785; blacksmiths increased from 10 to 89; and coopers increased from 42 to 154.[49] These could be dangerous jobs, but they paid better than farming. Some Black people seem to have been put off from moving to New Orleans because of disease. As freedwoman Lizzie Chandler recalled, "Country people don't get sick like they do in the city."[50] Thus, many more Black Louisianans saw better opportunities—and chances for longevity—farther afield than New Orleans. Some departed for Texas; about 6,000 Exodusters headed for Kansas in 1879, and thousands more left for that state in future years. Small numbers went to Liberia (where many suffered from yellow fever), and a later colonization scheme led by freedman William Ellis brought some Black people to Mexico.[51]

The New Acclimated Citizens

With immigration declining during Reconstruction, the New Orleans job market placed renewed value on the acclimation credential. White jobseekers filled newspapers with declarations of immunity, just as they had before the war. One "Practical business man of 45; energetic, steady, acclimated" sought a position in a New Orleans commission house, noting his willingness to travel to Central America and the West Indies. A "competent and acclimated book-keeper" with good references and a willingness to work for a very small salary sought any kind of job. Another acclimated and married man of "active business habits," good references, and familiarity with business "in Louisiana, Mississippi, Texas and Alabama" desired a position in a cotton house. He promised he could "influence consignments from a desirable class of shippers."[52] The message to job-seeking whites had not changed: only the acclimated need apply.

But what of the value of Black acclimation in New Orleans's new political and economic context? Before the war, enslaved Black people's disease risk and reward accrued to whites. This was no longer the case post-emancipation, nor was there consensus on whether innate racial immunity actually existed, what that meant for the future of labor and how agriculture should be organized, or whether immunity meant Blacks as well as whites deserved to be "citizens." Immediately after the war, some whites sought to rewrite all the rules about yellow fever and privilege. Black people had been immune before the war, they said, but were now—somehow—as liable to yellow fever as whites. "In old times," one writer in the *Picayune* claimed, "the negroes were accredited with an almost total exemption from yellow fever. Who ever heard of a darky having yellow fever? was the common remark." But after emancipation, the writer claimed that Black men, having been told "that among his 'constitutional rights' is the right to have yellow fever like a white man . . . is exhibiting everywhere a liability to take it."[53] This development, the writer said, was "truly astonishing." Some doctors agreed that *enslaved* people had enjoyed an "absolute exemption" from yellow fever or at least "very rarely" had it before 1853; but *freedmen* were proving "more and more subject to it." This "remarkable" development, as Dr. William Holcombe assured readers of the *Southern Literary Messenger,* was "quite a puzzle to medical philosophers." Holcombe's theory was that Black people's constitutions in the United States had gradually become "de-Africanized," a process that made freedpeople susceptible to yellow fever as well as many other diseases.[54]

Some whites claimed Black people's "new" susceptibility had nothing to do with "de-Africanization" and everything to do with emancipation. Tobias Gibson, a Mississippi-born cotton and sugar planter with thirty-six years of experience in Louisiana, testified in 1865 before the Smith-Brady Commission in Washington (investigating corruption in the South), "We never had the yellow fever or cholera on our plantations, because our police regulations were such that fewer negroes died than white men." Gibson believed this reflected well on him and the planter class in general; that white enslavers had proved skillful stewards of Black health. But it was also a tacit assertion that Black people were unprepared for freedom, untutored in how to preserve their own health, and would "die out" in time.[55]

This extinction hypothesis, put forward by Gibson and many others, was part of a much larger discourse surrounding emancipation and Black health during and after the Civil War. It was born of the fact, as shown in medical reports, that many freedpeople did suffer through staggering epidemics of smallpox and cholera. Many people's first experience of legal freedom, in fact, was accompanied by sickness and death because federal and state governments, as well as the Union army, shirked responsibility for Black health. Contraband camps were rife with disease and violence, housing conditions were everywhere cramped, and Black people were malnourished, immunosuppressed, and often not innoculated against smallpox. But these materially terrible conditions were manipulated by white ex-Confederates into a narrative about innate Black degeneracy and inferiority. One writer to the *Liberator,* the nation's most widely circulated anti-slavery newspaper, saw through this thinly veiled proslavery apologia, and described the true "paternity" of this extinction theory: "If the emancipation of the negro is destined to result only in his extinction, 'the sacred institution' is justified in its name, and its overthrow is not a blessing but a curse."[56]

Others rejected Holcombe's "de-Africanization" model, asserting that all Black people, in slavery or freedom, were extraordinarily resistant to yellow fever. Dr. Harvey L. Bird insisted in 1873 that "*black vomit*" could not infect "a genuine negro."[57] The president of the Louisiana Board of Health, Dr. Joseph Holt, maintained that Black people were "constitutionally" immune, remarking after the 1878 epidemic that "the exemption of the negro race" from yellow fever was striking, and noting that 569 whites had died in one district of New Orleans compared with "only twenty-nine" Black people. Dr. Chaillé turned to the census for answers. He concluded that Black people had been dying in greater numbers since emancipation, with Black mortality greater than white mortality in every instance "except during yellow fever epidemics."[58]

Black people's views on their own immunity (or lack thereof) extended across the spectrum. Freedman Henry Pettus from Georgia and later Arkansas, for example, remembered that yellow fever became more serious for Black people after emancipation. Earlier in his life, "chills was my worst worry in these swamps," Pettus recalled, but in 1875, "yellow fever come on. Black folks didn't have yellow fever at first but they later come to have it. Some died of it. White folks had died in piles." Walter Jones related that the "biggest thing" that ever happened to him was surviving yellow fever, in an epidemic that killed Black and white people alike: "Some of both color got well. A lot of people died." One formerly enslaved man remembered binding white yellow fever patients onto their beds as they went crazy when they fell ill, though Black victims had uniformly milder cases. Others insisted that Black people were entirely immune. Indeed, Rev. Ellis Jefson, who was born in Virginia, enslaved in Mississippi, and moved to Kansas after the war, came to this conclusion while nursing people for five months in Memphis during the epidemic of 1878. Jefson insisted that "Negroes didn't have it . . . I never heard of a case of Yellow Fever . . . [a]mong my race."[59]

After the war, many whites lost interest in trying to provide a rational explanation for innate Black immunity, though they still wanted to maintain a racialized labor hierarchy—and avoid the hardest physical labor themselves. To this end, whites sought new racial and ethnic others to replace Black slaves, and once again tried to use yellow fever to justify their prejudices. A few Louisiana planters imported "coolies" from the "overcrowded districts of Asia" to replace Black labor in cane fields. Held in abject, slavery-adjacent conditions, these "Chinamen" cost sugar planters $80 a year, far less than the thousands of dollars an enslaved person represented before the war. And as one editorialist claimed, coolies, who survive "principally on rice" and are "acclimated to the tropics," could be put to productive use in the sickliest swamps. As the sugar industry tapered off in Lower Louisiana by the 1880s (shifting mostly to Hawaii), however, coolies never constituted a major part of the Reconstruction-era labor force.[60]

Still other planters employed southern Europeans, particularly Sicilians who concentrated in New Orleans's "Little Palermo" neighborhood. Many turned to the most abundant group of outsiders: the Irish, now conveniently held up as impervious to fevers. "I have at last succeeded in getting all the white hands I want," said one planter returning from Vicksburg, "They are all, except one, Confederate soldiers, who went out in 1861, from Louisiana, Alabama, and Mississippi, and were in the ranks at the surrender." This man marveled that these Irishmen were acclimated and not "grog-blossomed or emaciated, with swamp fever." Instead, they were "quite sober, and only take a spree when whisky is convenient . . . They are a stout and stalwart set of pock-marked and bullet scarred veterans, full of spunk, fun and blarney." With labor scarce, J. D. B. De Bow claimed white labor was preferable to Black labor, "when acclimated men can be secured." He noted that a friend he visited employed "fifty blacks and twenty-five whites," and was delighted by the whites as they were "far more reliable than the negroes."[61]

But old habits—and prejudices—die hard. Most whites still maintained that Black people were "preferable, for this part of the country, to any other laborer." One planter described his preference for Black labor this way: "1. He is thoroughly acclimated, and enjoys an immunity from the local diseases which the white man, though native and to the manor born, can never hope to attain." And "2. He is of strong *physique,* inured, almost from his birth . . . to make a comfortable living by manual agriculture." Another white planter summarized the mood in 1866: Black people "can thrive and grow fat on a soil and under a sun where the white man must inevitably weaken and grow sickly."[62] As the old orthodoxy of Black acclimation no longer aligned with the political status quo of emancipation, there was never again a solid white party line on the immunity question. Instead, beliefs remained a muddled array of contradictions, with everyone claiming a scientific basis for their prejudice.

Slaughterhouse, Voting, and Violence

When a twenty-six year-old carpetbagger named Henry Clay Warmoth came to Louisiana and became governor in 1868, he was disgusted by New Orleans and its few paved streets, seeing it as a backward, primitive, once-great metropole that was now "a dirty, impoverished, and hopeless place." Styling himself a champion of free labor, infrastructure, and economic development, Warmoth vowed to repair the city's levees, build sewers, sanitize streets, and rid it of its numerous disgusting slaughterhouses.[63] While some businessmen might have embraced such modernization and believed in the "harmony of interests," others—especially Democrats and neo-Confederates—interpreted Warmoth's economic development plans as a Trojan horse for racial equality, and never accepted the legitimacy of his governorship. His Democratic opponents adopted a "rule or ruin" strategy in opposing his and other Republican's administrations. They used obstructionist lawsuits, racist propaganda, and racial violence—even staging a coup d'état in 1874 at Liberty Place that forced another Republican governor, William Kellogg, to flee the city—claiming at rallies that Radicals and their Black and carpetbagging acolytes were "public enemies trying to impoverish and enslave us."[64]

It was not long before some of Warmouth's reforms were challenged in the highest court in the nation, implicating not only his specific policies but all the Civil War Amendments. The US Supreme Court decided its first

Fourteenth Amendment case with the *Slaughterhouse* decision, handing it down on Easter Sunday 1873—the eighth anniversary of President Abraham Lincoln's assassination and the same day as the Colfax Massacre, in which a white supremacist mob murdered at least 165 Black people in Grant Parish, Louisiana. The seemingly benign *Slaughterhouse* case concerned white butchers, city filth, and unsanitary abattoirs. But as one historian bluntly put it in 1965, "the only thing slaughtered in the Slaughterhouse cases was the right of the Negro to equality."[65]

Slaughterhouse originated in March 1869, when the Louisiana state legislature, then controlled by Republicans, created a corporation to run a central slaughterhouse in New Orleans. Butchers had been a nuisance in the city since the eighteenth century. Animals were herded through the streets and slaughtered in the roads. Offal was then loaded onto leaky open carts that were driven to the "nuisance wharves" and dumped into the Mississippi. Cutting corners, many butchers just discarded bones and blood in their backyards, nearby canals, or street gutters and left them to rot, emitting a foul stench that proved offensive to almost everyone. The new law sought to rectify the nuisance by requiring all of the city's 150 butchers to move across the Mississippi River to a new "grand slaughterhouse" run by the Crescent City Live-Stock Landing & Slaughterhouse Co. Sanitationists lauded this move as excellent for the public's health. But the butchers were furious, and several associations accused the city of creating a monopoly that coerced the "involuntary servitude" of the butchers—in violation of the Thirteenth Amendment—and that it infringed their "right to pursue one's chosen calling" as guaranteed in the equal protection and due process clauses of the Fourteenth Amendment.[66]

How a debate about sanitation, entrails, and monopoly in New Orleans became a test of the federal government's ability to protect the rights of freedpeople was not immediately obvious. But the connection between public health and civil rights certainly fit with tradition in New Orleans. The butchers' case was argued before the US Supreme Court by John A. Campbell. Campbell—a doctor and former US Supreme Court justice himself who had concurred in the 1857 *Dred Scott* decision and resigned his position in 1861 to join the Confederate government—had become New Orleans's most distinguished racist, Reconstruction-hating attorney. Playing off the "wage slavery" trope, Campbell portrayed the white butchers as patriotic citizens who had been made into *slaves* through the reactionary heavy hand of an overzealous government. He was building on the philosophy, common among the prewar New Orleans elite, that viewed any state action aimed at improving the public's health as a tyrannical intrusion on personal and economic freedoms.

In a close 5–4 decision, the Supreme Court rejected the plaintiffs' challenge, maintaining that the purpose of the Thirteenth and Fourteenth Amendments had been to protect former slaves and guarantee their rights of citizenship—not those of white butchers. At the same time, however, it gutted much of the musculature of the Fourteenth Amendment, stating that "privileges and immunities . . . are left to the State government for security and protection, and not by this article placed under the special care of the federal government." This meant that the privileges and immunities clause was effectively removed as a basis for applying the Bill of Rights to the states. Though Campbell technically lost the case, the impact of the verdict was exactly what he had desired: it crippled the federal government's ability to guarantee almost any right of citizenship to Black former slaves. This meant that southern states had the Court's blessing to continue to subjugate freedpeople.[67]

The *Slaughterhouse* litigation was part of a larger campaign waged by Democrats against perceived overreach by the state—that is, by Republicans and carpetbaggers. And Democrats attacked carpetbaggers just as they had attacked Northern abolitionists in the 1850s, constructing them as ignorant outsiders rendered biologically and epidemiologically unwelcome in the South.[68] For example, when government offices in Alabama had to close on account of yellow fever in 1871 because many officials were "tempting food for the disease" (a shorthand for northern-born), one newspaper claimed this was a sign that the South should be returned to home rule. "Nature steps in here and administers a rebuke" to the Republicans, the editorialist wrote, "for sending men down to hold office in the South whom the very climate hates." The writer continued: "Who blames the acclimated Southron for scorning a fellow against whom nature protests and drives disease into his liver and disease into his heart?" The writer closed by claiming that there were plenty of white southern men who could execute the duties of office, who "have no waxed fingers when they handle money, and with whom malaria and yellow jack are on the best of terms."[69]

Democrats also sought to wrest back control at the ballot box, through violence and climate gerrymandering. Black men in the South exercised their suffrage in spite of extraordinary risks—thousands were killed and intimidated during the elections of 1868, 1872, and 1876.[70] But white Democrats again used yellow fever as a tactic of voter suppression, to prevent Black men and known white Republicans from voting. In New Orleans, multiple white and Black people noted that registration dates were moved or arbitrarily truncated throughout the 1860s and 1870s. Some years, registrations were only open in September and October, when yellow fever was present. Dr. Stanford Chaillé, a white man, tried to register in New Orleans on October 28, 1874, and testified that there were one hundred Black men lined up outside the office, some of whom had been waiting on line for nine hours—amid an epidemic. As it took at least fifteen minutes to register each man, some of the men he talked to had been trying and failing to register for seven days. Some simply gave up.[71]

In 1878 one Louisiana planter named J. D. McGill—who had owned 140 slaves before the war though he did not fight in it—told a congressional committee investigating voter suppression that the white people of Tensas Parish (mostly Democrats) had put up a quarantine for several days surrounding the Republican convention. It was "the impression of the [Black] people in the country—not mine particularly," said McGill, that it was a "got up" contrivance. Yellow fever was certainly a problem that summer, but the purpose of this quarantine had been to prevent Black people from participating in politics and get them back to work, dressed up as a health measure. McGill told the committee that Black people "had a habit of going to town, drinking whisky, and wasting their time and doing worse, when they ought to be in the field." Admittedly for selfish reasons, McGill supported this alleged public health measure, though "I was under the impression that it was a sort of a trick myself." This sham quarantine, however, caused much "dissatisfaction among the black people" as they firmly believed "that the quarantine was kept up for the purpose of preventing them from holding their convention; an angel from heaven could hardly convince them to the contrary." McGill concluded his testimony with the admission: "I do not blame them for thinking so."[72]

"Health Is Wealth" to the End of Reconstruction

Following *Slaughterhouse*—as well as multiple yellow fever outbreaks in the city in the 1870s—it was clear to many Americans that New Orleans's reputation for filth and fevers was deserved. Its apathetic city council still maintained ultimate responsibility for public health. Many health officers actively rejected sanitation, quarantine, and the bacteriological revolution overall. In short, the city's official response to disease was much the same as it always had been. But now, outsiders increasingly derided New Orleans's approach as retrograde, even senseless, with some critics noting that rampant disease was accelerating the city's demise. Moreover, *insiders*—white Deep Southerners—increasingly saw through the boosters' playbook: that is, to censor any whisper of yellow fever, lie when epidemics took hold, claim the city had never been healthier, publish sunny anecdotes about successful acclimations, and blame northerners for spreading false rumors. As the Alexandria-based *Louisiana Democrat*—a paper with the tagline "The World Is Governed Too Much"—pronounced in 1871: New Orleans behaved "disingenuously towards the rest of the world when ever the yellow fever makes its appearance in the city." The *Democrat* declared that if it was New Orleans's intention "to inoculate every unacclimated citizen with the disease, to entice to the city every stranger who never had it, and to spread it to all the neighboring towns, their conduct could not be very different from what it now is."[73]

Before the war, people in towns along the lower Mississippi or the Gulf of Mexico seldom criticized New Orleans's approach to health. Simply, New Orleans was the leviathan, and they required the port's services, credit, and products and (rightly) believed public criticism was pointless. But during Reconstruction, inland towns across a larger, railroad-linked Yellow Fever South—a little less reliant on New Orleans for news and trade—could push back. In 1871 Texas governor Edmund Davis established a quarantine at Galveston against vessels approaching from New Orleans, much to the chagrin of Louisiana's merchants. And people in proximate locales, who understood that their health was a function of official decisions made (or not made) in New Orleans, tired of boosters' typical bloviation and whataboutism. As the same Alexandria-based paper pleaded, "We don't care whether it is an indigenous or an imported disease; whether it depends on dirt or cleanliness; whether it is contagious or not; and we would not learn if we could the New Orleans method of determining when it is endemic or epidemic." Rather, "It is time that Medical men were settling down on something definite as to the nature of yellow fever, or else that they admit they know nothing about it."[74]

By Reconstruction's end, some critics *within* New Orleans castigated the city's see-no-evil approach to yellow fever, deriding the still-rigid hierarchy of acclimation—as well as the whole system of immunocapitalism—as antimodern, unsustainable, unnecessarily risky, and cruel. Before the war, acclimated "mechanics, physicians, merchants, [and] servants" the *New*

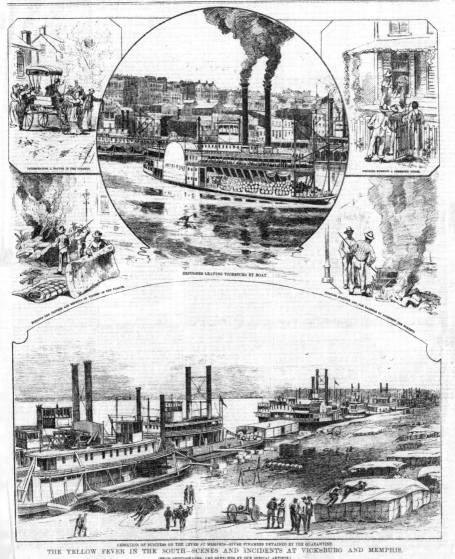

INTERRUPTING A DOCTOR IN THE STREETS.

REFUGEES ENTERING A DESERTED HOUSE.

BURNING THE CLOTHES AND BEDDING OF VICTIMS OF THE PLAGUE.

REFUGEES LEAVING VICKSBURG BY BOAT.

BURNING SULPHUR AND TAR BARRELS TO DISINFECT THE STREETS.

CESSATION OF BUSINESS ON THE LEVEE AT MEMPHIS—RIVER STEAMERS DETAINED BY THE QUARANTINE.

THE YELLOW FEVER IN THE SOUTH—SCENES AND INCIDENTS AT VICKSBURG AND MEMPHIS.

[FROM PHOTOGRAPHS, AND SKETCHES BY OUR SPECIAL ARTISTS.]

The Yellow Fever in the South—Scenes and Incidents at Vicksburg and Memphis, September 16, 1878. The Historic New Orleans Collection.

Orleans Republican opined in 1876, "enjoy[ed] a monopoly of employment, and prices ranged high." But that was during the halcyon days of slavery, booming immigration, steamboats, and cotton, when New Orleans occupied a secure commercial position at the outlet of the Mississippi. Back then, elites felt "no necessity for conciliation" to the urban masses, enslaved people, or to the inhabitants of its hinterlands because the dead could be replaced so easily. Everyone had to pay tribute to New Orleans, either in cotton or with their lives. Yellow fever thus "sustained" white elites' power, said the *Republican,* with the "monopolists return[ing] the compliment by constantly parading the terrors of [yellow fever] in the ears of the unacclimated." Tens of thousands had been lured to their deaths through boosters' deceit, the *Republican* charged. Doctors had likewise acted disingenuously, with "the rich harvest of a yellow fever year . . . too great a temptation for their integrity." Worse, officials derided quarantines, spurned sanitation, and forced the unacclimated to toe the party line that their city was a health spa. To even speak of yellow fever in the antebellum city, in fact, had been considered a slanderous protest against the merchants. Why, the *Republican* asked, would this system be worthy of continuance?[75]

In 1877 all remaining federal troops left New Orleans as Reconstruction ended. By now the anti-infrastructure, anti-public-health factions in power in the city and state governments were confronted by the obvious decline of their position relative to other southern cities. Immigration had all but ended. The city was receiving health criticism from nearby cities upon which, to the merchants' horror, New Orleans was now increasingly dependent. Some merchants grumbled that they would even have agressively court northern capital or face ruination.

Then in 1878, calamity hit. Yet another massive epidemic of yellow fever struck New Orleans and unfurled across the region—reaching towns like Memphis, Tennessee, and Grenada, Mississippi—places that had never had a case of yellow fever before. Approximately 20,000 people died across the Mississippi Valley, 5,000 of them in New Orleans. A further 25,000 people fled. In August—a month into the epidemic—the board of health finally installed a quarantine below New Orleans. "Everyone is caught up in the panic," Ellen Shields of Natchez wrote, even "the negroes, always heretofore fatalists, have caught up; it is frightful the suffering people are going through."[76]

The US House of Representatives estimated that the epidemic of 1878 had cost New Orleans over $12 million. This figure included the cost of ten days of sickness per victim at $3 per day, the cost of funerals at $25 each, the capital value of those who died, commercial losses from paralyzed trade, and trade diversions to other cities. In total, the nation had lost $30 million. But the greatest damage done was to New Orleans's civic credit, a fact city elites could no longer choose to ignore said Ernst von Hesse-Wartegg, an Austro-German aristocrat who published an account of his journeys through the United States in 1879. If New Orleans continued to ignore health, Hesse-Wartegg warned, its once golden reputation as "the proud Queen of the South" would be entirely squandered and replaced with the epithet: "the whore of pestilence, the breeder of Yellow Jack."[77]

Within New Orleans's city government the finger pointing started. The battle was pitched on a Republican–Democratic axis, with Republicans castigated as weak-willed, spendthrift scalawags and Democrats derided as indifferent to disease to the point of manslaughter. The Republican-leaning *Chicago Tribune* reported on these political divisions, declaring that "epidemics only occur under Democratic administration." The last major epidemic in 1867 had happened under Mayor John. R. Conway, a Democrat; the current epidemic could be entirely attributed to the recklessness of the current mayor, Edward Pilsbury, also a Democrat, who had slashed the city's budget and placed his "inexperienced" cronies on the health board, refusing to appoint anyone who had held a commission under a "Radical" governor. The result, the *Tribune* tallied, was that 5,000 people were made unemployed by the epidemic, the region was in chaos, and New Orleans's civic credit was depleted. It also broke the scandal that the Chamber of Commerce and the Cotton Exchange—conservative organizations of mostly Democratic businessmen—had pressured and bribed quarantine officials to push their mail through ahead of all other packages. "States' rights in quarantine matters," the *Tribune* concluded, "have lost their charms to their victims in Louisiana."[78]

Well practiced at deflecting blame, and resolutely opposed to change, Democrats and immunocapitalists insisted that "croakers" and "penny-a-liners" in New York had exaggerated the extent of the epidemic of 1878 to unrecognizable levels. They said outside critics were using this particular disaster to further subjugate the South, extend Reconstruction, and trample their constitutional rights.[79] The *Picayune* responded to the *Chicago Tribune,* noting, "It is true that the City Council might have done better with ampler means." But, practically bellowing from the page, it continued, "The history of the Radical Boards of Health, their attorneys, coal oil inspectors, quarantine physicians and sanitary inspectors" was a history of corruption and overreach, with "the moral odor of the carpet-baggers' dynasty" pervading the city and spoiling what remained of its commercial prospects. The *Picayune* closed with the following: "If, as alleged, there were no epidemics under Radical misrule, it may be counted a dispensation of a merciful Providence that spared us from a double calamity."[80]

But as in 1853, the 1878 epidemic proved too disruptive to sweep under the rug or justify as an act of God. Permanent damage had been done. Now New Orleans was seen as a risky and reckless backwater that few sane outsiders would travel to or invest in. On March 31, 1879, approximately 200 men representing a variety of businesses and religious institutions across New Orleans organized the Auxiliary Sanitary Association, which adopted the Sanitarians' motto as its maxim: "Public Health Is Public Wealth." Their address, "To the Citizens of New Orleans," signed by Dr. E. D. Fenner as well as a shipping agent, a bank president, a tobacco merchant, and an insurance company president, opened with the bold declaration, "Health is capital for a man. It is also capital for a community." The pamphlet unfolded as a call to action. If the city remained unhealthy, its future was in jeopardy, because no metropolis could continue "under the reputation of unhealthiness and hope to prosper." The address tiptoed around accepting blame for the epidemic of 1878, conceding, "It is felt abroad, too, that our city is in a great degree responsible . . . Right or wrong, New Orleans is credited with it all." The Sanitary Association called for a citizen's committee to work with the city council and board of health to promote public health, declaring that citizens should be aware of the "great interest on which the well-being, not only of New Orleans, but of a large part of the Mississippi valley, depends . . . It is the part of philanthropy, of common sense, and of self-interest." These words acknowledged facts that had been all too plain to city residents since the eighteenth century. But they were just words. And they were far too little, and came much too late.[81]

EPILOGUE

Fever and Folly

The privately funded Sanitary Association could not meet the complex requirements of regulating health in a large port city, nor could it act as a liaison between apathetic municipal bodies, the state government, and the commercial sector. Nor was it the proper intermediary for the federal government. In the aftermath of the 1878 epidemic, Congress established the National Board of Health, a new body empowered to investigate sickness and recommend the installation of quarantine in any American port. It faced stringent opposition in New Orleans, especially from the hypersensitive and egotistical president of Louisiana's Board of Health Joseph Jones (a. YF 1878), a professor of chemistry and clinical medicine at the University of Louisiana and one of the city's foremost authorities on yellow fever.

Jones was not anti-quarantine *per se,* but he was against federal power. He said that any federally administered quarantines were "vicious . . . destructive at once of commerce and the best interest of the city." He refused to cooperate with inspectors, calling them "federal spies" hell-bent on damaging New Orleans's reputation. Cities and towns along the Mississippi criticized Jones and his pugilistic approach. One health officer from Memphis called New Orleans "a standing menace to the country," its medical establishment content to elevate the commercial interests of a narrow sliver of city elites above the health of the entire Deep South. Brushing aside such criticism, Jones insisted he was immune to the "threats or demands of citizens, however numerous" and refused to back down. And when in 1883 the quarantine powers of the National Board expired and Congress did not renew its grant of authority, Jones—along with the bulk of New Orleans's businessmen—rejoiced. Stringent quarantine measures were, and would remain, a nonstarter in New Orleans.[1]

Likely because fewer unacclimated immigrants were arriving in New Orleans each year after 1878, yellow fever was not declared officially epidemic again until the 1890s. The editor of the *New Orleans Medical and Surgical Journal*—half pleased, half apprehensive—remarked in 1890 that it had been such a long time since yellow fever had been epidemic, that younger doctors had "never seen a case of yellow fever in their lives."[2] Despite this stretch of improved health, New Orleans continued to lose ground in the cotton market to Atlanta, St. Louis, Memphis, and other interior cities. Its rail network remained unfinished, and when in the 1880s the city completed its rail connection to the prime cotton lands of East Texas, other lines carrying goods, people, and capital elsewhere were already dominant and offered better rates.[3]

Feeling powerless to claw back the cotton market—or perhaps resigned to larger market trends—New Orleans's elites realigned around a curious combination of nostalgia for bygone days and hyper-boosterism. They derided railroads as artificial and rallied people around the symbol of the Mighty Mississippi, the lifeblood that had sustained the South for centuries. "It is a *big* river; it *does* drain the most productive area of the United States," said the *Picayune.* Moreover, the Mississippi was "always open," meaning that it could not "fall into the hands of [railroad] monopolists." Although it was "true that the Mississippi route is the longer one," the *Picayune* reasoned, "it is clear that the element of cheapness must become a superior consideration over that of time." In 1879 the Army Corps of Engineers had completed a new system of jetties at the mouth of the Mississippi, dredging the channel below New Orleans to allow larger oceangoing ships to reach the city. Because of this development, "the time is not far distant," the *Picayune* prophesied, "when through bills of lading for European ports via New Orleans will be signed as far up the Mississippi as St. Paul and Minneapolis." Boosters even predicted a reorientation of the entire Mississippi Valley trade from an east–west to a north–south axis, with farmers and factories in the Upper Mississippi Valley forgoing European and eastern markets and refocusing on South America and Mexico. As traveler Ernst von Hesse-Wartegg wrote, "What New Orleans lacks would magnify the city's increased prosperity: a direct line to South America, especially Brazil."[4] Louisiana's boosters asked Congress to subsidize a steamship line between New Orleans and South America. But this new southern orientation never bore the fruits that city merchants desired.

What is most striking—after a century, and thousands upon thousands of deaths across the region—was how little most self-styled experts knew about yellow fever, even still. One writer in 1883 called yellow fever truly "the opossum of diseases," prevaricating that it "is supposed, on very slender grounds, to be contagious. Its contagion, however, like everything else about it, is very queer. It is very contagious to some people, and not at all contagious to other people." Most doctors had a more complex understanding of the virus than this, but even tropical medicine experts had difficulty understanding how the disease spread, manifested, and killed. Some physicians still insisted that yellow fever was only a more serious manifestation of a generic fever; others that its worst symptoms could be checked by quinine or calomel. All, however, conceded that acclimation remained the only sure-fire protection. By the 1890s—with no cure or vaccination in sight—Dr. Edmond Souchon recommended that the medical profession rebrand yellow fever "yellowoid," a more scientific-sounding ailment that would defang people's dread of the virus. Other doctors saw this correctly as a ridiculous and bombastic effort to curb public fear through empty linguistic tricks.[5]

By this time New Orleans's trade had dropped off so significantly that it could no longer claim to be the great entrepôt of the west. In 1860, New Orleans had handled over two-thirds of all US cotton; by the 1880s it was handling just a quarter, almost no sugar, and very little tobacco. The bustle of the antebellum levee had dissipated. New Orleans had been the fourth-largest city in the country in 1840. By 1900 it was twelfth in population and fourteenth in the value of its real estate.[6] This was due to many factors. But US Supreme Court Justice Samuel Freeman Miller, who had been on the court during *Slaughterhouse*, attributed some of the city's decline to persistent, unchecked yellow fever. Miller recalled a recent past when northern capitalists, like "Englishmen returning from India," had been proud of surviving a season in New Orleans—boasting of their acclimation, and imagining immunity as an insider's badge to the Cotton Kingdom. But after the war, Louisiana's "ostracism or fanaticism"—politically and epidemiologically—had made northerners weary. No longer was doing business in New Orleans worth risking death. The city was thus, as Miller wrote, "delivered over to yellow fever . . . and folly."[7]

But what of New Orleans's once-proud "acclimated citizens," those men who had gambled their lives for immunocapital? Some people—especially sailors and dockworkers—relocated elsewhere, acclimation certificate in hand. Well into the twentieth century, a certifiably acclimated workman in Havana or Panama could demand a higher wage. Within the city, it remained essential for white businessmen and employees to declare their acclimation (through certificates, witnesses, and promises) in order to prove they were legitimate, naturalized southerners. Credit reporters like Dun & Bradstreet still listed length of residence in New Orleans, and therefore hinted at acclimation, as a determinant of creditworthiness. Acclimation still mattered in the Jim Crow Deep South, not least because it was still the best health protection available. And immunity still afforded some privileges for whites: better professional-level jobs and social recognition. But as economic opportunities dwindled, so did the value of yellow fever immunity. The core ingredients of New Orleans's immunocapitalism—slavery, immigration, and commercial dominance—had collapsed.[8]

At the end of the nineteenth century, yellow fever continued to strike New Orleans in small epidemics. Townspeople seemed increasingly immune to concern. As the carpetbagging police chief Algernon Badger, who remained in New Orleans after the Civil War, told his brother in October 1897, yellow fever caused him "little or no excitement." Like most "New Orleans folk," Badger had simply come to accept yellow fever's visitation "from time to time." Badger became even more sanguine after his young son "Algie" fell seriously ill with a "dreadful" case of yellow fever in November 1897 and survived—the last person in his family to become acclimated.[9]

The people's confidence in the face of epidemic disease grew once the *A. aegypti* mosquito was confirmed as yellow fever's vector. By the late 1890s the government fumigated the commercial districts, docks, and incoming boats—everything but fruit ships—in its battle to control urban mosquitoes. New Orleans experienced its last epidemic in 1905, which killed about 500 people, many of them Italians. Hereafter, acclimation ceased to be a powerful form of capital, organizing social principle, or method of class and racial dominance in New Orleans. On his tour of the South in 1905, President Teddy Roosevelt made a point of scheduling his last stop in New Orleans in late October, to signal to the nation that yellow fever was no longer to be feared and that New Orleans, perhaps, would rise again.[10] He was greeted by cheering crowds. The memories of wealthy, sickly, and indifferent New Orleans—a necropolis—became the stuff of ghost stories.

And in the tale of yellow fever in nineteenth-century New Orleans, as in most ghost stories, death was the leitmotif. In 1901 Dr. John McKowen wrote an entire book about the dangers of greed and disease in New Orleans. He titled it *Murder as a Money-Making Art,* labeling city politicians and doctors "murderers," bit-players in a multigenerational conspiracy to suppress the truth about yellow fever and generate disasters—always with the goal of preserving and expanding their capital.[11] McKowen opened and closed his book with a reminder that the dead were all around in New Orleans; that they could not be forgotten. Buried within the city limits, McKowen estimated, there were "three times as many dead as there are living inhabitants." Even as the twentieth century dawned, the corpses of thousands of unacclimated strangers—products of a brutal system that had made a few immensely rich at the cost of mass suffering—were still causing sorrow. Their "rotting flesh and bones," McKowen closed, added filth to New Orleans and promised to heap misery upon future generations.[12]

Abbreviations

AHR	*American Historical Review*
AMA	*Transactions of the American Medical Association*
Barings	The Baring Archive, London, UK
BHM	*Bulletin of the History of Medicine*
Clay Papers	*The Papers of Henry Clay,* ed. James F. Hopkins and Mary W. M. Hargreaves, 11 vols. (Lexington: University Press of Kentucky, 1959)
CLB	*Official Letterbooks of W.C.C. Claiborne, 1801–1816,* ed. Dunbar Rowland, 6 vols. (Jackson, Miss., 1917)
CVOP	New Orleans Conseil de Ville, Official Proceedings (translations), AB301, New Orleans Public Library
CVOR	New Orleans Conseil de Ville, Ordinances and Resolutions (translations), AB311, New Orleans Public Library
DBR	*De Bow's Review*
Duke	David M. Rubenstein Rare Book and Manuscript Library, Duke University, Durham, North Carolina
HAR	*Annual Reports,* ProQuest Historical Annual Reports Database from America's Corporate Foundation
HBS	Baker Library Historical Collections, Harvard Business School, Cambridge, Massachusetts
HNOC	Williams Research Center, The Historic New Orleans Collection, New Orleans
JAH	*Journal of American History*
JER	*Journal of the Early Republic*
JSH	*Journal of Southern History*
LH	*Louisiana History*
LHQ	*Louisiana Historical Quarterly*

ABBREVIATIONS

LRC	Louisiana Research Collection, Howard-Tilton Memorial Library Special Collections, Tulane University, New Orleans
LSM	Historical Center at the Louisiana State Museum, New Orleans
LSU	Louisiana and Lower Mississippi Valley Collections, Louisiana State University Libraries, Baton Rouge
MM	Mayor's Messages, New Orleans Conseil de Ville (translations), AA506, New Orleans Public Library
MOHS	The State Historical Society of Missouri, St. Louis, Missouri
MONY	The Mutual Life Insurance Company of New-York
NARA	National Archives and Records Administration
Newberry	Newberry Library, Chicago
NOMNHG	*New Orleans Medical News and Hospital Gazette*
NOMSJ	*New Orleans Medical and Surgical Journal*
NOPL	New Orleans Public Library
N-YHS	New-York Historical Society
NYL&T	New York Life & Trust
ORN	U.S. Navy Department, *Official Records of the Union and Confederate Navies in the War of the Rebellion,* 30 vols. (Washington, DC: US Government Printing Office, 1894–1922)
Rothschild	The Rothschild Archive, London, UK
RCH	*Report of the Board of Administration of the Charity Hospital* (New Orleans, 1842–1974), Tulane University Digital Library
RSC	*Report of the Sanitary Commission of New Orleans on the Epidemic Yellow Fever, of 1853* (New Orleans, Office of the Picayune, 1854)
SHC	Southern Historical Collection, The Wilson Library, University of North Carolina at Chapel Hill
Slave Narratives	*Born in Slavery: Slave Narratives from the Federal Writers' Project, 1936 to 1938,* Library of Congress
TPUS	*Territorial Papers of the United States,* comp. and ed. Clarence Edwin Carter, 28 vols. (Washington, DC, 1940)
UTA	Dolph Briscoe Center for American History, University of Texas at Austin

Notes

Introduction

1. John B. Johnson of Sussex County, New Jersey, is the basis for this opening vignette. I have supplemented this opening story with multiple sources, making him a historically grounded composite. John B. Johnson to Rebecca Johnson, May 5, 1825, ms. 2007.0257.19; William Vandergriff to Rebecca Johnson, August 10, 1825, ms. 2007.0257.21, HNOC; Baron Ludwig von Reizenstein, *The Mysteries of New Orleans,* 1854, ed. and trans. Steven Rowan (Baltimore: Johns Hopkins University Press, 2002), 507.

2. For the transformation of southwestern markets, see Walter Johnson, *River of Dark Dreams: Slavery and Empire in the Cotton Kingdom* (Cambridge, MA: Harvard University Press, 2013); Adam Rothman, *Slave Country: American Expansion and the Origins of the Deep South* (Cambridge, MA: Harvard University Press, 2005), 34–35; Scott P. Marler, *The Merchants' Capital: New Orleans and the Political Economy of the Nineteenth-Century South* (New York: Cambridge University Press, 2013); Thomas N. Ingersoll, *Mammon and Manon in Early New Orleans: The First Slave Society in the Deep South, 1718–1819* (Knoxville: University of Tennessee Press, 1999), 243–348; Sven Beckert, *Empire of Cotton: A New History of Global Capitalism* (New York: Knopf Doubleday, 2014), 214–215.

3. For descriptions of life early in an epidemic, see A Steam-Boat Clerk, "The Last Trip," *Knickerbocker,* July–December 1855, 604; Irene S. Di Maio, ed. and trans., *Gerstäcker's Louisiana: Fiction and Travel Sketches from Antebellum Times through Reconstruction* (Baton Rouge: LSU Press, 2006), 55; Joseph Holt Ingraham, *The South-West, by a Yankee* (New York: Harper and Brothers, 1835), 1:164; Charles Sealsfield, *The Americans as They Are; Described in a Tour through the Valley of the Mississippi* (London: Hurst, Chance and Co., 1828), 193–194.

4. Ingraham, *The South-West*, 2:27–28.

5. Conversation snippets constructed from Mary L. Bissell, *Ned Grant's Quest* (Boston: E.P. Dutton and Co., 1867), 166–167, 171; Bennet Dowler, *Tableau of the Yellow Fever of 1853 with Topographical, Chronological, and Historical Sketches of the Epidemics of New Orleans since Their Origin in 1796* (New Orleans: Office of the Picayune, 1854), 61; Alexander Mackay, *The Western World, or, Travels in the United States in 1846–47* (London: Richard Bentley, 1849), 2:302–304; "The Convalescent," *Daily Picayune,* September 18, 1853; "Talk about Town," *Daily Delta,* November 9, 1858; "History and Incidents of the Plague in New Orleans," *Harper's New Monthly Magazine,* June–November 1853, 803.

6. "Sketches of Character. No. LXIX. The Unacclimated Man," *Daily Delta,* July 29, 1853; John B. Johnson to Major Francis Donlery, July 16, 1825, ms. 2007.0257.20, HNOC.

7. For the loss of a job during epidemics, see Ralph Roanoke, "Random Leaf from the Life of Ralph Roanoke," *Knickerbocker,* September 1852, 196–203.

8. Roanoke, "Random Leaf," 201. For symptoms and treatment, see Max Neubling to Theodor Neubling, May 20, 1825, Max Neubling Letter Book, ms. 873, LSU.

9. "As to Yellow Fever," no date, George Washington Cable Papers, box 112, folder 30, ms. 2, LRC.

10. A Physician of New Orleans, *History of the Yellow Fever during the Summer of 1853* (Philadelphia and St. Louis: C.W. Kenworthy, 1854), 21. For New Orleans's Charity Hospital, see Austin Flint, *The Life and Labors of Laennec: An Introductory Address Delivered at the New Orleans School of Medicine, November 14, 1859* (New Orleans: Bulletin Book and Job Office, 1859), 3; John Salvaggio, *New Orleans' Charity Hospital: A Story of Physicians, Politics, and Poverty* (Baton Rouge: LSU Press, 1992), 35–40.

11. For yellow fever symptoms and treatment, see René La Roche, *Yellow Fever, Considered in Its Historical, Pathological, Etiological, and Therapeutic Relations,* 2 vols. (Philadelphia, 1855), 1:129–142; J. F. Beugnot, "An Essay on Yellow Fever . . . Read before the Louisiana Medico-Chirurgical Society, Sept. 1843," *NOMSJ* 1, no. 1 (May–July 1844): 1–28, esp. 10–12; Urmi Engineer Willoughby, *Yellow Fever, Race, and Ecology in Nineteenth-Century New Orleans* (Baton Rouge: LSU Press, 2017), 16–17.

12. "As to Yellow Fever"; William Vandergriff to Rebecca Johnson, August 10, 1825, ms. 2007.0257.21, HNOC.

13. Theodore Clapp, *Autobiographical Sketches and Recollections during a Thirty-Five Years' Residence in New Orleans* (Boston: Phillips, Sampson, and Co., 1857), 189–194, here 189.

14. John P. Ordway, *Let Me Kiss Him for His Mother: Song and Chorus, as Performed by Ordway's Æolians and Other Popular Bands* (Boston: E.H. Wade, ca. 1859); William Vandergriff to Mrs. Rebecca J. Johnson, August 10, 1825, ms. 2007.0257.21, HNOC.

15. For the "Good Death," see Drew Gilpin Faust, *This Republic of Suffering: Death and the Civil War* (New York: Knopf, 2008).

16. "Sketches of Character. No. LXX. The Acclimated Man," *Daily Delta*, August 1, 1853; "Sketches of Character. No. LXXV. The Anti-Panic Man," *Daily Delta*, August 13, 1853; "Sketches of Character. No. LXIX. The Unacclimated Man," *Daily Delta*, July 29, 1853.

17. Bennet Dowler, *Researches upon the Necropolis of New Orleans, with Brief Allusions to Its Vital Arithmetic* (New Orleans: Bills and Clark, 1850), 3–28.

18. For yellow fever storytelling, see Solomon Northup, *Twelve Years a Slave: Narrative of Solomon Northup, a Citizen of New-York, Kidnapped in Washington City in 1841, and Rescued in 1853* (Buffalo: Derby, Orton and Mulligan, 1853), 176–178; Erasmus Darwin Fenner, *The Epidemic of 1847: Or, Brief Accounts of the Yellow Fever, That Prevailed at New-Orleans, Vicksburg, Rodney, Natchez, Houston and Covington* (New Orleans, 1848). For Mary and Maria, see Mary Copes to Joseph Copes, September 18, 1853, Joseph S. Copes Papers, box 10, folder 9, ms. 733, LRC; Harry Careless, "A Tale of the Yellow Fever," *Knickerbocker,* November 1848, 433–439.

19. For excellent histories of yellow fever and public health in New Orleans, see Willoughby, *Yellow Fever,* 37–62; Jo Ann Carrigan, *The Saffron Scourge: A History of Yellow Fever in Louisiana, 1796–1905* (Lafayette: University of Louisiana at Lafayette Press, 1994); John Duffy, *Sword of Pestilence: The New Orleans Yellow Fever Epidemic of 1853* (Baton Rouge: LSU Press, 1966), 122–124; Margaret Humphreys, *Yellow Fever and the South* (Baltimore: Johns Hopkins University Press, 1992), 45–112; Benjamin Trask, *Fearful Ravages: Yellow Fever in New Orleans, 1796–1905* (Lafayette: University of Louisiana at Lafayette Press, 2005), 5–59.

20. Walter Scheidel, *The Great Leveler: Violence and the History of Inequality from the Stone Age to the Twenty-First Century* (Princeton, NJ: Princeton University Press, 2017).

21. J. R. McNeill, *Mosquito Empires: Ecology and War in the Greater Caribbean, 1620–1914* (Cambridge: Cambridge University Press, 2010), 2; Vincent Brown, *The Reaper's Garden: Death and Power in the World of Atlantic Slavery* (Cambridge, MA: Harvard University Press, 2008), 4. For disease determinism in Atlantic history, see Alfred W. Crosby, *Ecological Imperialism: The Biological Expansion of Europe, 900–1900* (Cambridge: Cambridge University Press, 1986); Terence Ranger and Paul Slack, eds., *Epidemics and Ideas: Essays on the Historical Perception of Pestilence* (Cambridge: Cambridge University Press, 1995); Philip Curtin, *Disease and Empire: The Health of European Troops in the Conquest of Africa* (Cambridge: Cambridge University Press, 1998).

22. For the long history of constructing biological otherness, see Geraldine Heng, *The Invention of Race in the European Middle Ages* (Cambridge: Cambridge University Press, 2018). For risk in the nineteenth century, see Jonathan Levy, *Freaks of Fortune: The Emerging World of Capitalism and Risk in America* (Cambridge, MA: Harvard University Press, 2009), 64–118.

23. For immunocapital, see Kathryn Olivarius, "Immunity, Capital and Power in Antebellum New Orleans," *AHR* 124, no. 2 (April 2019): 425–455.

24. Cenci, August 15, 1850, in *Letters of Cenci, Written Four Years Ago, on the Sanitary Reforms Needed in New Orleans and Re-Published by the Order of the City Council* (New Orleans: Isaac T. Hinton, 1853), 12, Wellcome Collection, London.

25. For Barton's quote, see *Daily Picayune,* November 26, 1841.

26. Jean-Louis-Marie Alibert, *A Treatise on Malignant Intermittents* (Philadelphia: Fry and Kammerer, 1807), 183.

27. Rana Hogarth, *Medicalizing Blackness: Making Racial Difference in the Atlantic World, 1780–1840* (Chapel Hill: University of North Carolina Press, 2017); Daina Ramey Berry, *The Price for Their Pound of Flesh: The Value of the Enslaved, from Womb to Grave, in the Building of a Nation* (New York: Beacon Press, 2017); Khary Oronde Polk, *Contagions of Empires: Scientific Racism, Sexuality, and Black Military Workers Abroad, 1898–1948* (Chapel Hill: University of North Carolina Press, 2020); Dea Boster, *African American Slavery and Disability: Bodies, Property, and Power in the Antebellum South, 1800–1860* (New York: Taylor and Francis, 2013).

28. For identity and belonging, see Conevery Bolton Valenčius, *The Health of the Country: How American Settlers Understood Themselves and Their Land* (New York: Perseus Books Group, 2002), 22–34.

29. For slaveholders' tax aversion, see Robin Einhorn, *American Slavery, American Taxation* (Chicago: University of Chicago Press, 2008).

30. For New Orleans's natural ecology, see Ari Kelman, *A River and Its City: The Nature of Landscape in New Orleans* (Berkeley: University of California Press, 2003), 1–4; Lawrence N. Powell, *The Accidental City: Improvising New Orleans* (Cambridge, MA: Harvard University Press, 2013); Christopher Morris, *The Big Muddy: An Environmental History of the Mississippi and Its Peoples from Hernando de Soto to Hurricane Katrina* (New York: Oxford University Press, 2012), 9–47.

31. Pierre-Louis Berquin-Duvallon, *Travels in Louisiana and the Floridas, in the Year 1802, Giving a Correct Picture of Those Countries* (New York: I. Riley and Co., 1806), 35.

32. John S. Kendall, *History of New Orleans* (Chicago: Lewis, 1922), 1:7; C. C. Robin, *Voyage to Louisiana, 1803–1805,* trans. Stuart O. Landry Jr. (New Orleans: Pelican, 1966), 31. Quote from Charles Gayarré, *History of Louisiana: The Spanish Domination* (New York: Redfield, 1854), 332.

33. Sugar did not grow easily in Louisiana, due to the nine-month growing season (in the Caribbean, sugar had fourteen months to grow). Edouard de Montulé, *Voyage to North America, and the West Indies in 1817* (London: Sir Richard Phillips and Co., 1821), 55; Richard Follett, *The Sugar Masters: Planters and Slaves in Louisiana's Cane World, 1820–1860* (Baton Rouge: LSU Press, 2005), 19.

34. W. C. C. Claiborne to Jonathan Dayton, March 18, 1802, William C. C. Claiborne Papers, folder 1, item 1, ms. 427, LRC; E. R. Mudge, *Report upon Cotton* (Washington, DC: US Government Printing Office, 1869), 28; Claiborne to Jefferson, July 10, 1806, *CLB,* 3:36.

35. Careless, "Tale of the Yellow Fever," 434; Estwick Evans, *Evans's Pedestrious Tour of Four Thousand Miles, through the Western States and Territories, during the Winter and Spring of 1818* (Concord, NH: Joseph S. Spear, 1819), 339.

36. Pierre Clément de Laussat, *Memoirs of My Life,* trans. Agnes-Josephine Pastwa, ed. Robert Bush (Baton Rouge: LSU Press, 1978), 103 (orig. pub. 1831).

37. Elizabeth Fussell, "Constructing New Orleans, Constructing Race: A Population History of New Orleans," *JAH* 94, no. 3 (December 2007): 846–855; Fredrick Mar Spletstoser, "The Impact of the Immigrants on New Orleans," in *A Refuge for All Ages: Immigration in Louisiana History,* Louisiana Purchase Bicentennial Series, vol. 10, ed. Carl Brasseaux (Lafayette: Center for Louisiana Studies, 1996), 287–322, 5–33; Peter McClelland and Richard Zeckhauser, *Demographic Dimensions of the New Republic: American Interregional Migration, Vital Statistics, and Manumissions, 1800–1860* (Cambridge: Cambridge University Press, 1982), table C-1, 138–139; Beckert, *Empire of Cotton,* 109, 215–216.

38. Michael Tadman, "Slave Trading in the Ante-Bellum South: An Estimate of the Extent of the Inter-Regional Slave Trade," *Journal of American Studies* 13, no. 2 (1979): 195–220; Rothman, *Slave Country,* 220; Walter Johnson, *Soul by Soul: Life inside the Antebellum Slave Market* (Cambridge, MA : Harvard University Press, 1999), 6; Steven Deyle, *Carry Me Back: The Domestic Slave Trade in American Life* (Oxford: Oxford University Press, 2006).

39. Beckert, *Empire of Cotton,* 103–104; Ingraham, *The South-West,* 2:91. For the "second slavery," see Dale W. Tomich, *Through the Prism of Slavery: Labor, Capital, and World Economy* (Lanham, MD: Rowman and Littlefield, 2004), esp. 56–71.

40. James Stirling, *Letters from the Slave States* (London: J.W. Parker and Son, 1857), 182; Lillian Foster, *Wayside Glimpses North and South* (New York: Rudd and Carleton, 1860), 168–169.

41. John Harrison, "Remarks on Yellow Fever," *NOMNHG* 2, no. 2 (April 1855): 51; Kelman, *A River and Its City,* xi.

42. John Eadie, "The First American Life Underwriters' Convention," *Assurance Magazine,* October 1859, 273.

43. "Yellow Jack," *Daily Picayune,* October 18, 1844.

44. William Holcombe, "Queer Things about Yellow Fever," *Southwestern Christian Advocate,* February 6, 1879.

45. Mariola Espinosa, *Epidemic Invasions: Yellow Fever and the Limits of Cuban Independence, 1878–1930* (Chicago: University of Chicago Press, 2009), chap. 4.

46. Wesley Bradshaw, *Angel Agnes: Or, The Heroine of the Yellow Fever Plague in Shreveport* (Philadelphia: Old Franklin Publishing House, 1873), 3. For profanity, see William Crenshaw to Nathaniel Bower, September 11, 1841, William Crenshaw Letters, ms. 46, NOPL.

47. Clapp, *Autobiographical Sketches,* 189.

48. Josiah Nott, "Life Insurance at the South," *DBR* 3, no. 5 (May 1847): 358–376, here 365.

49. For mistaken or dubious acclimation, see a debate among six doctors in E. D. Fenner, "The Yellow Fever of 1853," *DBR* 17, no. 1 (July 1854): 39–42, here 41.

50. Richard Henry Wilde to John Walker Wilde, August 4, 1847, in Edward L. Tucker, ed., "Richard Henry Wilde in New Orleans: Selected Letters, 1844–1847," *LH* 7, no. 4 (Autumn 1966): 333–356, here 355.

51. Pierre Bourdieu, *Outline of a Theory of Practice*, trans. Richard Nice (Cambridge: Cambridge University Press, 1977); Bourdieu, "The Forms of Capital," in *Handbook of Theory and Research for the Sociology of Education*, ed. John Richardson (Westport, CT: Greenwood Press, 1986), 241–258, quotes from 244, 249. See also Sven Beckert and Christine Desan, eds., *American Capitalism: New Histories* (New York: Columbia University Press, 2018); Geoffrey Martin Hodgson, *Conceptualizing Capitalism: Institutions, Evolution, Future* (Chicago: University of Chicago Press, 2015); Jonathan Levy, "Capital as Process and the History of Capitalism," *Business History Review* 91, no. 3 (2017): 483–510.

52. *Proceedings and Debates of the Convention of Louisiana, Which Assembled at the City of New Orleans January 14, 1844* (New Orleans: Besancon, Ferguson and Co., 1845), 19, 32.

53. Richard Claiborne, "Three Letters of Richard Claiborne to William Miller, 1816–1818," ed. Walter Prichard, *LHQ* 24, no. 3 (July 1941): 729–743, here 739.

54. Henry Anthony Murray, *Lands of the Slave and the Free: Or, Cuba, the United States, and Canada* (London: John W. Parker and Son, 1855), 1:248.

55. Samuel Cartwright, "On the Prevention of Yellow Fever," *NOMSJ* 10 (November 1853): 316.

56. For the "Second Middle Passage," see Ira Berlin, *Generations of Captivity: A History of African-American Slaves* (Cambridge, MA: Harvard University Press, 2003), chap. 4. Interview with Lizzie Barnett, Arkansas, 2:113, Slave Narratives.

57. Alejandro de la Fuente and Ariela J. Gross, *Becoming Free, Becoming Black: Race, Freedom, and Law in Cuba, Virginia, and Louisiana* (Cambridge: Cambridge University Press, 2020), table on 156.

58. Naomi Klein, *The Shock Doctrine: The Rise of Disaster Capitalism* (New York: Henry Holt, 2010).

59. For climatic defenses of slavery, see Mart Stewart, *"What Nature Suffers to Groe": Life, Labor, and Landscape on the Georgia Coast, 1680–1920* (Athens: University of Georgia Press, 2002).

60. "The Population of New Orleans and the Fever," *Tri-Weekly Commercial* (Wilmington, NC), August 23, 1853.

61. Edward Hall Barton, *RSC*, 8.

62. "Editorial and Miscellaneous," *NOMNHG* 2, no. 9 (November 1855): 418.

1. Patriotic Fever

1. Report of Joseph de Castanedo, CVOP, September 12, 1804, AB301, 176. For Davis's testimony, see CVOP, September 27, 1804, AB301, 184–185. See also Rashauna Johnson, *Slavery's Metropolis: Unfree Labor in New Orleans during the Age of Revolutions* (Cambridge: Cambridge University Press, 2016), chap. 1.

2. CVOP, June 27, 1804, 124; June 30, 1804, 127–127b; July 7, 1804, 129.

3. John Watkins to Claiborne, February 2, 1804, *CLB,* 2:5–9; CVOP, August 8, 1804, 150B; Peter Kastor, *The Nation's Crucible: The Louisiana Purchase and the Creation of America* (New Haven, CT: Yale University Press, 2004), 65; Adam Rothman, *Slave Country: American Expansion and the Origins of the Deep South* (Cambridge, MA: Harvard University Press, 2005), 104–105.

4. No. 183: "Remonstrance of the People of Louisiana against the Political System Adopted by Congress for Them," December 31, 1804, *American State Papers: Miscellaneous* (Washington, DC: Gales and Seaton, 1834) (hereafter cited as "Remonstrance"), 1:396–399.

5. John Clay to Henry Clay, July 6, 1804, *Clay Papers,* 1:139–140; Hilary Baker to Nathaniel Evans, July 7, 1804, Nathaniel Evans and Family Papers, box 1, folder 1, ms. 670, LSU.

6. Claiborne to Jefferson, September 13, September 18, and October 5, 1804, *TPUS,* 9:286–287, 298, 309.

7. "Petition of the Inhabitants & Colonists of Louisiana," September 17, 1804, *TPUS,* 9:297.

8. Claiborne to Jefferson, September 18, 1804, *TPUS,* 9:298.

9. Claiborne to Madison, December 17, 1809, *TPUS,* 9:860; Christina Vella, *Intimate Enemies: The Two Worlds of the Baroness de Pontalba* (Baton Rouge: LSU Press 1997), 9–10, 84; Pierre Clément de Laussat, *Memoirs of My Life,* trans. Agnes-Josephine Pastwa, ed. Robert Bush (Baton Rouge: LSU Press, 1978), 32.

10. Eberhard Faber, *Building the Land of Dreams: New Orleans and the Transformation of Early America* (Princeton, NJ: Princeton University Press, 2016), 140, 195–196.

11. Claiborne to Madison, January 4, 1805, and December 17, 1809, *TPUS,* 9:362, 860; Kastor, *The Nation's Crucible,* 223–224; Benjamin Trask, *Fearful Ravages: Yellow Fever in New Orleans, 1796–1905* (Lafayette: University of Louisiana at Lafayette Press, 2005), 10.

12. Claiborne to Jefferson, September 13 and October 5, 1804, *TPUS,* 9:286–287, 309. See also M. K. Beauchamp, *Instruments of Empire: Colonial Elites and U.S. Governance in Early National Louisiana, 1803–1815* (Baton Rouge: LSU Press, 2021).

13. For yellow fever's global impact in 1804, see William Augustus Shubert, *Yellow Fever: Its Origin, Improper Treatment, Prevention and Cure* (Savannah, GA: J.M. Cooper and Co., 1860), 9–10.

14. For Indigenous populations in the Mississippi Valley, see Daniel Usner, *Indians, Settlers, and Slaves in a Frontier Exchange Economy: The Lower Mississippi Valley before 1783* (Chapel Hill: University of North Carolina Press, 1992), 24–31; Kathleen DuVal, *The Native Ground: Indians and Colonists in the Heart of the Continent* (Philadelphia: University of Pennsylvania Press, 2006); Daniel Clark, "An Account of the Indian Tribes in Louisiana," September 29, 1803, *TPUS*, 9:63–64. For death in Virginia between 1620 and 1640, see Edmund Morgan, *American Slavery, American Freedom: The Ordeal of Colonial Virginia* (New York: W. W. Norton, 1975), chap. 8.

15. James Pitot, *Observations on the Colony of Louisiana from 1796 to 1802*, trans. Henry C. Pitot (Baton Rouge: LSU Press, 1979), 30–31.

16. Charles Caldwell, "Thoughts on the Probable Destiny of New Orleans, in Relation to Health, Population and Commerce," *Philadelphia Journal of the Medical and Physical Sciences* 6 (January 1823): 13; Claiborne to Jefferson, January 16, 1804, *TPUS*, 9:163.

17. Thomas Hamilton, *Men and Manners in America* (Edinburgh: William Blackwood, 1833), 2:212.

18. François Furstenberg, "The Significance of the Trans-Appalachian Frontier in Atlantic History," *AHR* 113, no. 3 (June 2008): 660–663.

19. "Memorial to Congress by Permanent Committee of the Natchez District," October 23, 1797, *TPUS*, 5: 9–11. For more on free Black life in New Orleans, see Kimberly S. Hanger, *Bounded Lives, Bounded Places: Free Black Society in Colonial New Orleans, 1769–1803* (Durham, NC: Duke University Press, 1997), 136–162.

20. J. E. Bryant, E. C. Holmes, and A. D. T Barrett, "Out of Africa: A Molecular Perspective on the Introduction of Yellow Fever Virus into the Americas," *PLoS Pathogens* 3, no. 5 (May 2007): e75; Yan Li and Zexiao Yang, "Adaptive Diversification between Yellow Fever Virus West African and South American Lineages: A Genome-Wide Study," *American Journal of Tropical Medicine and Hygiene* 96, no. 3 (March 2017): 727–734.

21. J. R. McNeill, *Mosquito Empires: Ecology and War in the Greater Caribbean, 1620–1914* (Cambridge: Cambridge University Press, 2010), 40–52; Philip Curtin, "'The White Man's Grave': Image and Reality, 1780–1850," *Journal of British Studies* 1, no. 1 (November 1961): 96–97; Billy Smith, *Ship of Death: A Voyage That Changed the Atlantic World* (New Haven, CT: Yale University Press, 2014), 187–193; Urmi Engineer Willoughby, *Yellow Fever, Race, and Ecology in Nineteenth-Century New Orleans* (Baton Rouge: LSU Press, 2017), 34–35.

22. For conditions on the transatlantic voyage, see Marcus Rediker, *The Slave Ship: A Human History* (New York: Viking, 2007).

23. McNeill, *Mosquito Empires*, 24–27; Willoughby, *Yellow Fever*, 13–17.

24. James D. Goodyear, "The Sugar Connection: A New Perspective on the History of Yellow Fever," *BHM* 52, no. 1 (Spring 1978): 11.

25. Richard Ligon, *A True & Exact History of the Island of Barbados* (London: Humphrey Moseley, 1657), 22; Munro S. Edmonson, trans., *The Ancient Future of the Itza: The Book of Chilam Balam of Tizimin* (Austin: University of Texas Press, 1982), 24; McNeill, *Mosquito Empires,* 64.

26. McNeill, *Mosquito Empires,* 106–109, 129–132, here 132. John Pinkerton, *Modern Geography: A Description of the Empires, Kingdoms, States, and Colonies* (London, 1811), iii.

27. McNeill, *Mosquito Empires,* 91–136, 144–168, 186; Willoughby, *Yellow Fever,* 13–36; Philip Curtin, *Death by Migration: Europe's Encounter with the Tropical World in the Nineteenth Century* (Cambridge: Cambridge University Press, 1989), 18.

28. Trevor Burnard, *Jamaica in the Age of Revolution* (Philadelphia: University of Pennsylvania Press, 2020), chap. 1, esp. 50–51.

29. Daniel Defoe, *The History of the Most Remarkable Life, and Extraordinary Adventures, of the Truly Honourable Colonel Jaque, Vulgarly Call'd Colonel Jack,* 2 vols. (Oxford: Basil Blackwell, 1927), 1:154. For violence as statecraft, see Vincent Brown, *The Reaper's Garden: Death and Power in the World of Atlantic Slavery* (Cambridge, MA: Harvard University Press, 2008), chap. 2; Vincent Brown, *Tacky's Revolt: The Story of an Atlantic Slave War* (Cambridge, MA: Harvard University Press, 2020).

30. Edward Long, *The History of Jamaica, Or, General Survey of the Antient and Modern State of That Island,* 3 vols. (London: T. Lowndes, 1774), 2:216; Andrew O'Shaughnessy, *An Empire Divided: The American Revolution and the British Caribbean* (Philadelphia: University of Pennsylvania Press, 2015), esp. chaps 2 and 3; Rediker, *The Slave Ship,* 252.

31. Rana Hogarth, *Medicalizing Blackness: Making Racial Difference in the Atlantic World, 1780–1840* (Chapel Hill: University of North Carolina Press, 2017), 19.

32. Trevor Burnard, "'The Countrie Continues Sicklie': White Mortality in Jamaica, 1655–1780," *Social History of Medicine* 12, no. 1 (1999): 46; Gerald N. Grob, *The Deadly Truth: A History of Disease in America* (Cambridge, MA: Harvard University Press, 2009), 76.

33. Willoughby, *Yellow Fever,* 30.

34. Ira Berlin, *Generations of Captivity: A History of African-American Slaves* (Cambridge, MA: Harvard University Press, 2003), 57; Stephanie Smallwood, *Saltwater Slavery: A Middle Passage from Africa to American Diaspora* (Cambridge, MA: Harvard University Press, 2008), 55, 145–146; Philip D. Curtin, "Epidemiology and the Slave Trade," *Political Science Quarterly* 83, no. 2 (June 1968): 190–216.

35. John Lining, *A Description of the American Yellow Fever, which prevailed at Charleston, in South Carolina, in the year 1748* (Philadelphia: Thomas Dobson, 1799), 7; Thomas Trotter, *Medicina Nautica: An Essay on the Diseases of Seamen* (London, 1797), 184; Robert Southey to Thomas Southey, February 11, 1804, in *The Life and Correspondence of Robert Southey,* ed. Charles Cuthbert Southey (London: Longman, Brown, Green and Longmans, 1849), 2:257.

36. Quoted from Richard S. Newman, *Freedom's Prophet: Bishop Richard Allen, the AME Church, and the Black Founding Fathers* (New York: NYU Press, 2009), 87–88; Matthew Carey, *A Short Account of the Malignant Fever, Lately Prevalent in Philadelphia* (Philadelphia: Printed by the author, 1793), 63.

37. Absalom Jones and Richard Allen, *A Narrative of the Proceedings of the Black People during the Late Awful Calamity in Philadelphia and a Refutation of Some Censures Thrown Upon Them in Some Late Publications* (Philadelphia: William W. Woodward, 1794), 11–15.

38. M. Perrin du Lac, *Travels through the Two Louisianas and among the Savage Nations of the Missouri* (London: Printed for Richard Phillips by J.G. Barnard, 1807), 7.

39. Laurent Dubois, *Avengers of the New World: The Story of the Haitian Revolution* (Cambridge, MA: Harvard University Press, 2004).

40. David Geggus, "Yellow Fever in the 1790s: The British Army in Occupied Saint Domingue," *Medical History* 23, no. 1 (January 1979): 50; McNeill, *Mosquito Empires,* 33, 252–259.

41. Paul LaChance, "Repercussions of the Haitian Revolution in Louisiana," in *The Impact of the Haitian Revolution in the Atlantic World,* ed. David Geggus (Columbia: University of South Carolina Press, 2001), 210.

42. Jefferson to Robert Livingston, April 18, 1802, in *The Writings of Thomas Jefferson,* ed. Paul Leicester Ford (New York: G.P. Putnam Sons, 1892–1899), 8:143–147; Alexander Hamilton, "Purchase of Louisiana," *New-York Evening Post,* July 5, 1803.

43. Alexander Hamilton to the College of Physicians, September 11, 1793, in *The Papers of Alexander Hamilton,* ed. Harold C. Syrett (New York: Columbia University Press, 1979), 15:331–332.

44. Smith, *Ship of Death,* 211–217; J. H. Powell, *Bring Out Your Dead: The Great Plague of Yellow Fever in Philadelphia in 1793* (Philadelphia: University of Pennsylvania Press, 1949), x, 107–108; Hogarth, *Medicalizing Blackness,* 17.

45. Jo Ann Carrigan, *The Saffron Scourge: A History of Yellow Fever in Louisiana, 1796–1905* (Lafayette: University of Louisiana at Lafayette Press, 1994), 15–19; George Washington Cable, *The Creoles of Louisiana* (New York: Charles Scribner's Sons, 1884), 291. See also Guillermo Náñez Falcón, ed., *Favrot Family Papers: Documentary Chronicle of Early Louisiana* (New Orleans: Howard Tilton Memorial Library, Tulane, 1988), 1:247–248.

46. Quoted from John Duffy, "Pestilence in New Orleans," in *The Past as Prelude: New Orleans, 1718–1968,* ed. Hodding Carter et al. (Gretna, LA: Pelican, 1968), 100.

47. René La Roche, *Yellow Fever, Considered in Its Historical, Pathological, Etiological, and Therapeutic Relations* (Philadelphia: Blanchard and Lea, 1855), 2:64–103; Carrigan, *Saffron Scourge,* 23–29.

48. "Census of the City of New Orleans," 1803, New Orleans Municipal Records, ms. 16, LRC.

49. For population and demographics, see Elizabeth Fussell, "Constructing New Orleans, Constructing Race: A Population History of New Orleans," *JAH* 94, no. 3 (December 2007): 846–855; Nathalie Dessens, *Creole City: A Chronicle of Early American New Orleans* (Gainesville: University of Florida Press, 2015), 188–189; Sybil Kein, *Creole: The History and Legacy of Louisiana's Free People of Color* (Baton Rouge: LSU Press, 2000), 62–64.

50. Faber, *Building the Land of Dreams*, 46–49, quote on 48; Kastor, *The Nation's Crucible*, 3; Jon Kukla, *A Wilderness So Immense: The Louisiana Purchase and the Destiny of America* (New York: Knopf Doubleday, 2004), 4–5.

51. Rothman, *Slave Country*, 34–35; James E. Scanlon, "A Sudden Conceit: Jefferson and the Louisiana Government Bill of 1804," *LH* 9, no. 2 (Spring 1968): 139–162.

52. If the outcome of a person's experience with yellow fever is known, I note it like so: (d. YF 1847) means a person died from yellow fever in 1847; (a. YF 1847), means a person was infected with yellow fever in 1847 but survived and is "acclimated."

53. Captain James Sterrett to Nathaniel Evans, October 22, 1804, Nathaniel Evans and Family Papers, ms. 670, LSU; James Wilkinson to Jefferson, "Characterization of New Orleans Residents," July 1, 1804, *TPUS*, 9:248–258; Claiborne to Madison, January 2, 1804, *CLB*, 1:326–327.

54. Claiborne to Jefferson, April 15, 1804, *TPUS*, 9:222. Watkins's first wife died of yellow fever in 1795. Jerah Johnson, "Dr. John Watkins, New Orleans' Lost Mayor," *LH* 36, no. 2 (Spring 1995): 187–196; John Watkins to John Graham, September 6, 1805, *TPUS*, 9:504.

55. Jefferson to Henry Dearborn, September 6, 1804, *TPUS*, 9:291.

56. Pierre August Derbigny, *Esquisse de la situation politique et civil de la Louisiane* (New Orleans: Beleurgey & Renard, 1804); Boré to Jefferson, February 10, 1804, *TPUS*, 9:185; Claiborne to Jefferson, April 15, 1804, *TPUS*, 9:222.

57. Fidelis, "A Dream," *Louisiana Gazette*, February 8, 1805. Fidelis was the pen name of Robert Sterry, a Rhode Islander who arrived in New Orleans in 1803. Claiborne to Jefferson, February 17, 1805, *TPUS*, 9:393–394; Julien Vernet, *Strangers on Their Native Soil: Opposition to United States' Governance in Louisiana's Orleans Territory, 1803–1809* (Jackson: University Press of Mississippi, 2013), 33, 91–92.

58. Gwendolyn Midlo Hall, *Africans in Colonial Louisiana: The Development of Afro-Creole Culture in the Eighteenth Century* (Baton Rouge: LSU Press, 1992), 278; S. Charles Bolton, *Fugitivism: Escaping Slavery in the Lower Mississippi Valley, 1820–1860* (Fayetteville, University of Arkansas Press, 2019), 36–38; T. Lindsay Baker and Julie P. Baker, eds., *The WPA Oklahoma Narratives* (Norman: Oklahoma University Press, 1996), 82.

59. Thomas Ashe, *Travels in America, Performed in 1806, For the Purpose of Exploring the Rivers Alleghany, Monongahela, Ohio, and Mississippi* (London: Richard Phillips, 1808), 3:228.

60. Samuel Henry Dickson, "On the Blending and Conversion of Types of Fever," *AMA* 5 (1852): 148; McNeill, *Mosquito Empires,* 45, n89.

61. For the mechanics of the interior African slave trade, see Paul E. Lovejoy, *Transformation in Slavery: A History of Slavery in Africa* (Cambridge: Cambridge University Press, 2012); Gwendolyn Midlo Hall, *Slavery and African Ethnicities in the Americas: Restoring the Links* (Chapel Hill: University of North Carolina Press, 2009), 58, 98–100.

62. John Watkins to Secretary Graham, September 6, 1805, *TPUS,* 9:503; Paul Lachance, "The Politics of Fear: French Louisianans and the Slave Trade, 1786–1809," *Plantation Society* 1 (June 1979): 164–182; Hall, *Africans in Colonial Louisiana,* append. A, 382–384; Curtin, "Epidemiology and the Slave Trade," 190–216, here 215; Gregory O'Malley, "Beyond the Middle Passage: Slave Migration from the Caribbean to North America, 1619–1807," *William and Mary Quarterly* 66, no. 1 (January 2009): 125–172; Adam Rothman, "The Domestication of the Slave Trade in the United States," in *The Chattel Principle: Internal Slave Trades in the Americas,* ed. Walter Johnson (New Haven, CT: Yale University Press, 2004), 37.

63. Quoted from Lachance, "The Politics of Fear," 175; Jean-Pierre Le Glaunec, "Slave Migrations and Slave Control in Spanish and Early American New Orleans," in *Empires of the Imagination: Transatlantic Histories of the Louisiana Purchase,* ed. Peter J. Kastor and Francois Weil (Charlottesville: University of Virginia Press, 2009), 204–238.

64. See Edward Rugemer's discussion of the "Edwards Thesis." Rugemer, *The Problem of Emancipation: The Caribbean Roots of the American Civil War* (Baton Rouge: LSU Press, 2008), 42–65.

65. Order issued by the Baron de Carondelet, New Orleans, to the city steward Juan de Castanedo, June 20, 1795, LRC; LaChance, "Repercussions," 211.

66. C. C. Robin, *Voyage to Louisiana, 1803–1805,* trans. Stuart O. Landry Jr. (New Orleans: Pelican, 1966), 53–54; John Craig Hammond, *Slavery, Freedom, and Expansion in the Early American West* (Charlottesville: University of Virginia Press, 2007), 34; Rothman, *Slave Country,* 32.

67. Quoted from Lachance, "The Politics of Fear," 162; Sarah Russell, "Ethnicity, Commerce, and Community on the Lower Louisiana's Plantation Frontier, 1803–1828," *LH* 40, no. 4 (Autumn 1999): 391–398.

68. "Memorial to Congress by Permanent Committee of the Natchez District," October 23, 1797, *TPUS,* 5:9–10; Meriwether Lewis to Jefferson, December 28, 1803, in *Letters of the Lewis and Clark Expedition with Related Documents, 1783–1854,* ed. Donald Jackson (Urbana: University of Illinois Press, 1962), 153.

69. William Plumer, *William Plumer's Memorandum of the Proceedings of the United States Senate, 1803–1807,* ed. Everett Somerville Brown (New York: n.p., 1923), 120, Hillhouse quote on 118.

70. Plumer, *Memorandum,* 119, 114, 1225. See also Ira Berlin, *Many Thousands Gone: The First Two Centuries of Slavery in North America* (Cambridge, MA: Harvard University Press, 1998), 333.

71. John Craig Hammond, "'Uncontrollable Necessity': The Local Politics, Geopolitics, and Sectional Politics of Slavery's Expansion," in *Contesting Slavery: The Politics of Bondage and Freedom in the New American Nation,* ed. John Craig Hammond and Matthew Mason (Charlottesville: University of Virginia Press, 2011), 141.

72. Richard Kilbourne, *A History of the Louisiana Civil Code: The Formative Years, 1803–1839* (Baton Rouge: LSU Press, 1987), 13; Hatch Dent to James H. McCulloch, July 14, 1804, *TPUS,* 9:265–266.

73. "Remonstrance."

74. Thomas Paine, "To the French Inhabitants of Louisiana," in *The Political Works of Thomas Paine,* 2 vols. (London: W.T. Sherwin, 1819), 2:155.

75. "Discontent in Louisiana," *National Intelligencer,* August 24, 1804; "United States, Louisiana," *Connecticut Gazette,* May 30, 1804.

76. John Watkins to Claiborne, February 2, 1804, *CLB,* 2:3–10; Hammond, "Uncontrollable Necessity," 141–144. See also Captain James Sterrett to Nathaniel Evans, October 29, 1804, Nathaniel Evans and Family Papers, ms. 670, LSU.

77. Section 10, "An Act for the Organization of Orleans Territory and the Louisiana District," March 26, 1804, *TPUS,* 9:209. It was only after 1815 that the domestic slave trade met the demands of Louisiana planters. Berlin, *Many Thousands Gone,* 338–357; Rothman, *Slave Country,* 34, 83–95.

78. John Adair to James Wilkinson, February 14, 1804, Edward Alexander Parsons Collection, folder 2, 3E477, UTA.

79. James Brown to Henry Clay, February 27, 1806, *Clay Papers,* 1:220; *Annals of Congress,* 9th Congress, 1st Sess. (1805–1806): 928.

80. John Wilds, *Collectors of Customs at the Port of New Orleans* (Washington, DC: Department of the Treasury, 1991), here 7, 141; Gautham Rao, *National Duties: Custom Houses and the Making of the American State* (Chicago: University of Chicago Press, 2016), 4–14.

81. Hore Browse Trist to Mary Trist, January 7, 1803, Nicholas Philip Trist Family Papers, ms. 2104, SHC.

82. Trist to Trist, May 14, 1803, Trist Family Papers, SHC.

83. Captain James Sterrett to Nathaniel Evans, November 18 and December 2, 1809, Nathaniel Evans and Family Papers, ms. 670, LSU; John Bristed, *The Resources of the United States of America* (New York: James Eastburn and Co., 1818), 80; John Clark, *New Orleans, 1719–1812: An Economic History* (Baton Rouge: LSU Press, 1970), 279.

84. Claiborne to Madison, November 19, 1809, *TPUS,* 9:858.

85. Gurley, born in Connecticut, died in a duel in 1808, at age twenty-eight. His wife Grace had died from yellow fever in New Orleans in 1804. *Louisiana Gazette,* March 4, 1808.

86. John Breckenridge to Wilson Cary Nichols, August 17, 1803, folder 11, 3E477, UTA; Allan Bowie Magruder to unknown, March 5, 1806, Opelousas Letter, ms. 558,

Newberry Library, Chicago; Civil Appointments, December 31, 1806, *TPUS,* 9:700–702; Rothman, *Slave Country,* 42–45.

87. Philip Grymes to the Secretary of the Treasury, May 22, 1809, *TPUS,* 9:839–840.

88. Philip Grymes, Judge Lewis, and Secretary Robertson to the Secretary of the Treasury, January 8, 1810; Columbus Lawson to the Secretary of the Treasury, June 21, 1811, *TPUS,* 9:861–863, 890–900, 937–938.

89. Claiborne to Jefferson, November 25, 1804, *TPUS,* 9:340; Faber, *Building the Land of Dreams,* 170; Claiborne to Jefferson, October 22, 1804, *TPUS,* 9:311.

90. William Kernan Dart, "The Justices of the Supreme Court," *LHQ* 4, no. 1 (January 1921): 113; Claiborne to Madison, November 26, 1804, in *Interim Appointment: W.C.C. Claiborne Letter Book, 1804–1805,* ed. Jared W. Bradley (Baton Rouge: LSU Press, 2002), 103–104.

91. Claiborne to Jefferson, December 2, 1804, *TPUS,* 9:344–346; William Kenner to Major Stephen Minor, November 1, 1804, William Kenner Papers, box 1a, folder 1a, mss. 1477, 1491, LSU.

92. Mark F. Fernandes, "New Orleans, a Tale of Two Cities: The Legal System That Wasn't," *LH* 51, no. 4 (Fall 2010): 389–403; Faber, *Building the Land of Dreams,* 372n39.

93. Jefferson to Claiborne, January 7, 1805, *TPUS,* 9:363; Samuel Groner, "Louisiana Law: Its Development in the First Quarter-Century of America Rule," *Louisiana Law Review* 8 (1947–1948): 369–370; George Mathews to Madison, April 20, 1806, *TPUS,* 9:626.

94. Washington Irving, *Knickerbocker's History of New York* (Chicago: W.B. Conkey Co., 1809), bk. 5, chap. 9.

95. Claiborne to Jefferson, May 20, 1807, *TPUS,* 9:736; Wilds, *Collectors of Customs,* 6–13; George Dargo, *Jefferson's Louisiana: Politics and the Clash of Legal Traditions* (Cambridge, MA: Harvard University Press, 1975), 174.

96. Eleanor Stauman to her aunt, September 9, 1820, Ker and Texada Papers, folder 1, ms. 545, LRC; Thomas Robertson to William Robertson, September 12, 1820, Walter Prichard Papers, ms. 2509, LSU; CVOP, April 4, 1805, 1–6, April 19, 1809, 49–52.

97. Laussat, *Memoirs of My Life,* 88–90. Bishop Davenport, *A New Gazetteer: Or Geographical Dictionary of North America and the West Indies* (Baltimore: George M'Dowell and Son, 1833), 121; Richard Follett, *The Sugar Masters: Planters and Slaves in Louisiana's Cane World, 1820–1860* (Baton Rouge: LSU Press, 2005), 8; Clark, *New Orleans,* 300–305.

98. Paul Alliot, "Historical and Political Reflections on Louisiana," in *Louisiana under the Rule of Spain, France, and the United States, 1785–1807: Social, Economic, and Political Conditions of the Territory Represented in the Louisiana Purchase,* ed. and trans. James A. Robertson (Cleveland: Arthur H. Clark, 1911), 1:65–67.

99. CVOP, June 17, 1807, 211–213; Pitot, *Observations,* 30–31.

100. CVOP, August 20, 1806, 103–109; Walter Johnson, *River of Dark Dreams: Slavery and Empire in the Cotton Kingdom* (Cambridge, MA: Harvard University Press, 2013), 85–87; Rothman, *Slave Country,* xi.

101. "Statement of Stephen, a Free Negro, to Governor Claiborne," January 23, 1806, *TPUS,* 9:575–576.

102. CVOP, April 4, 1805, 1–6.

103. François-Xavier Martin, *A General Digest of the Acts of the Legislatures of the Late Territory of Orleans, and the State of Louisiana* (New Orleans: Peter K. Wagner, 1816), 616, 640–642; Craig Colten, *An Unnatural Metropolis: Wresting New Orleans from Nature* (Baton Rouge: LSU Press, 2005), 331; Judith Schafer, *Slavery, the Civil Law, and the Supreme Court of Louisiana* (Baton Rouge: LSU Press, 1994), 25; Alejandro de la Fuente and Ariela J. Gross, *Becoming Free, Becoming Black: Race, Freedom, and Law in Cuba, Virginia, and Louisiana* (Cambridge: Cambridge University Press, 2020), 123–127.

104. Shirley Elizabeth Thompson, *Exiles at Home: The Struggle to Become American in Creole New Orleans* (Cambridge, MA: Harvard University Press, 2009), 27.

105. For genesis stories, see Vincent Nolte, *Fifty Years in Both Hemispheres; or, Reminiscences of the Life of a Former Merchant* (New York: Redfield, 1854), 91–92; Maunsel White, "The Olden Time in New-Orleans and Yellow Fever," *DBR* 6, no. 2 (1848): 156–158; Scott P. Marler, *The Merchants' Capital: New Orleans and the Political Economy of the Nineteenth-Century South* (New York: Cambridge University Press, 2013), 28; Bennet Dowler, *Tableau of the Yellow Fever of 1853 with Topographical, Chronological, and Historical Sketches of the Epidemics of New Orleans since Their Origin in 1796* (New Orleans: Office of the Picayune, 1854), 8.

106. Johann Joachim Lagemann to brother, March 1, 1801, Johan Joachim Lagemann Letters, ms. 77-1, NOPL.

107. Erwin Ackerknecht, *History and Geography of the Most Important Diseases* (New York: Hafner, 1972), 52; James Brown to Henry Clay, February 27, 1806, *Clay Papers,* 1:220.

108. *Dewees v. Morgan,* 1 Mart. (o.s.) 1 (La. 1809).

109. For the other case, see *Cornish v. Shelton,* 12 LA. Ann. 415 (1857).

110. Colten, *An Unnatural Metropolis,* 345; Daniel Rasmussen, *American Uprising: The Untold Story of America's Largest Slave Revolt* (New York: Harper, 2011); Johnson, *River of Dark Dreams,* chap. 1; Peter Regnier to Seth Lewis, January 19, 1811, Peter Regnier Letter, MISC:R, LSU; CVOP, January 12, 1811, 1–3.

111. O'Shaughnessy, *An Empire Divided.*

112. Claiborne to Madison, October 8, 1811, *TPUS,* 9:947–948; see also, Bartlet and Cox to Henry Clay, November 11, 1811, *Clay Papers,* 1: 595–596; *Constitution of the State of Louisiana,* January 22, 1812.

113. Kimbrough Owen, "The Need for Constitutional Revision in Louisiana," *Louisiana Law Review* 8, no. 1 (November 1947): 86.

2. Danse Macabre

1. Liliane Crété, *Daily Life in Louisiana, 1815–1830*, trans. Patrick Gregory (Baton Rouge: LSU Press, 1981), 157.

2. Ralph Randolph Gurley, *Life an Eloquence of the Rev. Sylvester Larned: First Pastor of the First Presbyterian Church in New-Orleans* (New York: Wiley and Putnam, 1844), 66; Mary L. Bissell, *Ned Grant's Quest* (Boston: E.P. Dutton and Co., 1867), 168.

3. Drew Gilpin Faust, *This Republic of Suffering: Death and the Civil War* (New York: Knopf, 2008); John Macaulay, *Unitarianism in the Antebellum South: The Other Invisible Institution*, 2nd ed. (Tuscaloosa: University of Alabama Press, 2016), 49.

4. Bennet Dowler estimated the mortality at 2,190, noting that this applied "only to the city proper." British naturalist Thomas Nuttal estimated that between 5,000 and 6,000 died. Dowler, *Tableau of the Yellow Fever of 1853 with Topographical, Chronological, and Historical Sketches of the Epidemics of New Orleans since Their Origin in 1796* (New Orleans: Office of the Picayune, 1854), 15–16; Thomas Nuttal, *A Journal of Travels into the Arkansa Territory, during the Year 1819* (Philadelphia: Thos. H. Palmer, 1821), 243.

5. Christina Vella, *Intimate Enemies: The Two Worlds of the Baroness de Pontalba* (Baton Rouge: LSU Press 1997), 10–11; Lawrence N. Powell, *The Accidental City: Improvising New Orleans* (Cambridge, MA: Harvard University Press, 2013), 207; Thomas Hamilton, *Men and Manners in America* (Edinburgh: William Blackwood, 1833), 2:215; "New-Orleans," *Orleans Gazette and Commercial Advertiser*, October 25, 1819.

6. "Died at New-Orleans," *Mississippi Herald & Natchez Gazette*, September 2, 1806.

7. Theodore Clapp, *Autobiographical Sketches and Recollections during a Thirty-Five Years' Residence in New Orleans* (Boston: Phillips, Sampson, and Co., 1857), 71–72; John Russell Hutchinson, *Reminiscences, Sketches and Addresses Selected from My Papers during a Ministry of Forty–Five Years in Mississippi, Louisiana and Texas* (Houston: E.H. Cushing, 1874), 169–170.

8. Clapp, *Autobiographical Sketches*, 71–72; Gurley, *Life an Eloquence of the Rev. Sylvester Larned*, 92–97; Physico-Medical Society, *Report of the Committee of the Physico-Medical Society of New Orleans on the Epidemic of 1820* (New Orleans: C.W. Duhy, 1821), append., case 3; John K. Bettersworth, "Protestant Beginnings in New Orleans," *LHQ* 21, no. 3 (July 1938): 839; "Extract of a Letter from the Correspondent of the Mirror," *Connecticut Courier*, October 11, 1820; "Death of Mrs. Sarah Wyn Larned," *Mothers' Journal and Family Visitant*, September 1848, 262.

9. Timothy F. Reilly, "Parson Clapp of New Orleans: Antebellum Social Critic, Religious Radical, and Member of the Establishment," *LH* 16, no. 2 (Spring 1975): 169; Theodore Clapp, *Parson Clapp of the Strangers' Church of New Orleans*, ed. John Duffy (Baton Rouge: LSU Press, 1957), 119.

10. Clapp, *Autobiographical Sketches*, 189–202. For the larger religious transformations of the early nineteenth century, see Kathryn Gin Lum, *Damned Nation: Hell in*

America from the Revolution to Reconstruction (Oxford: Oxford University Press, 2014), chap. 2.

11. Philo Tower, *Slavery Unmasked: Being a Truthful Narrative of a Three Years' Residence and Journeying in Eleven Southern States* (Rochester, NY: E. Darrow and Brother, 1856), 288.

12. Henry Tudor, *Narrative of a Tour in North America: Comprising Mexico, the Mines of Real del Norte, the United States, and the British Colonies* (London: James Duncan, 1834), 2:64–65; Adam Hodgson, *Letters from North America, Written during a Tour in the United States and Canada* (London: Hurst, Robinson, and Co., 1824), 2:260; Harriet Martineau, *Retrospect of Western Travel* (London: Saunders and Oatley, 1838), 1:125.

13. "A Visit to the Cemetery," *Camden Weekly Journal* (Camden, SC), August 23, 1853.

14. For poetry and songs, see Julia Knapp Chandler, "Broken Hearted: An O'er True Tale of the Fever" (New Orleans, 1878), ms. PS1289.C45 B7 1878, HNOC.

15. Baron Ludwig von Reizenstein, *The Mysteries of New Orleans*, 1854, ed. and trans. Steven Rowan (Baltimore: Johns Hopkins University Press, 2002), 430–431; Charles Lyell, *A Second Visit to the United States of North America* (London, 1849), 2:98; Hugh Murray, *Historical Account of Discoveries and Travels in North America* (London: Longman, Rees, Orme, Brown and Green, 1829), 2:427.

16. Reizenstein, *Mysteries of New Orleans*, 3.

17. Jo Ann Carrigan, "Yellow Fever in New Orleans, 1853: Abstractions and Realities," *JSH* 25, no. 3 (August 1959): 339–355.

18. Dupuy de Chambery, "A Historical Sketch of the Endemic Yellow Fever, Which Prevailed in the City of New-Orleans in the Summer and Autumn of 1819," in *The Medical Repository of Original Essays and Intelligence, Relative to Physic, Surgery, Chemistry, and Natural History*, vol. 6 (New York: William A. Mercein, 1821), 19; Ashbel Smith, *An Account of the Yellow Fever Which Appeared in the City of Galveston, Republic of Texas, in the Autumn of 1839, with Cases and Dissections* (Houston: Hamilton Stuart, 1839), 33.

19. John Bell, ed., *The Eclectic Journal of Medicine*, vol. 1 (Philadelphia: Haswell, Barrington, and Haswell, 1837): 249–250; Urmi Engineer Willoughby, *Yellow Fever, Race, and Ecology in Nineteenth-Century New Orleans* (Baton Rouge: LSU Press, 2017), 64–65; Nancy Stepan, *Picturing Tropical Nature* (Chicago: University of Chicago Press, 2001), 153.

20. Daniel Drake, *A Systematic Treatise, Historical, Etiological and Practical, on the Principal Diseases of the Interior Valley of North America* (Cincinnati: Winthrop B. Smith and Co., 1850), 102. For foul airs, see Melanie Kiechle, *Smell Detectives: An Olfactory History of Nineteenth-Century Urban America* (Seattle: University of Washington Press, 2017).

21. Margaret Brashear to Walter Brashear Jr., January 18, 1830, Brashear and Lawrence Family Papers, series 1, folder 4, ms. 3355, SHC.

22. William Darby, *A Geographical Description of the State of Louisiana,* 2nd ed. (New York: James Olmstead, 1817), 267. Postl's pen name was Charles Sealsfield. Charles Sealsfield, *The Americans as They Are: Described in a Tour through the Valley of the Mississippi* (London: Hurst, Chance and Co., 1828), 194–195; Benjamin Henry Latrobe, *The Journal of Latrobe: Being the Notes and Sketches of an Architect, Naturalist and Traveler in the United States from 1796 to 1820* (New York: D. Appleton and Co., 1905), 234; Arthur Singleton, *Letter from the South and West* (Boston, 1824), 130.

23. J. R. McNeill calculated historical mortality rates as ranging from 38 to 69 percent; Slosek's calculation was 50 to 94.5 percent. J. R. McNeill, *Mosquito Empires: Ecology and War in the Greater Caribbean, 1620–1914* (Cambridge: Cambridge University Press, 2010), 33–40, esp. 37–38; J. Slosek, "*Aedes aegypti* Mosquitoes in the Americas: A Review of Their Interactions with the Human Population," *Social Science & Medicine* 23, no. 3 (1986): 249–257, here 249; Steven Stowe, *Doctoring the South: Southern Physicians and Everyday Medicine in the Mid-Nineteenth Century* (Chapel Hill: University of North Carolina Press, 2004), 5–6.

24. One doctor related that the youngest case of yellow fever he had ever seen was a "white infant aged *five weeks.*" E. D. Fenner, "Report on the Epidemics of Louisiana, Mississippi, Arkansas, and Texas, in the Year 1853," *AMA* 7 (1854): 468. Some epidemiologists suggest that dengue fever and Japanese encephalitis, other flaviviruses, confer on those who survive some cross-immunity to yellow fever. Kenneth Kiple, ed., *The Cambridge Historical Dictionary of Disease* (Cambridge: Cambridge University Press, 2003), 366.

25. For male bias, see Dowler, *Tableau,* 14; Records of Deaths, Interments, Lafayette Cemetery, 1841–1843, vol. 2, 11–19, LM430, NOPL.

26. *Report of the Committee Appointed to Investigate the Causes and Extent of the Late Extraordinary Sickness and Mortality in the Town of Mobile* (Philadelphia: S. Potter and Co., 1820), 8–10; Latrobe, *Journal,* 244.

27. A Physician of New Orleans, "The Unburied Daughter," in *History of the Yellow Fever in New Orleans, during the Summer of 1853* (Philadelphia: C.W. Kenworthy, 1854): 75–77; "History and Incidents of the Plague in New Orleans," *Harper's Monthly,* June–November 1853, 797–798.

28. For Benedict's activities, see Epidemic of 1858, Gribble, ms. 900, HNOC. Henry Didimus, *New Orleans as I Found It* (New York: Harper and Brothers, 1845), 43–45.

29. J. S. McFarlane, "A Review of the Yellow Fever, Its Causes, &c.," in *The Epidemic Summer: List of Interments in All the Cemeteries of New Orleans* (New Orleans: Proprietor of the True Delta, 1853), viii; Charles Caldwell, "Thoughts on the Probable Destiny of New Orleans, in Relation to Health, Population and Commerce," *Philadelphia Journal of the Medical and Physical Sciences* 6 (January 1823): 5.

30. Jonathan Pritchett and İnsan Tunali, "Strangers' Disease: Determinants of Yellow Fever Mortality during the New Orleans Epidemic of 1853," *Explorations in Economic History* 32, no. 4 (1995): 517–539, here 518–520. Edward Barton suggested in

1853 that mortality was about 6¾ per 100, conceding that this was probably an under-estimate as it was derived from "official *published* sources." Barton, *RSC*, 222; "The Mortality of New Orleans," *DBR* 9, no. 2 (August 1850): 245–246.

31. J. Smith Homans, ed., *A Cyclopedia of Commerce and Commercial Navigation* (New York: Harper and Brothers, 1858), 1066; Bennet Dowler, *Researches upon the Necropolis of New Orleans, with Brief Allusions to Its Vital Arithmetic* (New Orleans: Bills and Clark,1850), 13–15.

32. Barton, *RSC*, 185–188. John Nau suggested that 35,000 yellow fever victims were interred between 1853 and 1855 alone, most of them European immigrants. John Nau, *The German People of New Orleans, 1850–1900* (Leiden, Netherlands: E. J. Brill, 1958), 7n1, 15–16; Richard Dunn, *Sugar and Slaves: The Rise of the Planter Class in the English West Indies, 1624–1713* (Chapel Hill: University of North Carolina Press, 1972), 302. See also John O'Hanlon, *The Irish Emigrant's Guide for the United States* (Boston, 1851), 31, 116–117.

33. Historians have long debated hereditary resistance. See Kenneth Kiple and Virginia King, *Another Dimension to the Black Diaspora: Diet, Disease, and Racism* (Cambridge: Cambridge University Press, 1981), 39; Todd Savitt, *Medicine and Slavery: The Diseases and Health Care of Blacks in Antebellum Virginia* (Urbana: University of Illinois Press, 1978), 241; McNeill, *Mosquito Empires,* 46. Espinosa believes that "there is no evidence" to support hereditary immunity, and that "it is time for historians to discard it." Watts entirely rejects hereditary immunity. Mariola Espinosa, "The Question of Racial Immunity to Yellow Fever in History and Historiography," *Social Science History* 38, no. 3–4 (January 2014): 437–453, here 437; Sheldon Watts, "Yellow Fever Immunities in West Africa and the Americas in the Age of Slavery and Beyond: A Reappraisal," and Watts, "Response to Kenneth Kiple," *Journal of Social History* 34, no. 4 (Summer 2001): 955–967, 975–976.

34. Physico-Medical Society, *Report of the Committee of the Physico-Medical Society of New Orleans on the Epidemic of 1820* (New Orleans: C.W. Duhy, 1821), 17–27 (append.); James Stark, *Vital Statistics of New Orleans* (Edinburgh: Robert Inches, 1851), 10; Kiple and King, *Another Dimension,* 42.

35. *RSC,* table between pages 460 and 461. "The City: Mortuary," *Daily Picayune,* October 12, 1858.

36. De Chambery, "Historical Sketch," 17; Edward Jenner Coxe, *Practical Remarks on Yellow Fever, Having Special Reference to the Treatment* (New Orleans: Morgan, 1859), 43; C. R. Fassitt, "Yellow Fever in the Country," *NOMNHG* 2, no. 9 (November 1855): 407.

37. Josiah Nott, "Unity of the Human Race," *Southern Quarterly Review* 9, no. 17 (January 1846): 9; Samuel Cartwright, "On the Prevention of Yellow Fever," *NOMSJ* 10 (November 1853): 316; Philip Tidyman, "A Sketch of the Most Remarkable Diseases of the Negroes in the Southern States," *Philadelphia Journal of the Medical and Physical Sciences* 12 (1826): 325.

38. A. Perlee, "An Account of the Yellow Fever in Natchez," *Philadelphia Journal of the Medical and Physical Sciences* 3 (1821): 7–8, 10; Armand Allard to Guy Allard Duplantier, March 5, 1801, Armand Duplantier Family Letters, series 2, ms. 5060, LSU.

39. William Holcombe, *Yellow Fever and Its Homeopathic Treatment* (New York, 1856), 12; William Wells Brown, *Clotel, Or the President's Daughter* (London: Partridge and Oakley, 1853), 203–204.

40. Lauren E. Blake and Mariano A. Garcia-Blanco, "Human Genetic Variation and Yellow Fever Mortality during 19th Century U.S. Epidemics," *mBio* 5, no. 3 (2014): 1–6, here 2.

41. Willoughby, *Yellow Fever*, 85–94.

42. Susan Sontag, *Illness as Metaphor* (New York: Farrar, Straus and Giroux, 1978), 1–10; Charles E. Rosenberg, "What Is an Epidemic? AIDS in Historical Perspective," *Daedalus* 118, no. 2 (Spring 1989): 1–17, here 2; Keith Wailoo, "Spectacles of Difference: The Racial Scripting of Epidemic Disparities," *BHM* 94, no. 4 (Winter 2020); Jo Ann Carrigan, *The Saffron Scourge: A History of Yellow Fever in Louisiana, 1796–1905* (Lafayette: University of Louisiana at Lafayette Press, 1994), 34.

43. The most cited compendiums of yellow fever mortality remain John Gayle Aiken and George Augustin. Aiken estimated that about 42,147 people died between 1817 and 1899; Augustin estimated it was about 38,052. For some years there is a wide range in the authors' estimates; neither cited their sources. See George Augustin, *History of Yellow Fever* (New Orleans: AMS Press, 1909); John Gayle Aiken, "The Medical History of New Orleans," in *Standard History of New Orleans, Louisiana,* ed. Henry Rightor (Chicago: Lewis, 1900).

44. "Editorial and Miscellaneous," *NOMNHG* 2, no. 4 (June 1855): 187.

45. CVOR, January 20, 1824, 8; "1824 New Orleans City Directory," Orleans Parish, Louisiana Division, NOPL.

46. David R. Goldfield, "The Business of Health Planning: Disease Prevention in the Old South," *JSH* 42, no. 4 (November 1976): 566; M. Morton Dowler, "Letter on Yellow Fever," *NOMSJ* 11, no. 1 (July 1854): 425.

47. "Board of Health," *NOMSJ* 1, no. 2 (July 1844): 96–97; J. C. Simonds, *An Address on the Sanitary Condition of New Orleans* (New Orleans: D. Davies, Son, and Co., 1851), 30.

48. Lafayette was a suburb of New Orleans annexed in 1852. Diary entries for October 17 and 26, 1846, in Abner Phelps Diaries, vol. 2, ms. 1064, LRC.

49. A. Oakey Hall, *The Manhattaner in New Orleans: Or, Phases of "Crescent City" Life* (New York: J.S. Redfield, 1851), 67; Simonds, *Address,* 14, 19.

50. Latrobe, *Journal,* 241–242; "Our City," *Daily Picayune,* August 31, 1837; "The Yellow Fever at New Orleans," *Glasgow Herald,* September 5, 1853; Irene S. Di Maio, ed. and trans., *Gerstäcker's Louisiana: Fiction and Travel Sketches from Antebellum Times through Reconstruction* (Baton Rouge: LSU Press, 2006), 55.

51. Thomas Ashe, *Travels in America, Performed in 1806, For the Purpose of Exploring the Rivers Alleghany, Monongahela, Ohio, and Mississippi* (London: Richard Phillips, 1808), 3: 242; Dowler, *Tableau*, 15–16; *Orleans Gazette and Commercial Advertiser*, December 30, 1819.

52. A. Perlu letter, July 3, 1828, ms. 2979, LSU.

53. Maria Inskeep to Fanny Hampton, October 28, 1832, Fanny Leverich Eshleman Craig Collection, box 1, folder 13, ms. 225, LRC; Statistics Charity Hospital of New Orleans, Charity Hospital Papers, box 2, folder 4156b, ms. RG29, LSM.

54. Edward Barton, *Account of the Epidemic Yellow Fever Which Prevailed in New Orleans during the Autumn of 1833* (Philadelphia: Joseph R.A. Skerrett, 1834), 65; Simonds, *Address*, 13; Erasmus Darwin Fenner, *The Epidemic of 1847: Or, Brief Accounts of the Yellow Fever, That Prevailed at New-Orleans, Vicksburg, Rodney, Natchez, Houston and Covington* (New Orleans, 1848), 189–206; Simonds, *Address*, 4.

55. Chart Exhibiting the Annual Mortality of New Orleans," in *RSC*, 315; Henry Sigerist, "The Cost of Illness to the City of New Orleans in 1850," *BHM* 15 (January 1944): 503–505; "List of Mortality," *NOMNHG* 2, no. 7 (September 1855): 336; T. M. Coan, "Some Peculiarities of Yellow Jack," *Harper's Monthly*, December 1878, 126–130.

56. Hall, *The Manhattaner*, 66–67; "False Alarm about the Yellow Fever," *New York Times*, December 19, 1853.

57. "Lauderdale White Sulphur Spring," *Daily Picayune*, June 6, 1856; Pontchartrain Railroad Company minutes, 1829–1837, Railroad Documents Collection, box 1, folder 4, ms. 526, LRC.

58. Maria Inskeep to Fanny G. Hampton, October 28, 1832, Fanny Leverich Eshleman Craig Collection, box 1, folder 13, ms. 225, LRC; "The Population of New Orleans and the Fever," *Tri-Weekly Commercial*, August 23, 1853; *National Advocate*, September 22, 1823.

59. "The Sickness," *True American*, August 29, 1839; "Letter from the First Private," *Daily Delta*, September 28, 1853; Faust, *This Republic of Suffering*, 148.

60. Elisha Bartlett, *The History, Diagnosis, and Treatment of the Fevers of the United States* (Philadelphia: Lea and Blanchard, 1856), 504; "Domestic Occurrences—Mississippi," *American Monthly Magazine and Critical Review*, December 1817, 140; Carl Kohn Letter Book, September 23, 1833, ms. 269, HNOC.

61. Charles J. Daron to Rothschild & Sons in London, August 13, 1853, XI / 38 / 164, Rothschild; Circular Letter concerning Yellow Fever, 1820, ms. 98-42-L, HNOC; "Our City," *The Picayune*, September 6, 1837.

62. Louisiana Accounts, July 29, 1830, Barings Bank Records, item 18, North America series HC5.7.6, Barings.

63. Thomas Gale to Benjamin Johns, October 25, 1817, Gale and Polk Family Papers, ms. 266, SHC; William Kenner to Major John Minor, October 24, 1820, William

Kenner Papers, box 2, folder 11, mss. 1477, 1491, LSU. For the disruption to banks' operation, see Julia Mansfield, "Sickness and Stagnation: The Interplay of Disease and Markets in 1819," *JER* 40, no. 4 (Winter 2020): 703–708.

64. *Daily Picayune*, September 6, 1837.

65. Vella, *Intimate Enemies*, 10; George to Samuel Fennell, March 1838, ms. 152, HNOC; *True American*, August 27 and 29, October 5, 1839; Joseph Holt Ingraham, *The South-West, by a Yankee* (New York: Harper and Brothers, 1835), 1:164; A Steam-Boat Clerk, "The Last Trip," *Knickerbocker* 46 (July–December 1855): 602–604; William Crenshaw to Nathaniel Bower, September 11 and 14, 1841, William Crenshaw Letters, ms. 46, NOPL.

66. Joseph Bieller to Jacob Bieller, August 27, 1827, Alonzo Snyder Papers, box 1, folder 1, ms. 655, LSU; "Sickness on the Mississippi," *Providence Patriot* (Providence, RI), November 24, 1819.

67. Quotes from Franklin L. Riley, ed., "Diary of a Mississippi Planter, January 1, 1830, to April 1836," *Publications of the Mississippi Historical Society* 10 (1909): 334.

68. John North to Eliza Bowman Lyons, June 30, 1850, Bowman-Turnbull Family Papers, ms. 5059, LSU.

69. Moses Liddell to John Liddell, August 30, 1847, Moses and St. John Richardson Liddell Family Papers, ms. 531, LSU.

70. Brown, *Clotel*, 204, 86.

71. Solomon Northup, *Twelve Years a Slave: Narrative of Solomon Northup, a Citizen of New-York, Kidnapped in Washington City in 1841, and Rescued in 1853* (Buffalo, NY: Derby, Orton and Mulligan, 1853), 167, 183, 177–178; Mark Fiege, *The Republic of Nature: An Environmental History of the United States* (Seattle: University of Washington Press, 2012), 132–133.

72. C. C. Robin, *Voyage to Louisiana, 1803–1805*, trans. Stuart O. Landry Jr. (New Orleans: Pelican, 1966), 248; Joseph Roach, *Cities of the Dead: Circum-Atlantic Performance* (New York: Columbia University Press, 1995), 60. See also James H. Sweet, *Recreating Africa: Culture, Kinship, and Religion in the African-Portuguese World, 1441–1770* (Chapel Hill: University of North Carolina Press, 2003), 178.

73. Latrobe, *Journal*, 191–192, 230, 241. On mourning and burial rituals in the Black Atlantic, see Jason R. Young, *Rituals of Resistance: African Atlantic Religion in Kongo and the Lowcounty South in the Era of Slavery* (Baton Rouge: LSU Press, 2007), 126; Lafcadio Hearn, *Gombo Zhèbes: Little Dictionary of Creole Proverbs, Selected from Six Creole Dialects* (New York: Will H. Coleman, 1885), 18.

74. Latrobe, *Journal*, 232; Roach, *Cities of the Dead*, 61–63. See also Londa Schiebinger, *Secret Cures of Slaves: People, Plants, and Medicine in the Eighteenth-Century Atlantic World* (Stanford, CA: Stanford University Press, 2017).

75. "The City," *Daily Picayune*, January 2, 1858; John Dunlap to Beatrice Dunlap, October 4, 1847, John G. and Beatrice A. Dunlap Family Correspondence, box 1, folder 6, ms. 631, LRC.

76. "City Intelligence: Grave Merchandise," *Daily Picayune*, October 18, 1855; Ned Sublette, *The World That Made New Orleans: From Spanish Silver to Congo Square* (Chicago: Lawrence Hill Books, 2008),109–110; Stephanie Camp, *Closer to Freedom: Enslaved Women and Everyday Resistance in the Plantation South* (Chapel Hill: University of North Carolina Press, 2004), 7.

77. L. H. Peters letter, March 22, 1833, ms. 222, LSU; William Kenner to John Minor, November 24, 1817, William Kenner Papers, mss. 1477, 1491, LSU.

78. "Editorial and Miscellaneous," *NOMNHG* 2, no. 9 (November 1855): 418; "New Goods! New Goods!," *Daily Picayune*, November 8, 1854; "All Saints Day," *Daily Picayune*, October 22, 1858; "Michon & Desportes," *New Orleans Crescent*, November 3, 1859; "Grave Merchandise," *Daily Picayune*, October 18, 1855; William Kingsford, *Impressions of the West and South during a Six Weeks' Holiday* (Toronto: A.H. Armour and Co., 1858), 58.

79. *Mississippi State Gazette,* December 4, 1819; J. B. Warren to Aaron Warren, November 18, 1837, John Bliss Warren Letters, folder 5, ms. RG447, LSM; Mary Copes to Joseph Copes, November 15, 1847, Joseph S. Copes Papers, ms. 733, LRC.

80. Nancy Brown Phelps to Almira Louise Phelps, September 3, 1858, Nancy Brown Phelps Letters, folder 3, ms. 384, HNOC; Reizenstein, *Mysteries of New Orleans,* 430; diary entry for December 27, 1849, Eliza Ann Marsh Robertson Papers, ms. 1181-z, SHC.

81. Quoted from Roulhad Toledano, "Louisiana's Golden Age: Valcour Aime in St. James Parish," *LH* 10, no. 3 (Summer 1969): 211–222.

82. William L. Robinson, *The Diary of a Samaritan: By a Member of the Howard Association of New Orleans* (New York: Harper and Brothers, 1860), 284–285.

83. "A Song Written for and Sung at the Abovenamed Ball on the 12th Inst.," October 14, 1839, Edward Turner and Family Papers, folder 9, ms. 1403, LSU; A Physician of New Orleans, *History of the Yellow Fever in New Orleans, during the Summer of 1853* (Philadelphia: Kenworthy, 1854), 99.

84. *Daily Picayune*, November 13, 1841.

85. George Fennell to brother, March 1838, George Fennell Letters, ms. 152, HNOC.

86. Live burials rarely, if ever, happened. See interviews with Olivier Blanchard, Texas, and interview with Lizzie Barnett, Arkansas, 16:91–92, 2:113, Slave Narratives.

87. *Harper's New Monthly Magazine,* June–November 1853, 846; Willard Glazier, *Peculiarities of American Cities* (Philadelphia: Hubbard Brothers, 1885), 274.

88. "The Destiny of New Orleans," *DBR* 10 (April 1851): 441; "The Moral Advance of New Orleans," *DBR* 2 (November 1846): 349.

89. James Robb, *Speech of James Robb, Esqr., in the South-Western Railroad Convention* (New Orleans: Alex Levy and Co., 1852), 24–25, 18; Robin, *Voyage to Louisiana,* 36, 56.

90. Murray, *Historical Account,* 2:429; James Wyche to O. A. Otey, January 26, 1857, Wyche and Otey Family Papers, folder 9, ms. 1608, SHC; W. L. Gunnels to sister, September 30, 1855, Yellow Fever Correspondence, ms. 699, HNOC.

91. "The Plague in the Southwest," *DBR* 15, no. 6 (December 1853): 598.

92. L. H. Peters letter, March 22, 1833, ms. 222, LSU.

93. *A General Digest of the Acts of the Legislature of Louisiana: Passed from the Year 1804, to 1827* (New Orleans: Benjamin Levy, 1828), 238.

94. *The Laws of the Territory of Louisiana. Comprising All hose Which Are Now Actually In Force Within The Same* (St. Louis [L.]: Joseph Charless, 1808), 19, Newberry; CVOP, April 4, 1805, 2–3; Charles E. Wynes, "Dr. James Durham, Mysterious Eighteenth-Century Black Physician: Man or Myth?," *Pennsylvania Magazine of History and Biography* 103, no. 3 (July 1979): 325–333, quote on 331.

95. *Biennial Report of the Louisiana State Board of Health, 1883–4* (New Orleans: Leon Jastremski, 1884), 139.

96. J. L. E. W. Shecut, *An Essay on the Prevailing, or Yellow Fever of 1817* (Charleston: A.E. Miller, 1817), 29–30; William Dosité Postell, "The Principles of Medical Practice in Louisiana during the First Half of the Nineteenth Century," *Bulletin of the Medical Library Association* 30, no. 3 (April 1942).

97. George Lewis, *Impressions of America and the American Churches* (Edinburgh: W.P Kennedy, 1845), 172–173; Crété, *Daily Life,* 181–182.

98. John Duffy, ed., *The Rudolph Matas History of Medicine in Louisiana* (Baton Rouge: LSU Press, 1958), 1:271; John Salvaggio, *New Orleans' Charity Hospital: A Story of Physicians, Politics, and Poverty* (Baton Rouge: LSU Press, 1992), 30–31.

99. John Duffy, "Pestilence in New Orleans," in *The Past as Prelude: New Orleans, 1718–1968,* ed. Hodding Carter et al. (Gretna, LA: Pelican, 1968), 103–105.

100. "Yellow Fever," *Daily Picayune,* August 17, 1841; E. B. Harris, "Cases of the Epidemic Yellow Fever Prevalent at New Orleans in the Summer and Fall of 1833," *American Journal of the Medical Sciences* 14, no. 27 (May 1834): 46–74.

101. "False Alarm."

102. Samuel Gray to Samuel Merrill, January 1, 1848, Samuel Gray Collection, ms. 233, HNOC; "Sanitary Conditions of the City," *Transcripts Relating to the Medical History of Texas,* vol. 8, *Yellow Fever in Texas, 1839–58,* 25–28, 32, 2R345, UTA.

103. "The Yellow Fever at New Orleans," *The Standard* (London), October 16, 1833; "Necrology," *NOMNHG* 2, no. 7 (September 1855): 334.

104. Crété, *Daily Life,* 183–184.

105. Latrobe, *Journal,* 243; Juanita to Gertrude Calder, September 19, 1905, Gertrude Calder Papers, folder 9, ms. 128, LRC.

106. Reizenstein, *Mysteries of New Orleans,* 422; A. H. Mann, "Life in New Orleans," *Wisconsin Express,* November 9, 1847.

107. "Fever & Ague and Intermittent Fever Cured," *Mississippi State Gazette,* August 15, 1818; "R.R.R.," *Daily Picayune,* September 24, 1856; "Dr. Stillman's Card," *Daily Picayune,* June 15, 1842; "Song of the Yellow Fever Demons," *Daily Picayune,* September 27, 1842; Account Book, 1841–1842, Circus Street Infirmary, ms. 171, NOPL;

Mary Campbell to Joseph Copes, August 3, 1847, Copes Family Papers, box 7, folder 8, ms. 733, LRC.

108. Claiborne to Madison, January 4, 1805, *TPUS*, 9:362; Johann Joachim Lagemann to brother, May 30, 1806, Johann Joachim Lagemann Letters, ms. 77-1, NOPL; George Devol, *Forty Years a Gambler on the Mississippi* (Cincinnati: Devol and Haines, 1887), 20; Cenci to Editors of Crescent, August 26, 1850, in *Letters of Cenci, Written Four Years Ago, on the Sanitary Reforms Needed in New Orleans* (New Orleans: Isaac T. Hinton 1853), 20.

109. Lyell, *A Second Visit*, 2:98; Max to Theodor Neubling, May 11, 1824, and May 20, 1825, Max Neubling Letter Book, ms. 873, LSU.

110. William Crenshaw to Nathaniel Bower, September 11, 1841, William Crenshaw Letters, ms. 46, NOPL.

111. See "Inventory of John Dick's Estate," May 29, 1824, in *General Index of All Succession, Opened in the Parish of Orleans, from the Year 1805, to the Year 1846*, ed. P. M. Bertin (New Orleans: Yeomans and Fitch, 1849), 60.

112. "Embalming the Dead," *Houma Ceres*, April 11, 1857; Reizenstein, *Mysteries of New Orleans*, 530; "My Old Street," *Daily Picayune*, November 28, 1855; CVOR, September 16, 1819, 138, AB311; W. H. Rainey, comp., *A. Mygatt & Co.'s New Orleans Directory for 1857* (New Orleans: L. Pesson and B. Simon, 1857), 22.

113. *Collins v. Graves*, 13 La. Ann. 95 (1858); MM, October 31, 1832, 117.

114. Juanita to Gertrude Calder, September 19, 1905, Gertrude Calder Papers, folder 9, ms. 128, LRC.

115. Alfred Hunt, *Haiti's Influence on Antebellum America: Slumbering Volcano in the Caribbean* (Baton Rouge: LSU Press, 1988), 65–66.

116. Notebook, Christian Miltenberger Papers, box 4, folder 44, vol. 5, ms. 513, SHC; William Dosite Postell, "The Medical Societies of Louisiana Prior to the War between the States," *NOMSJ* 93 (August, 1940): 69–72; Francois Weil, "The Purchase and the Making of French Louisiana," in *Empires of the Imagination: Transatlantic Histories of the Louisiana Purchase*, ed. Peter J. Kastor and Francois Weil (Charlottesville: University of Virginia Press, 2009), 310.

117. "Doit Mr. Miltenberger pour son habitation du Detours des Anglais, au Dr. Allain," June–October 1825; Journal of Christian Miltenberger; Fire Insurance, Louisiana State Insurance Company, Christian Miltenberger Papers, ms. 513, SHC; Rainey, *A. Mygatt & Co.'s New Orleans Business Directory*, 215.

118. G. W. Campbell and E. D. Fenner reports, Louisiana, vol. 9, 49, R. G. Dun & Co. credit report volumes, ms. 791, D8978, HBS.

119. Samuel Cartwright, "Alcohol and the Ethiopian," *NOMSJ* 10 (September 1853): 162; Martha Carolyn Mitchell, "Health and the Medical Profession in the Lower South, 1845–1860," *JSH* 10, no. 4 (November 1944): 435; Salvaggio, *New Orleans' Charity Hospital*, 40. See entries 128, 130, and 153 in Admission Book of the Truro Infirmary,

1855, mf# GS36-214, NOPL; Katherine Kemi Bankole, *Slavery and Medicine: Enslavement and Medical Practices in Antebellum Louisiana* (New York: Routledge 1998), append. B, 183.

120. Eugene Genovese, "The Medical and Insurance Costs of Slaveholding in the Cotton Belt," *Journal of Negro History* 45, no. 3 (July 1960): 141; Bill for Doctor's Care, March 1, 1814, Edward J. Gay Family Papers, box 1, ms. 1295, LSU.

121. Appointment of P. A. Lambert as a member of the Eastern Medical Board, March 10, 1843, Lambert Family Papers, OSF 1, ms. 244, LRC.

122. William Chambers, "Yellow Jack," *Chamber's Journal of Popular Literature, Science and Arts* 17, no. 449 (August 1862): 96.

123. Joshua D. Rothman, *Flush Times and Fever Dreams: A Story of Capitalism and Slavery in the Age of Jackson* (Athens: University of Georgia Press, 2010), 122–123.

124. Thomas Hersey, ed., *The Thomsonian Recorder; Or, Impartial Advocate of Botanic Medicine,* vol. 1 (Columbus, OH: Jarvis Pike and Co., 1833), 144.

125. "The Moving Panorama," *Weekly Comet,* September 11, 1853; *Acts Passed at the First Session of the Fourth Legislature of the State of Louisiana* (New Orleans: Thierry, Printer of the State of Louisiana, 1819), 123.

126. "Remedy for Yellow Fever," *Tri-Weekly Commercial,* August 23, 1853; George Washington Cable, "The Dance at Place Congo," *Century Magazine* 31, no. 4 (1886): 519–532; Carolyn Morrow Long, *A New Orleans Voudou Priestess: The Legend and Reality of Marie Laveau* (Gainesville: University Press of Florida, 2006); "Madame Virginica," *New Orleans Daily Crescent,* May 7, 1859; "Madame Caprell," *Daily Picayune,* April 11, 1859. Quote about Laveaux from Emily Suzanne Clark, "Nineteenth-Century New Orleans Voudou: An American Religion," *American Religion* 2, no. 1 (Fall 2020): 149.

127. Régine Latortue and Gleason R. W. Adams, eds. and trans., *Les Cenelles: A Collection of Poems by Creole Writers of the Early Nineteenth-Century* (Boston: G.K. Hall, 1979), xiv.

128. H. S. Fulkerson, *Random Recollections of Early Days in Mississippi* (Vicksburg, MS: Vicksburg Printing and Publishing Co., 1885), 38–40.

129. Margaret Brashear to Thomas Tilton Barr, June 19, 1824, Brashear and Lawrence Family Papers, ms. 3355, SHC; Thomas to William Robertson, August 7, 1823, Walter Prichard Collection, ms. 2509, LSU; Savitt, *Medicine and Slavery,* 20; J. E. to J. B. Craighead, September 11, 1847, Edward J. Gay Family Papers, ms. 1295, LSU.

130. Rosalie Priour, *The Adventures of a Family of Emmigrants Who Emmigrated to Texas in 1834: An Autobiography,* 60–62, 65–68, 2R154, UTA.

131. "The Harvest of Death," *New York Times,* September 26, 1853; Robinson, *Diary of a Samaritan,* 239; Marisa Fuentes, *Dispossessed Lives: Enslaved Women, Violence, and the Archive* (Philadelphia: University of Pennsylvania Press, 2016), 94–97.

132. Interview with Harriet Barrett, Texas, 15:49–50, Slave Narratives; Hearn, *Gombo Zhèbes,* 26; interview with Ceceil George, in *Mother Wit: The Ex-Slave Narratives*

of the Louisiana Writers' Project, ed. Ronnie Clayton (New York: P. Lang, 1990), 85–86. For more on sickness and slavery, see Sharla Fett, *Working Cures: Healing, Health, and Power on Southern Slave Plantations* (Chapel Hill: University of North Carolina Press, 2002).

133. Interview with Alice Douglass, Oklahoma, 13:73, Slave Narratives. For the key role of African practitioners of medicine, see Manuel Barcia, *The Yellow Demon of Fever: Fighting Disease in the Nineteenth-Century Transatlantic Slave Trade* (New Haven, CT: Yale University Press, 2020), chap. 5.

3. Immunocapital

1. Vincent Nolte, *Fifty Years in Both Hemispheres; or, Reminiscences of the Life of a Former Merchant* (New York: Redfield, 1854), 90–91. See also "Reviews, *Fifty Years in Both Hemispheres*," *Athenaeum Journal of Literature, Science, and the Fine Arts*, no. 1399 (August 1854): 1009–1013.

2. Edward E. Baptist, *The Half Has Never Been Told: Slavery and the Making of American Capitalism* (New York: Basic Books, 2014), 85–87, here 89. For Nolte's career, see Thomas N. Ingersoll, *Mammon and Manon in Early New Orleans: The First Slave Society in the Deep South, 1718–1819* (Knoxville: University of Tennessee Press, 1999), 279; Scott P. Marler, *The Merchants' Capital: New Orleans and the Political Economy of the Nineteenth-Century South* (New York: Cambridge University Press, 2013), 19–21; Sven Beckert, *Empire of Cotton: A New History of Global Capitalism* (New York: Knopf Doubleday, 2014), 214.

3. Nolte, *Fifty Years*, 91.

4. For the status of Nolte's loans to the city, see MM, May 6, 1826, 30; April 19, 1828, 29.

5. "The History of a Cosmopolite," *Putnam's Monthly Magazine*, July–December 1854, 325–330; Benjamin Henry Latrobe, *The Journal of Latrobe: Being the Notes and Sketches of an Architect, Naturalist and Traveler in the United States from 1796 to 1820* (New York: D. Appleton and Co., 1905), 209–210.

6. Nolte, *Fifty Years*, 91; Conevery Bolton Valenčius, *The Health of the Country: How American Settlers Understood Themselves and Their Land* (New York: Perseus Books Group, 2002), 22–34, here 32.

7. John Palfrey to John Gorham Palfrey, April 18, 1810, ms. 333, LSU.

8. John Clark, *New Orleans, 1719–1812: An Economic History* (Baton Rouge: LSU Press, 1970), 308; quote from Adam Rothman, *Slave Country: American Expansion and the Origins of the Deep South* (Cambridge, MA: Harvard University Press, 2005), 52–53.

9. John Palfrey to Beverly Chew and Richard Relf, April 15, 1812, Palfrey Family Papers, ms. 333, LSU.

10. Palfrey to Chew and Relf, April 15, 1812; Palfrey to Isaac Baldwin, September 2 and October 14, 1815, Palfrey Family Papers, box 1, folder 7, ms. 333, LSU; Gwendolyn

Midlo Hall, "Afro-Louisiana History and Genealogy, 1718–1820," database, record for "Maria," https://www.ibiblio.org/laslave/individ.php?sid=63912.

11. Rothman, *Slave Country,* 184.

12. John G. Palfrey, "The Inter-State Slave Trade," *Anti-Slavery Tracts. No. 5* (Boston, 1855), 3.

13. Jonathan Levy, *Freaks of Fortune: The Emerging World of Capitalism and Risk in America* (Cambridge, MA: Harvard University Press, 2009), 1–4.

14. For the many risks of New Orleans, see Calvin Schermerhorn, *The Business of Slavery and the Rise of American Capitalism, 1815–1860* (New Haven, CT: Yale University Press, 2015), 100; Walter Johnson, *River of Dark Dreams: Slavery and Empire in the Cotton Kingdom* (Cambridge, MA.: Harvard University Press, 2013), 73–96; Arwen Mohun, *Risk: Negotiating Safety in American Society* (Baltimore: Johns Hopkins University Press, 2013), 1–5; Jessica Lepler, *The Many Panics of 1837: People, Politics, and the Creation of a Transatlantic Financial Crisis* (Cambridge: Cambridge University Press, 2013), chaps. 6 and 7.

15. Alexander Mackay, *The Western World, or, Travels in the United States in 1846–47* (London: Richard Bentley, 1849), 2:88. See also Billy Smith, *Ship of Death: A Voyage That Changed the Atlantic World* (New Haven, CT: Yale University Press, 2014), 236–237.

16. *Bulletin* quoted in "Fever," *New-York Daily Tribune,* September 13, 1842.

17. Louis P. Masur, "'Age of the First Person Singular': The Vocabulary of the Self in New England, 1780–1850," *Journal of American Studies* 25, no. 2 (August 1991): 189–211. See also Daniel Howe, *Making the American Self* (Cambridge, MA: Harvard University Press, 1997), 114–117.

18. For personality "faults" leading to failure, see Scott Sandage, *Born Losers: A History of Failure in America* (Cambridge, MA: Harvard University Press, 2005), chap. 2; Ann Fabian, *The Unvarnished Truth: Personal Narratives in Nineteenth-Century America* (Berkeley: University of California Press, 2002), chap. 1.

19. *Daily Picayune,* November 26, 1841.

20. "The Theory of Acclimation," *Natchez Daily Courier,* August 20, 1853. For various uses of the term "acclimation," see Hans Sloane, *A Voyage to the Islands Madera, Barbados, Nieves, S. Christophers and Jamaica* (London: B.M., 1707), 1:xcvii; Thomas Dancer, *The Medical Assistant, or Jamaica Practice of Physic* (Kingston, Jamaica: Alexander Aikman, 1809), 89–90.

21. Adjective: E. D. Fenner, "The Yellow Fever Quarantine at New Orleans," *AMA* 2 (1849): 604, 624, 628. Noun: Erasmus Darwin Fenner, *The Epidemic of 1847: Or, Brief Accounts of the Yellow Fever, That Prevailed at New-Orleans, Vicksburg, Rodney, Natchez, Houston and Covington* (New Orleans, 1848), 207; James Wynne, *Report on the Vital Statistics of the United States, Made to the Mutual Life Insurance Company of New York* (New York: H. Baililiere, 1857), 198. Verb: "The Season," *Daily Picayune,* October 25, 1842.

22. "Acclimated Cows," *Daily Picayune*, September 7, 1858.

23. E. D. Fenner, "General Report on the Medical Topography and Meteorology of New Orleans," *Southern Medical Reports*, vol. 1 (New Orleans: B.M. Norman, 1849–1850), 32; Philip Tidyman, "A Sketch of the Most Remarkable Diseases of the Negroes of the Southern States, with an Account of the Method of Treating Them, Accompanied by Physiological Observations," *Philadelphia Journal of the Medical and Physical Sciences* 12 (May and August 1826): 306–338, here 326; Bennet Dowler, review of Daniel Drake, *A Systematic Treatise*, in *NOMSJ* 7, no. 1 (1850): 67.

24. Nicholas Gerardin, *Mémoires sur la fièvre jaune: Considérée dans sa nature et dans ses rapports avec les gouvernements* (Paris: Mequignon-Marvais, 1820), 13, 15, my translations.

25. "Mortality of the Last Sickly Season," *Daily Picayune*, November 19, 1841. For the fear of losing acclimation, see T. M. Coan, "Some Peculiarities of Yellow Jack," *Harper's Monthly*, December 1878, 126–130. For "northern acclimatization," see Anya Zilberstein, *A Temperate Empire: Making Climate Change in Early America* (Oxford: Oxford University Press, 2016), chap. 3. African, Panamanian, and Congo fever were alleged to be particularly virulent manifestations. "Panama Fever," *Daily Picayune*, September 22, 1853; H., "The Fever," *Daily Picayune*, August 6, 1853.

26. Mark Twain, *The Gilded Age: A Tale of To-Day* (Hartford, CT: American, 1874), 153.

27. For national debates surrounding yellow fever's etiology, see Thomas A. Apel, *Feverish Bodies, Enlightened Minds: Science and the Yellow Fever Controversy in the Early American Republic* (Stanford, CA: Stanford University Press, 2016), 3–25.

28. Andrew Ellicott, *The Journal of Andrew Ellicott* (Philadelphia: William Fry, 1814), 288.

29. "Anonymous Letter about Yellow Fever," November 17, 1847, ms. 1808, LSU.

30. A Returned Immigrant, "Liberty and Slavery in America," *New Monthly Magazine and Literary Journal* (London) 1 (1836): 326.

31. "The Season," *Daily Picayune*, October 25, 1842.

32. James McMartin to Peter McMartin, June 15, 1849, Peter McMartin Papers, N-YHS.

33. Fenner, *The Epidemic of 1847*, 206.

34. Edward Jenner Coxe, *Practical Remarks on Yellow Fever, Having Special Reference to the Treatment* (New Orleans: Morgan, 1859), 42–44.

35. George Washington Cable, *The Creoles of Louisiana* (New York: Charles Scribner's Sons, 1884), 292.

36. J. S. McFarlane, "A Review of the Yellow Fever, Its Causes, &c.," in *The Epidemic Summer: List of Interments in All the Cemeteries of New Orleans* (New Orleans: Proprietor of the True Delta, 1853), ix–x.

37. Charles Deléry, *Précis historique de la fièvre jaune* (New Orleans, 1859), 8; Jean Charles Faget, *Mémoires et lettres sur la fièvre jaune et la fièvre paludéenne* (New Orleans,

1864). See also Shirley Elizabeth Thompson, *Exiles at Home: The Struggle to Become American in Creole New Orleans* (Cambridge, MA: Harvard University Press, 2009), 37–38.

38. Barton quoted in Wynne, *Report on the Vital Statistics,* 200, emphasis in the original. For more on the difficulty of differentiating malaria from yellow fever, see John Duffy, "The Impact of Malaria on the South," in *Disease and Distinctiveness in the American South,* ed. Todd L. Savitt and James Harvey Young (Knoxville: University of Tennessee Press, 1988), 29–54, here 33–35; Samuel Henry Dickson, "On the Blending and Conversion of Types in Fever," *AMA* 5 (1852): 127–161, here 148.

39. Nott, "Life Insurance at the South," *DBR* 3, no. 5 (May 1847): 366; Josiah Nott and George Gliddon, *Indigenous Races of the Earth; Or, New Chapters of Ethnological Inquiry* (Philadelphia: J. B. Lippincott & Co., 1857), 376.

40. Elizabeth Trist to unknown recipient, March 1, 1806, Nicholas Philip Trist Papers, box 1, folder 8, ms. 2104, SHC; Robeson DeHart to Sarah B. Evans, September 21, 1839, Nathaniel Evans and Family Papers, box 1, folder 14, ms. 6701, LSU; M. Morton Dowler, "Letters on Yellow Fever," *NOMSJ* 11, no. 4 (January 1855): 499.

41. Élisée Reclus, *Correspondance* (Paris: Librairie Schleicher Frères, 1911), 1:78–81; "Later from Liberia," *Daily Picayune,* October 14, 1851.

42. George Washington Cable, *The Grandissimes: A Story of Creole Life* (New York, 1880), 46; E. H. Barton, *Introductory Lecture on Acclimation, Delivered at the Opening of the Third Session of the Medical College of Louisiana* (New Orleans: Commercial Bulletin Print, 1837), 4.

43. Stanford Chaillé, "Acclimatisation, or Acquisition of Immunity from Yellow Fever," *NOMSJ* 33 (August 1880): 101–136, here 132.

44. Richard Clague to Mayor John Minor, August 24, 1820, William Kenner Papers, mss. 1477, 1491, LSU; Charles Watts to Family, June 5, 1825, Charles Watts Papers, New Orleans, RL.10958, Duke; Isaac H. Charles to John Edward Siddall, September 18, 1847, Isaac H. Charles Letters, ms. 621, LSU.

45. "The Epidemic," *Daily Picayune,* October 6, 1843; *Daily Picayune,* November 26, 1841; Charles Caldwell, "Thoughts on the Probable Destiny of New Orleans, in Relation to Health, Population and Commerce," *Philadelphia Journal of the Medical and Physical Sciences* 6 (January 1823): 12; George Washington Cable, *Dr. Sevier* (Boston, 1883), 280. For more on prejudice, see Jo Ann Carrigan, "Privilege, Prejudice, and the Strangers' Disease in Nineteenth-Century New Orleans," *JSH* 36, no. 4 (November 1970): 568–578, here 570–573.

46. Diary entry for September 24, 1858, Thomas Kelah Wharton Diaries and Sketchbook, ms. 3306, New York Public Library Archives and Manuscripts; "More Subjects for the Fever," *The Picayune,* September 14, 1837; "Now," *Daily Picayune,* October 9, 1855; "Don't Go to New Orleans," *Republican Banner and Nashville Whig,* September 27, 1853; "To Young Men at a Distance," *Daily Picayune,* September 21, 1837.

47. *Daily Picayune*, October 7, 1845. For rents, see L. H. Peters Letter, March 22, 1833, ms. 222, LSU; "Editorial and Other Items," *New Orleans Times*, September 27, 1866.

48. Ralph Roanoke, "Random Leaf from the Life of Ralph Roanoke," *Knicker-bocker*, September, 1852, 200, 201.

49. "Sketches of Character. No. LXX. The Acclimated Man," *Daily Delta*, August 1, 1853; "The Convalescent," *Daily Picayune*, September 18, 1853.

50. "Some Banquet Hall Deserted," *Daily Delta*, July 28, 1853; "The Convalescent," *Daily Picayune*, September 18, 1853; "Talk about Town," *Daily Delta*, November 9, 1858; "New Years," *Daily Picayune*, January 1, 1858; A. Oakey Hall, *The Manhattaner in New Orleans: Or, Phases of "Crescent City" Life* (New York: J.S. Redfield, 1851), esp. 66; "History and Incidents of the Plague in New Orleans," *Harper's Monthly*, June–November 1853, 803; Barton, *RSC*, 180, 223.

51. "Situation Wanted," *New-Orleans Commercial Bulletin*, December 18, 1844; "To Dry Good Merchants," *Daily Picayune*, October 25, 1843; "Situation Wanted," *Daily Picayune*, June 23, 1838; "Wanted," *Daily Picayune*, September 5, 1839; "Wants," *Daily Picayune*, December 16, 1857; *Daily Picayune*, November 20, 1839; "Situation Wanted," *Daily Picayune*, August 13, 1840.

52. *Daily Picayune*, August 30, 1846; "Wanted," *Daily Picayune*, June 20, 1839; *Daily Picayune*, August 14, 1853. For acclimation's value in Charleston, see Michael D. Thompson, *Working on the Dock of the Bay: Labor and Enterprise in an Antebellum Southern Port* (Columbia: University of South Carolina Press, 2015), esp. chap. 5.

53. For acclimation certificates, see "Arrival of Steamship Philadelphia," *Daily Picayune*, August 15, 1857; "Health and Acclimation Certificate," in *Annual Report for the Supervising Surgeon-General of the Marine-Hospital Service of the United States for the Fiscal Year 1899* (Washington, DC: US Government Printing Office, 1893), 493. Eliza Breedam to Louisa Millard, September 3, 1833, Taylor Miles and Family Papers, box 1, folder 1:1a, ms. 1378, LSU.

54. Gustav Dresel, *Gustav Dresel's Houston Journal: Adventures in North America and Texas, 1837–1841*, ed. and trans. Max Freund (Austin: University of Texas Press, 1954), 21–22; *Daily Picayune*, November 6, 1858.

55. A Returned Emigrant, "Liberty and Slavery in America," *New Monthly Magazine and Literary Journal* 46, pt. 1 (1836): 321–334, here 326. For mistaken acclimation, see Fenner, "The Yellow Fever of 1853," *DBR* 17, no. 1 (1854): 41.

56. "A Brilliant Chance," *Daily Picayune*, September 19, 1846.

57. "False Alarm about the Yellow Fever," *New York Times*, December 19, 1853; John Palfrey to Henry Palfrey, October 4, 1819, Palfrey Family Papers, ms. 333, LSU.

58. "Information Wanted," *Daily Picayune*, June 15, 1842; "Information Wanted," *Daily Picayune*, February 2, 1839.

59. Theodore Clapp, *Parson Clapp of the Strangers' Church of New Orleans*, ed. John Duffy (Baton Rouge: LSU Press, 1957), 97, 108–109; "Southern Intelligence," *Baltimore Sun*, September 13, 1847.

60. George Fennell to Samuel Fennell, March 1838, George Fennell Letters, ms. 152, HNOC; H. J. Masson to James Emile Armor, September 25, 1837, and September 28, 1841, James Emile Armor Papers, box 1, folder 1, ms. 100, NOPL.

61. See any listing for Dun & Bradstreet in Louisiana, vol. 9, R. G. Dun & Co. credit report volumes, ms. 791, D8978, HBS.

62. "Cards," *Daily Picayune*, September 4, 1842.

63. D. G., "Our Public Schools," *Daily Picayune*, October 6, 1847.

64. "The Rev. Joel Parker," *Daily Picayune*, January 3, 1838.

65. F. A. Farley, "The Unitarian Church in New Orleans," *Daily Picayune*, May 10, 1868; John B. Warren to Aaron Warren, November 24, 1835, John Bliss Warren Letters, ms. RG447, LSM.

66. "Spirit of the Press," *Daily Delta*, October 28, 1854.

67. Maunsel White, "The Olden Time in New-Orleans and Yellow Fever," *DBR* 6, no. 2 (1848): 156–158, quote from 157. For more on White's life, see "Maunsel White, Merchant, of New-Orleans," *DBR* 14, no. 1 (1853): 85; Marler, *The Merchants' Capital*, 28; David T. Gleeson, *The Irish in the South, 1815–1877* (Chapel Hill: University of North Carolina Press, 2001), 122.

68. White, "The Olden Time," 157–158; Mary Louise Marshall, "Samuel A. Cartwright and States' Rights Medicine," *NOMSJ* 93 (July 1940–June 1941): 74–78, here 75. For an excellent account of Black women's medical expertise, see Deirdre Cooper Owens, *Medical Bondage: Race, Gender, and the Origins of American Gynecology* (Athens: University of Georgia Press, 2017).

69. William Holcombe, "Queer Things about Yellow Fever," *Southwestern Christian Advocate*, February 6, 1879.

70. "The Population of New Orleans and the Fever," *Tri-Weekly Commercial* (Wilmington, NC), August 23, 1853; McFarlane, "Review of the Yellow Fever," viii.

71. For wishful thinking, see the entry for June 10, 1832, in Carl Kohn Letterbook, ms. 269, HNOC.

72. Richard Campanella, *Time and Place in New Orleans: Past Geographies in the Present Day* (Gretna, LA: Pelican, 2002), 70; Richard Follett, *The Sugar Masters: Planters and Slaves in Louisiana's Cane World, 1820–1860* (Baton Rouge: LSU Press, 2005), 85–87, 90–91.

73. Tyrone Power, *Impressions of America: During the Years 1833, 1832, and 1835* (London: Richard Bentley, 1836), 2:242. For unionization, see Roger W. Shugg, *Origins of Class Struggle in Louisiana: A Social History of White Farmers and Laborers during Slavery and After, 1840–1875* (Baton Rouge: LSU Press, 1939), 113–120.

74. Charles Gayarré, *History of Louisiana: The American Domination* (New York: William J. Widdleton, 1866), 636.

75. T. P. Thompson, "Early Financing in New Orleans—Being the Story of the Canal Bank—1831–1915," *Publications of the Louisiana Historical Society* 7 (1913–1914): 27.

76. Barton, *RSC,* 247–248.

77. Cable, *The Creoles of Louisiana,* 292.

78. Eleanor Stauman to her aunt, September 9, 1820, Ker-Texada Paper, folder 1, ms. 545, LRC; James Copes to Joseph Copes, October 3, 1835, Joseph. S. Copes Papers, box 1, folder 24, ms. 733, LRC; Mahala Roach Diary, entries for September 1855, Roach-Eggleston Family Papers, vol. 52, folder 59, ms. 2614, SHC.

79. Thomas Gale to Benjamin Johns, June 1, 1817, Gale and Polk Family Papers, box 1, folder 1, ms. 266, SHC.

80. *Daily Picayune,* October 12, 1838.

81. Paul Lachance, "Intermarriage and French Cultural Persistence in Late Spanish and Early American New Orleans," *Histoire sociale / Social History* 15, no. 29 (1982): 75–77.

82. *Daily Picayune,* October 12, 1838.

83. Thomas Butler Gunn Diaries, October 19, 1858, vol. 9, MOHS; Eliza Breedam to Louisa Millard, September 3, 1833, Taylor Miles and Family Papers, box 1, folder 1:1a, ms. 1378, LSU; "Later from Texas," *Tennessean,* October 12, 1853.

84. Quotes from "Feverish Love," *Des Moines Register,* November 20, 1879; Dick Lester, "John Dick of New Orleans," *LH* 34, no. 3 (Summer 1993): 363.

85. William Augustus Shubert, *Yellow Fever: Its Origin, Improper Treatment, Prevention and Cure* (Savannah: J.M. Cooper and Co., 1860), 46–47; Elizabeth Trist to Nicholas Trist Jr., June 3, 1810, Nicholas Philip Trist Papers, folder 10, ms. 2104, SHC. For the widowocracy of colonial Virginia, see Edmund Morgan, *American Slavery, American Freedom: The Ordeal of Colonial Virginia* (New York: W. W. Norton, 1975), 166–179.

86. Baron Ludwig von Reizenstein, *The Mysteries of New Orleans,* 1854, ed. and trans. Steven Rowan (Baltimore: Johns Hopkins University Press, 2002), 434. For poor white women's experience of yellow fever, see Rosalie Priour, *The Adventures of a Family of Emmigrants Who Emmigrated to Texas in 1834: An Autobiography,* chaps. 25–27, UTA; "History and Incidents of the Plague in New Orleans," *Harper's Monthly,* June–November 1853, 805.

87. William L. Robinson, *The Diary of a Samaritan: By a Member of the Howard Association of New Orleans* (New York: Harper and Brothers, 1860), 239–240.

88. Richard Tansey, "Prostitution and Politics in Antebellum New Orleans," in *History of Women in the United States,* vol. 9: *Prostitution,* ed. Nancy Cott (London: K.G. Saur, 1993), 47; Cynthia Tolbert, "Alms for the Poor: An Historical Analysis of a System of Disgrace," *Loyola Poverty Law Journal* 1 (Spring 1995): 60–61. For acclimated wet nurses, see "Wanted," *Daily Picayune,* September 22, 1839.

89. David Eltis, Frank D. Lewis, and David Richardson, "Slave Prices, the African Slave Trade, and Productivity in the Caribbean, 1674–1807," *Economic History Review* 58, no. 4 (November 2005): 679.

90. The "second slavery" refers to the expansion and refashioning of Atlantic slavery during the nineteenth century, when chattel slavery proved compatible with

industrial capitalism. In the United States, Cuba, and Brazil, slavery's physical footprint and economic importance grew even as even as slavery declined, stagnated, or was abolished elsewhere. Anthony E. Kaye, "The Second Slavery: Modernity in the Nineteenth-Century South and the Atlantic World," *JSH* 75, no. 3 (August 2009): 627–650; Ira Berlin, *Generations of Captivity: A History of African-American Slaves* (Cambridge, MA: Harvard University Press, 2003), 169–171.

91. Ingersoll, *Mammon and Manon,* 278; Steven Deyle, *Carry Me Back: The Domestic Slave Trade in American Life* (Oxford: Oxford University Press, 2006), 140. For price fluctuations according to age, gender, skills, and many other factors, see Daina Ramey Berry, *The Price for Their Pound of Flesh: The Value of the Enslaved, from Womb to Grave, in the Building of a Nation* (New York: Beacon Press, 2017).

92. Interview with Ceceil George, in *Mother Wit: The Ex-Slave Narratives of the Louisiana Writers' Project,* ed. Ronnie Clayton (New York: P. Lang, 1990), 85–86; John Evans to Sarah Evans, January 25, 1834, and May 28, 1833, Nathaniel Evans Papers, box 1, folder 12, ms. 670, LSU; Henry McCall, "History of Evan Hall Plantation," Henry McCall's Evan Hall Plantation Book, ms. 2347, SHC; Charles Rosenberg, *The Cholera Years: The United States in 1832, 1849, and 1866* (Chicago: University of Chicago Press, 1962), 36–38.

93. Sharon Ann Murphy, "Securing Human Property: Slavery, Life Insurance, and Industrialization in the Upper South," *JER* 25, no. 4 (Winter 2005): 624–625.

94. Josiah Nott, "Statistics of Southern Slave Population with Especial Reference to Life Insurance," *DBR* 4, no. 3 (November 1847): 286–287.

95. Murphy, "Securing Human Property," 643. See also Berry, *Price for Their Pound,* 210–211.

96. John Knight to William M. Beall, May 22, 1843, and February 1 and August 12, 1844, Knight Family Papers, RL.11553, Duke.

97. Walter Johnson, *Soul by Soul: Life inside the Antebellum Slave Market* (Cambridge, MA: Harvard University Press, 1999), chap. 2; Berry, *Price for Their Pound,* 24–25.

98. *Louisiana Advertiser,* October 7, 1826; "For Sale," *New Orleans Crescent,* September 3, 1850; "For Sale," *Louisiana State Gazette,* March 11, 1825.

99. Joseph Holt Ingraham, *The South-West, by a Yankee* (New York: Harper and Brothers, 1835), 2:29–30; "Slave for Sale," *Daily Picayune,* January 21, 1854.

100. Martin quoted in Bennet Dowler, *Tableau of the Yellow Fever of 1853 with Topographical, Chronological, and Historical Sketches of the Epidemics of New Orleans since their Origin in 1796* (New Orleans: Office of the Picayune, 1854), 15. For fetishization in the slave market, see Edward Baptist, "'Cuffy,' 'Fancy Maids,' and 'One-Eyed Men': Rape, Commodification and the Domestic Slave Trade of the United States," *AHR* 106, no. 5 (December 2001): 1619–1650; John S. Kendall, "Shadow over the City," *LHQ* 22, no. 1 (January 1939): 142–165; Ingraham, *The South-West,* 2:243–245.

101. Deyle, *Carry Me Back,* 135–136, 159; Johnson, *Soul by Soul,* 139–140.

102. Benjamin Drew, *A North-Side View of Slavery: The Refugee: Or, The Narrative of Fugitive Slaves in Canada* (Boston, 1856), 84.

103. Joseph T. Hicks to Samuel Smith Downey, February 27, 1836, Samuel Smith Downey Papers, box 4, RL.00323, Duke; *Argus* quoted in Theodore Weld, *American Slavery as It Is: Testimony of a Thousand Witnesses* (New York, 1839), 162.

104. Herman Freudenberger and Jonathan B. Pritchett, "The Domestic United States Slave Trade: New Evidence," *Journal of Interdisciplinary History* 21, no. 3 (1991): 447–477, here 463–464; Laurence J. Kotlikoff, "The Structure of Slave Prices in New Orleans, 1804–1862," *Economic Inquiry* 17, no. 4 (1979): 496–518, here 503–506.

105. Kotlikoff, "Structure of Slave Prices," 503; Waters & Co. to W. K. Lathin, August 4, 1846, Snyder Collection, MOHS; William Kenner to John Minor, November 15, 1822; William Kenner to Katharine Minor, September 29, 1817, William Kenner Papers, mss. 1477, 1491, LSU. See also Deyle, *Carry Me Back*, 57.

106. Frederick Law Olmsted, *The Cotton Kingdom: A Traveller's Observations on Cotton and Slavery in the American Slave States* (New York: Mason Brothers, 1861), 1:276.

107. For the white / Black labor calculus, see Follett, *The Sugar Masters*, 85–93; Kotlikoff, "Structure of Slave Prices," 503.

108. Ariela Gross, *Double Character: Slavery and Mastery in the Antebellum Southern Courtroom* (Princeton, NJ: Princeton University Press, 2000), 122–130.

109. Judith K. Schafer, "'Guaranteed against the Vices and Maladies Prescribed by Law': Consumer Protection, the Law of Slave Sales, and the Supreme Court in Antebellum Louisiana," *American Journal of Legal History* 31, no. 4 (October 1987): 311–312; *Dewees v. Morgan*, 1 Mart. (o. s.) 1 (La., 1809).

110. *Acts Passed at the Second Session of the Seventh Legislature of the State of Louisiana* (New Orleans: James M. Bradford, 1826), 114–118.

111. A Creole, "Mr. Editor," *Louisiana Advertiser*, March 16, 1827; Johnson, *Soul by Soul*, 12, 169–170, 183–186.

112. Testimony of Peter Ryas, Texas, 16:274–277, here 277, Slave Narratives.

113. John B. Wyeth, *Oregon: Or, a Short History of a Long Journey from the Atlantic Ocean to the Pacific by Land* (Cambridge, MA, 1833), 72–74.

114. For free Black status in New Orleans, see Ira Berlin, *Slaves without Masters: The Free Negro in the Antebellum South* (New York: Pantheon, 1974), chap. 4; Laura Foner, "The Free People of Color in Louisiana and St. Domingue: A Comparative Portrait of Two Three-Caste Slave Societies," *Journal of Social History* 3, no. 4 (1970): 406–430, here 426–427; Paul Lachance, "The Limits of Privilege: Where Free Persons of Colour Stood in the Hierarchy of Wealth in Antebellum New Orleans," *Slavery and Abolition* 17, no. 1 (1996): 65–84, here 65–67.

115. Loren Schweniger, "Prosperous Blacks in the South, 1790–1880," *AHR* 95, no. 1 (1990): 39.

116. Robert C. Reinders, "The Free Negro in the New Orleans Economy, 1850–1860," *LH* 6, no. 3 (1965): 273–285.

117. For free women of color, see Rashauna Johnson, *Slavery's Metropolis: Unfree Labor in New Orleans during the Age of Revolutions* (Cambridge: Cambridge University Press, 2016), 94–110. For the displacement of Black workers by white European migrants, see Ira Berlin and Herbert G. Gutman, "Natives and Immigrants, Free Men and Slaves: Urban Workingmen in the Antebellum American South," *AHR* 88, no. 5 (December 1983): 1175–1200.

118. For the diversity of New Orleans's free Black population, see Alejandro de la Fuente and Ariela J. Gross, *Becoming Free, Becoming Black: Race, Freedom, and Law in Cuba, Virginia, and Louisiana* (Cambridge: Cambridge University Press, 2020), table on 156, 166–167; Ingersoll, *Mammon and Manon*, 346–348.

119. "Reveries of a Convalescent," *New Orleans Weekly Delta,* September 15, 1853.

120. September 23, 1833, in Carl Kohn Letterbook, ms. 269, HNOC.

121. Entries for September 1833 through the end of 1834, in Carl Kohn Letterbook, ms. 269, HNOC.

4. Public Health, Private Acclimation

1. John B. Wyeth, *Oregon: Or, a Short History of a Long Journey from the Atlantic Ocean to the Pacific by Land* (Cambridge, MA, 1833), 72–77.

2. Wyeth, *Oregon,* 72–77. Some of the 10,000 deaths were from cholera though it is impossible to disaggregate cholera from yellow fever deaths. John Ellis, "Businessmen and Public Health in the Urban South during the Nineteenth Century: New Orleans, Memphis, and Atlanta," *BHM* 44, no. 3 (May–June 1970): 204.

3. Henry P. Dart, introduction to Laura Porteous, trans., "Sanitary Conditions in New Orleans under the Spanish Regime, 1799–1800," *LHQ* 15, no. 4 (October 1932): 611.

4. Erasmus Darwin Fenner, *The Epidemic of 1847: Or, Brief Accounts of the Yellow Fever, That Prevailed at New-Orleans, Vicksburg, Rodney, Natchez, Houston and Covington* (New Orleans, 1848), 13; Edward H. Barton, *Annual Report of the Board of Health for 1849* (New Orleans, 1849), 13; J. C. Simonds, *An Address on the Sanitary Condition of New Orleans* (New Orleans: D. Davies, Son, and Co., 1851), 42.

5. Barton quoted in the *Bee* quoted in Barton, *The Cause and Prevention of Yellow Fever, Contained in the Report of the Sanitary Commission of New Orleans* (Philadelphia: Lindsay and Blakiston, 1855), 12. For classic accounts on the relationship between politics and prophylaxis, see Erwin Ackerknecht, "Anticontagionism between 1821 and 1867," *BHM* 22, no. 5 (September–October 1948): 567; Peter Baldwin, *Contagion and the State in Europe, 1830–1930* (Cambridge: Cambridge University Press, 1999), 12–13.

6. John Duffy, "Nineteenth Century Public Health in New York and New Orleans: A Comparison," *LH* 15, no. 4 (Autumn 1974): 325–337; Jo Ann Carrigan, *The*

Saffron Scourge: A History of Yellow Fever in Louisiana, 1796–1905 (Lafayette: University of Louisiana at Lafayette Press, 1994), 1–49; Margaret Humphreys, *Yellow Fever and the South* (Baltimore: Johns Hopkins University Press, 1992), 77–79, 150–178; Robert Reinders, *End of an Era: New Orleans, 1850–1860* (Gretna: Pelican, 1998), 105–106.

7. Leonard Curry, *The Corporate City: The American City as a Political Entity, 1800–1850* (Westport, CT: Greenwood Press, 1997), 125; Robin Einhorn, *American Slavery, American Taxation* (Chicago: University of Chicago Press, 2008), 6–8.

8. M. Morton Dowler, "Letters on Yellow Fever," *NOMSJ* 11, no. 3 (November 1854): 425; Bennett H. Wall, *Louisiana: A History* (Wheeling, IL: Harlan Davidson, 1990), 237. The city expended large sums on its quasi-military police force, which was tasked primarily with surveilling slaves. See CVOR, May 18, 1805, 33–41, esp. articles 23, 24, 25; December 14, 1805, 78. For strengthened surveillance laws, see October 15, 1817, 136–140.

9. William Novak, *The People's Welfare: Law and Regulation in Nineteenth-Century America* (Chapel Hill: University of North Carolina Press, 2000), 1–3, 9, and esp. chap. 6; *Gibbons v. Ogden*, 22 U.S. 1, 79 (1824); John Fabian Witt, *American Contagions: Epidemics and the Law from Smallpox to COVID-19* (New Haven, CT: Yale University Press, 2020), 22–24, 36–37; Kathryn Olivarius, "Data, Death, and Denial in Antebellum New Orleans," *Harvard Library Bulletin, The Contagion Project* (2021).

10. CVOR, June 7, 1816, 70; *Milne v. Davidson*, 5 Mart. (n.s.) 409 (1827).

11. "The Quarantine," *Daily Picayune*, June 7, 1857.

12. John C. McKowen, *Murder as a Money-Making Art* (Baton Rouge: Benton Print, 1901).

13. Shannon Lee Dawdy described New Orleans's eighteenth-century culture of "rogue colonialism," with residents contemptuous of government authority. Scott Marler suggested the city's lack of public health was a failure of politician's civic virtue. See Shannon Lee Dawdy, *Building the Devil's Empire: French Colonial New Orleans* (Chicago: University of Chicago Press, 2008), chap. 6; Scott P. Marler, *The Merchants' Capital: New Orleans and the Political Economy of the Nineteenth-Century South* (New York: Cambridge University Press, 2013), 25–26.

14. Andrea Mehrländer, *The Germans of Charleston, Richmond and New Orleans during the Civil War Period* (Berlin: De Gruyter, 2011), 53.

15. CVOR, October 16, 1833, 159–165; MM, October 3–31, 1833, 106–120.

16. *A Digest of the Ordinances, Resolutions, By-Laws and Regulations of the Corporation of New Orleans* (New Orleans: Gaston Brusle, 1836), 305. For the mayor–council tightrope, see CVOR, April 2, 1805, 7–8; Gordon Gilson, "Louisiana: Pioneer in Public Health," *LH* 4, no. 3 (Summer 1963): 210–211; John Duffy, *Sanitarians: A History of American Public Health* (Champaign: University of Illinois Press, 1992), 60; John Duffy, ed., *The Rudolph Matas History of Medicine in Louisiana* (Baton Rouge: LSU Press, 1958), 160–161.

17. Dowler, "Letters on Yellow Fever," 428.

18. Abdiel Crossman report March 1853, Louisiana, vol. 9, p. 28, R. G. Dun & Co. credit report volumes, ms. 791, D8978, HBS.

19. John M. Sacher, *A Perfect War of Politics: Parties, Politicians, and Democracy in Louisiana, 1824–1861* (Baton Rouge: LSU Press, 2003), 194–207, esp. 206; Henry M. McKiven Jr., "The Political Construction of a Natural Disaster: The Yellow Fever Epidemic of 1853," *JAH* 94, no. 3 (2007): 734–742; James Wynne, *Report on the Vital Statistics of the United States, Made to the Mutual Life Insurance Company of New York* (New York: H. Baililiere, 1857), 165–168.

20. Christina Vella, *Intimate Enemies: The Two Worlds of the Baroness de Pontalba* (Baton Rouge: LSU Press 1997), 84–86, quote from 85; "History and Incidents of the Plague in New Orleans," *Harper's Monthly,* June–November 1853, 797–801. For absenteeism among the upper classes, see Claiborne to Jefferson, December 2, 1804, *TPUS,* 9:344–346.

21. "Night Watch, September 17, 1840," Day Police and Night Watch of the Second Municipality, 1840–1852, TDK205 261, NOPL.

22. A. Oakey Hall, *The Manhattaner in New Orleans: Or, Phases of "Crescent City" Life* (New York: J.S. Redfield, 1851), 68; "Police Board," *Daily Picayune,* September 22, 1854; Dennis Rousey, *Policing the Southern City: New Orleans, 1805–1889* (Baton Rouge: LSU Press, 1996).

23. Cenci, September 12, 1850, *Letters of Cenci, Written Four Years Ago, on the Sanitary Reforms Needed in New Orleans and Re-Published by the Order of the City Council* (New Orleans: Isaac T. Hinton, 1853), 25–26; Benjamin Henry Latrobe, *The Journal of Latrobe: Being the Notes and Sketches of an Architect, Naturalist and Traveler in the United States from 1796 to 1820* (New York: D. Appleton and Co., 1905), 242.

24. Jerah Johnson, "Dr. John Watkins, New Orleans' Lost Mayor," *LH* 36, no. 2 (Spring 1995): 187–196. For cancelled meetings, see CVOP, August–November records in 1804, 1805, 1807, and 1811.

25. CVOR, May 18, 1810, 197; CVOP, September 23 and 27, 1817, 53 and 57; MM, September 28, 1822, 90–91.

26. "Journals of Minutes and Proceedings," New Orleans Common Council, Board of Assistant Aldermen, vol. 2, AB300, mf 89-338, NOPL. For canceled meetings, see "City Intelligence," *The Daily Bee,* July 29, 1853.

27. Duffy, "Nineteenth Century Public Health," 335–336.

28. *New-Orleans Commercial Bulletin,* July 12, 1853. See also "Why New-Orleans Does Not Advance," *DBR* 11, no. 4–5 (October–November 1851): 387–389.

29. "The Pandelly Case," *Evening Picayune,* October 26, 1853. See also Shirley Elizabeth Thompson, *Exiles at Home: The Struggle to Become American in Creole New Orleans* (Cambridge, MA: Harvard University Press, 2009), 27.

30. John Duffy, "Yellow Fever in the Continental United States during the Nineteenth Century," *Bulletin of the New York Academy of Medicine* 44 (June 1968): 690–691,

quote on 691; A Physician of New Orleans, *History of the Yellow Fever during the Summer of 1853* (Philadelphia: C. W. Kenworth, 1854), 18.

31. De Bow, "The Plague at the Southwest," *DBR* 15, no. 6 (December 1853): 609–611, 620.

32. Ari Kelman, *A River and Its City: The Nature of Landscape in New Orleans* (Berkeley: University of California Press, 2003), xi; "Testimony of Dr. S. W. Dalton," *RSC*, 17.

33. CVOP, March 1, 1805, 250.

34. CVOR, August 11, 1815, 343–344; Sacher, *Perfect War*, 206.

35. Daniel Walker Howe, *The Political Culture of the American Whigs* (Chicago: University of Chicago Press, 1979), 32–35; Richard Follett, *The Sugar Masters: Planters and Slaves in Louisiana's Cane World, 1820–1860* (Baton Rouge: LSU Press, 2005), 26–44.

36. Joseph G. Treagle Jr., *Louisiana in the Age of Jackson: A Clash of Cultures and Personalities* (Baton Rouge: LSU Press, 1999); Michael F. Holt, "The Politics of Impatience: The Origins of Know Nothingism," *JAH* 60, no. 2 (September 1973): 309–331.

37. *Proceedings and Debates of the Convention of Louisiana, Which Assembled at the City of New Orleans January 14, 1844* (New Orleans: Besancon, Ferguson and Co., 1845), 19–22, 32.

38. Cited from Sacher, *Perfect War*, 194. Quoted from Edward L. Tucker, ed., "Richard Henry Wilde in New Orleans: Selected Letters, 1844–1847," *LH* 7, no. 4 (Autumn 1966): 353–355.

39. "The Law of Parish Elections," *Daily Picayune*, September 1, 1854.

40. "False Alarm about the Yellow Fever," *New York Times*, December 19, 1853.

41. *Daily Picayune*, August 30, 1838; "Yellow Jack," *True American*, August 9, 1838.

42. Unlike the national party, the Louisiana Know-Nothings were not anti-Catholic. Reinders, *End of an Era*, 55–59.

43. Curry, *The Corporate City*, 62–74; David R. Goldfield, "The Business of Health Planning: Disease Prevention in the Old South," *JSH* 42, no. 4 (November 1976): 557–570, here 559.

44. Charles Rosenberg, *The Cholera Years: The United States in 1832, 1849, and 1866* (Chicago: University of Chicago Press, 1962), 83; Melanie Kiechle, *Smell Detectives: An Olfactory History of Nineteenth-Century Urban America* (Seattle: University of Washington Press, 2017), 22.

45. For Philadelphia, see Simon Finger, *The Contagious City: The Politics of Public Health in Early Philadelphia* (Ithaca, NY: Cornell University Press, 2012), 148. For New York, see John Duffy, *History of Public Health in New York City, 1626–1866* (New York: Columbia University Press, 1968), chap. 5; Duffy, "Nineteenth Century Public Health," 326–330, 337; Richard Bayley, *Letters from the Health Office, Submitted to the Common Council, of the City of New-York* (New York: John Furman, 1799), 20–40, 54–74; William Chambers, "Yellow Jack," *Chamber's Journal of Popular Literature,*

Science and Arts 17, no. 449 (August 1862): 95; "Quarantine and the Health of the Port," *New York Times*, August 23, 1860.

46. For Baltimore, see Seth Rockman, *Scraping By: Wage Labor, Slavery, and Survival in Early Baltimore* (Baltimore: Johns Hopkins University Press, 2009), 78–81, 171–183. For Charleston, see David Ramsay, *The Charleston Medical Register for the Year 1802* (Charleston, SC: W.P. Young, 1803), 1–22; Joseph I. Waring, "Charleston Medicine, 1800–1860," *Journal of the History of Medicine and Allied Sciences* 31, no. 3 (1976): 320–334; "Yellow or Stranger's Fever," *Hazard's United States Commercial and Statistical Register* 2, no. 1 (January–July 1840): 11–12.

47. Samuel Choppin, "History of the Importation of Yellow Fever into the United States," in *Public Health Reports and Papers . . . Presented at the Meetings of the American Public Health Association in the Years 1877–1878* (Boston: Houghton, Osgood, and Co., 1880), 4:190–206, quote from 206; Melanie Kiechle, "'Health Is Wealth': Valuing Health in the Nineteenth Century," *Journal of Social History* 54. no. 3 (2021): 1–24.

48. W. M. Carpenter, *Sketches from the History of Yellow Fever: Showing Its Origin, Together with Facts and Circumstances Disproving Its Domestic Origin, and Demonstrating Its Transmissibility* (New Orleans: J.B. Steel, 1844), 4.

49. Quoted from William Rucker, "Chervin, a Pioneer Epidemiologist: An Early Study of the Contagiousness of Yellow Fever," *LHQ* 8, no. 3 (July 1925): 441–443; Nicolas Chervin, *Examen des principes de l'administration en matière sanitere* (Paris: F. Didot, 1827), 15.

50. "Spurious Yellow Fever," *Vicksburg Daily Whig*, October 30, 1855; Chambers, "Yellow Jack," 96.

51. "Extract of a Letter from New-Orleans," *Daily National Intelligencer*, September 23, 1817; "Letter from the Secretary of War, Communicating, in Obedience to Law, Information in Relation to Quarantine on the Southern and Gulf Coasts," in *Senate Executive Documents for the Third Session of the Forty-Second Congress of the United States of America* (Washington, DC: US Government Printing Office, 1873), 46; Humphreys, *Yellow Fever and the South*, 12–14.

52. "Speech of Mr. Rouffinac in Answer to the Observations of Dr. Ker," *Orleans Gazette and Commercial Advertiser*, March 25, 1820.

53. Robert B. S. Hargis, ed., "On Endemicity," in *Yellow Fever: Its Ship Origin and Prevention* (New Orleans: D.G. Brinton, 1880): 59; Ackerknecht, "Anticontagionism," 567.

54. John Monette, *Observations on the Epidemic Yellow Fever of Natchez, and of the South-West* (Louisville, KY: Prentice and Weissinger, 1842); Carpenter, *Sketches*, 55; B. B. Strobel, *An Essay on the Subject of Yellow Fever, Intended to Prove Its Transmissibility* (Charleston, 1840).

55. H., "The Fever," *Daily Picayune*, August 6, 1853.

56. "To the Editor of the National Advocate," *New York Evening Post*, October 11, 1821; "Hear Both Sides," *New York Evening Post*, November 20, 1821.

57. "The Vanda," *Daily Picayune*, September 27, 1843; "Origin of Yellow Fever," *Baltimore Sun*, August 14, 1855.

58. Samuel Cartwright, "The Yellow Fever at Natchez in All Its Bearings on the Quarantine Question and Yellow Fever at New Orleans," *NOMNHG* 2, no. 1 (March 1855): 1; Dowler, "Letters on Yellow Fever," 424–426; M. Morton Dowler, "On the Reputed Causes of Yellow Fever, and the So Called Sanitary Measures of the Day," *NOMSJ* 11, no. 1 (July 1854): 55.

59. "Mobile, Aug. 18," *Daily National Journal*, September 5, 1829; "Health Regulations at Mobile," *Daily Picayune*, July 3, 1858; "Testimony of Dr. L. P. Blackburn," *RSC*, 534; "Revelation of the Conspiracy to Introduce Pestilence," *New York Times*, May 26, 1865.

60. See Monette, *Observations*, 102–111; "Health Regulations at Mobile," *Daily Picayune*, July 3, 1858; *Pennsylvania Gazette*, August 9, 1829; "Quarantine," *United States' Telegraph*, September 2, 1834; "Quarantine at Genoa," *Daily Picayune*, August 19, 1855.

61. E. H. Barton, *Report to the Louisiana State Medical Society, on the Meteorology, Vital Statistics, and Hygiene of the State of Louisiana* (New Orleans: Davies, Son and Co., 1851), 43; "Editorial and Miscellaneous," *NOMNHG* 2, no. 9 (November 1855): 418; Veritas, "For the Orleans Gazette," *Orleans Gazette and Commercial Advertiser*, October 29, 1819.

62. Board of Aldermen, *Report upon the Wealth, Internal Resources, and Commercial Prosperity of the City of New Orleans* (New Orleans: Bulletin Book and Job Office, 1855), 6–7.

63. William Kingsford, *Impressions of the West and South during a Six Weeks' Holiday* (Toronto: A.H. Armour and Co., 1858), 60.

64. Kiechle, *Smell Detectives*, 22.

65. CVOP, June 8, 1804, 111–112, July 25, 1804, 143, and April 26, 1809, 54.

66. "Quarantine and Yellow Fever," *Daily Picayune*, August 26, 1853.

67. Barton, *Report to the Louisiana State Medical Society*, 35–36; Harriet Martineau, *Retrospect of Western Travel* (London: Saunders and Oatley, 1838), 1:257.

68. "Public Health," *Daily Picayune*, April 22, 1855.

69. CVOR, April 26, 1817, 35.

70. Physician, "Editorial and Miscellaneous," *NOMNHG* 2, no. 4 (June 1855): 186.

71. "The Health of the City," *Daily Picayune*, March 25, 1849; "Health of New Orleans," *Weekly National Intelligencer*, September 30, 1854.

72. Richard Campanella, *Time and Place in New Orleans: Past Geographies in the Present Day* (Gretna, LA: Pelican, 2002), 7–9, 118; Campanella, "An Ethnic Geography of New Orleans," *JAH* 94, no. 3 (December 2007): 704–715; Amy R. Sumpter, "Segregation of the Free People of Color and the Construction of Race in Antebellum New Orleans," *Southeastern Geographer* 48, no. 1 (May 2008): 26.

73. CVOR, August 16, 1817, 66; June 19, 1819, 81–85.

74. CVOR, May 6, 1816, 82–85; July 12, 1817, 57; June 30, 1818, 63–64.

75. "New Orleans," *The North American,* September 10, 1839.

76. CVOR, January 3, 1829, 1.

77. A Resident of Said Street, but Unacclimated, "Communicated?," *New-Orleans Commercial Bulletin,* August 16, 1833; Liliane Crété, *Daily Life in Louisiana, 1815–1830,* trans. Patrick Gregory (Baton Rouge: LSU Press, 1981), 58; CVOR, July 31, 1827, 55.

78. "The Plague in the Southwest," *DBR* 15, no. 6 (December 1853): 600; Reinders, *End of an Era,* 104; Kiechle, *Smell Detectives,* 36–39.

79. *New Orleans Commercial Bulletin,* July 12, 1853; Goldfield, "Business of Health Planning," 557–560.

80. Thomas Kelah Wharton Diary, April 25, 1854, 359, ms. 807, LSU.

81. Simonds, *An Address,* 10, 31, 35–37.

82. Henry Sigerist, "The Cost of Illness to the City of New Orleans in 1850," *BHM* 15 (January 1944): 498–507; Simonds, *An Address,* 45–46.

83. "Statistics Charity Hospital of New Orleans," Charity Hospital Papers, box 2, folder 4156b, ms. RG29, LSM.

84. "New Orleans Charity Hospital," Charity Hospital Papers, 4096b, ms. RG29, LRC; *Report of the Board of the Administrators, Charity Hospital* (New Orleans: Emile La Sere, 1850, 1851, 1852); "Sickness at New-Orleans," *Louisville Public Advertiser,* December 18, 1819; "New-Orleans," *Daily National Intelligencer,* July 2, 1818.

85. For the abysmal inventory and care-giving capacities of the Hospital, see "Inventory Derived from Year 1801," Medical Documents Collection, box 1, folder 3, ms. 589, pp. 1–8, LRC.

86. John Castellanos, *The Early Charity Hospital* (New Orleans, 1897), 143.

87. Chase quoted in John Salvaggio, *New Orleans' Charity Hospital: A Story of Physicians, Politics, and Poverty* (Baton Rouge: LSU Press, 1992), 38.

88. "Certificate of John J. Ker," *Proceedings of the Physico-Medical Society of New Orleans: In Relation to the Trial and Expulsion of Charles A. Luzenberg* (New Orleans, 1838), 25; "The Yellow Fever at New Orleans," *Glasgow Herald,* September 5, 1853.

89. James Mather to W. C. C. Claiborne, October 12, 1811, William C. C. Claiborne Papers, box 2, folder 8, ms. 427, LRC.

90. "Council of Administration of the Charity Hospital of New Orleans, Friday, 3d of May, 1816," *Journal of the Twenty Seventh House of Representatives of the Commonwealth of Pennsylvania Commenced at Harrisburg* (Harrisburg: James Peacock, 1816–1817), 25–26.

91. *The Josefa Segunda,* 23 U.S. (10 Wheat.) 312 (1825); *RCH,* 1843, 1–4 and 1848–1849, 1–16.

92. Gerald L. Neuman, *Strangers to the Constitution: Immigrants, Borders, and Fundamental Laws* (Princeton, NJ: Princeton University Press, 1996), 30; *Daily Picayune,* June 11, 1843; Francis Burns, "Twenty-Five Dollars or Thirty Days," *Loyola Law Journal* 9, no. 2 (1928): 68–78; "Charity Hospital Passenger Tax," *Daily Picayune,* June 10, 1853.

To avoid the head tax, ships dumped their passengers upriver, downriver, or across-river from New Orleans. *RCH*, 1843, 8.

93. *RCH*, 1850, 1–19.

94. This was in addition to $315 in city tax and $200 in state tax levied on theaters. "Taxes on Theatres," *Daily Picayune*, November 25, 1856; Duffy, *Rudolph Matas*, 1:203.

95. For "gaping abyss," see MM, January 12, 1822, 3. Curry, *The Corporate City*, 37; CVOR, January 14, 1829, 5; Treagle, *Louisiana in the Age of Jackson*, 57; Henry A. Bullard, ed., *A New Digest of the Statute Laws of the State of Louisiana, from the Change of Government to the Year 1841, Inclusive* (New Orleans: E. Johns, 1842), 699–735; Marler, *Merchants' Capital*, 216–218; *Acts Passed at the First Session of the Seventeenth Legislature of the State of Louisiana* (New Orleans: Magne and Weisse, 1845), 65.

96. *Annual Report of the State Treasurer, to the Legislature of the State of Louisiana* (New Orleans, 1857), 1–14. For the uses of the sinking fun, see MM April 19 1828, 29.

97. CVOP, November 28, 1810, 246–247.

98. For Nolte's loan, see MM, May 6, 1826, 30–31; CVOR, July 25, 1829. 76. For the Baring loan, see August 28, 1830, Barings Bank Records, North America series HC5.7.3, Barings; Vincent Nolte, *Fifty Years in Both Hemispheres; or, Reminiscences of the Life of a Former Merchant* (New York: Redfield, 1854), 298–299.

99. Elna C. Green, *Before the New Deal: Social Welfare in the South, 1830–1930* (Athens: University of Georgia Press, 1999), 81–99.

100. "City Intelligence," *Daily Picayune*, August 31, 1847; "The Howards' Visit to Mobile," *Daily Picayune*, September 20, 1853.

101. John Blassingame, *Black New Orleans, 1860–1880* (Chicago: University of Chicago Press, 1973), 13; Dianne Batts Morrow, *Persons of Color and Religious at the Same Time: The Oblate Sisters of Providence, 1828–1860* (Chapel Hill: University of North Carolina Press, 2002), 117–118.

102. "Record Book, 1816–1822," Natchez Children's Home Records, folder 2, 3B33, UTA; Thomas N. Ingersoll, *Mammon and Manon in Early New Orleans: The First Slave Society in the Deep South, 1718–1819* (Knoxville: University of Tennessee Press, 1999), 272–273.

103. Priscilla Clement, "Children and Charity: Orphanages in New Orleans, 1817–1914," *LH* 27, no. 4 (Autumn 1986): 340–348; Laura D. Kelley, "Children of Refuge: Irish Immigrant Families and Catholic Orphanages in New Orleans; A Case Study of Survival Strategy," *LH* 52, no. 1 (Winter 2011): 70, 77–78.

104. Emily Suzanne Clark, *A Luminous Brotherhood: Afro-Creole Spiritualism in Nineteenth-Century New Orleans* (Chapel Hill: University of North Carolina Press, 2016), 89–90.

105. Julien Poydras Document, April 16, 1822, ms. 351, LSU; *National Advocate* (New York), August 21, 1824.

106. *Daily Orleanian*, April 2, 1851; Richard Tansey, "Prostitution and Politics in Antebellum New Orleans," in *History of Women in the United States*, vol. 9: *Prostitution*, ed.

Nancy Cott (London: K.G. Saur, 1993), 62; Eberhard Faber, *Building the Land of Dreams: New Orleans and the Transformation of Early America* (Princeton, NJ: Princeton University Press, 2016), 124. For a fictional account of McDonogh, see Baron Ludwig von Reizenstein, *The Mysteries of New Orleans*, 1854, ed. and trans. Steven Rowan (Baltimore: Johns Hopkins University Press, 2002), 430. "$500 Reward," *Daily Picayune*, November 7, 1850.

107. Vincent Nolte, *Fifty Years in Both Hemispheres; or, Reminiscences of the Life of a Former Merchant* (New York: Redfield, 1854), 87.

108. *McDonogh v. Murdoch*, 56 U.S. 367, 14 L. Ed. 732, 1853. Ellis, "Businessmen and Public Health," 202; Judith Schafer, *Brothels, Depravity, and Abandoned Women: Illegal Sex in Antebellum New Orleans* (Baton Rouge: LSU Press, 2009), 12; *The Last Will and Testament of John McDonogh, Late of McDonoghville, State of Louisiana* (New Orleans: Job Office of the Daily Delta, 1851), 38.

109. "Public Charities," *Daily Picayune*, March 2, 1860; Ellis, "Businessmen and Public Health," 202–205.

110. CVOP, March 15, 1817, 134, and February 15, 1817, 126.

111. Cynthia Tolbert, "Alms for the Poor: An Historical Analysis of a System of Disgrace," *Loyola Poverty Law Journal* 1 (Spring 1995): 60–61; CVOP, November 11, 1815, 109–110.

112. "City Council of New-Orleans," New Orleans Scrapbook, 1813–1865, 10, ms. 920, LSU; Henry J. Leovy and C. H. Luzenberg, *The Laws and General Ordinances of the City of New Orleans* (New Orleans: Simmons and Co., 1870), 320.

113. Simonds, *An Address*, 10.

114. *Comptroller's Report, Embracing a Detailed Statement of the Receipts and Expenditures of the City of New Orleans, From Jan. 1st, 1860, to July 1st, 1860* (New Orleans: Bulletin Book and Job Office, 1860), 9–11.

115. "The Population of New Orleans and the Fever," *Tri-Weekly Commercial* (Wilmington, NC), August 23, 1853.

116. *Proceedings and Debates of the Convention of Louisiana, Which Assembled at the City of New Orleans January 14, 1844* (New Orleans: Besancon, Ferguson and Co., 1845), 19–20, 32; Board of Aldermen, *Report upon the Wealth* (1855), 9–11; Katherine Newman and Rourke O'Brien, *Taxing the Poor: Doing Damage to the Truly Disadvantaged* (Berkeley: University of California Press, 2011), 3.

117. Einhorn, *American Slavery, American Taxation*, 225–226; Sacher, *Perfect War*, 217; "Relief of the State Treasury," *Daily Picayune*, April 10, 1853; Tansey, "Prostitution and Politics," 51. New York tax figures cited from Elizabeth Blackmar, "Housing and Property Relations in New York City, 1785–1850" (PhD diss., Harvard University, 1980), 584.

118. *Comptroller's Report, 1860*, 9–11.

119. "Coffeehouse License for the Second Municipality," New Orleans Municipal Records, 1782–1925, folder 15b, ms. 16, LRC; Louisiana, *Revised Statues* (1856), 459–461. For taxes on coffee and liquor houses, see CVOR, November 24, 1829, 122.

120. Tansey, "Prostitution and Politics," 57.

121. Schafer, *Brothels*, 147; *Comptroller's Report*, 1860, 20.

122. "Board of Assistant Aldermen," *Daily Picayune*, February 2, 1859; Tansey, "Prostitution and Politics," 74; *New Orleans Daily Crescent*, January 31, 1856.

123. "Official," *Daily Picayune*, August 16, 1854; Judith Schafer, "Slaves and Crime: New Orleans, 1846–1862," in *Local Matters: Race, Crime, and Justice in the Nineteenth-Century South*, ed. Christopher Waldrep and Donald G. Nieman (Athens: University of Georgia Press, 2001), 53–54.

124. Reinders, *End of an Era*, 165–166.

125. John S. Kendall, *History of New Orleans* (Chicago: Lewis, 1922), 112; CVOR, August 14, 1829, 85–86; "Record Book of Licenses, Bakers' Declarations, and Statements of Public Works, 1812," AA420, mf 89-236, NOPL; "No Place of Abode," *Daily Picayune*, August 26, 1852.

126. "Police Matters," *Daily Picayune*, January 21, 1857, September 18, 1858.

127. "Second Municipality Council," *Daily Picayune*, September 2, 1846; "Recorder Seuzeneau's Court," *Daily Picayune*, May 11, 1852; Henry Watkins Allen, *The Travels of a Sugar Planter or, Six Months in Europe* (New York: J.F. Trow, 1861), 236.

128. *Daily Picayune*, September 7, 1841; "Fines for December," *Daily Picayune*, January 9, 1859. See also: "Quiet Times," *Daily Picayune*, January 1, 1853; "Fined," *Daily Picayune*, November 10, 1854; *Daily Picayune*, July 24, 1855; "First District Court," *Daily Picayune*, July 19, 1855.

129. CVOR, November 27, 1816, 104–106.

130. Crété, *Daily Life*, 58; Burns, "Twenty-Five Dollars or Thirty Days," 74.

131. Schafer, *Brothels*, 145–146; Tansey, "Prostitution and Politics," 49, 60.

132. Schafer, *Brothels*, 19; "Police Matters," *Daily Picayune*, September 5, 1856. Bridget Malony landed in New Orleans with her husband Thomas in 1851 from County Galway, Ireland. He died about a week after landing. Evidently, she fell on hard times and died from yellow fever during the 1853 epidemic. For the 24 women, see "Police Matters," *Daily Picayune*, February 15, 1857; "Police Matters," *Daily Picayune*, August 27, 1857.

133. "Police Matters," *Daily Picayune*, October 11, 1858.

134. CVOR, October 27, 1827, 92; September 12, 1829, 88. Crété, *Daily Life*, 57; "The City Workhouse," *Daily Picayune*, January 10, 1857.

135. Commissioners, *Report of a General Plan for the Promotion of Public and Personal Health* (Boston: Dutton and Wentworth, 1850), 254.

5. Denial, Delusion, and Disunion

1. "Health, Mortality, &c.," *NOMSJ* 9, no. 3 (November 1852): 415–417; Jo Ann Carrigan, *The Saffron Scourge: A History of Yellow Fever in Louisiana, 1796–1905* (Lafayette: University of Louisiana at Lafayette Press, 1994), 58–59; Ari Kelman, *A River and*

Its City: The Nature of Landscape in New Orleans (Berkeley: University of California Press, 2003), 87–88; Urmi Engineer Willoughby, *Yellow Fever, Race, and Ecology in Nineteenth-Century New Orleans* (Baton Rouge: LSU Press, 2017), 71.

2. "Testimony of Dr. M. M. Dowler and Mr. Ebbinger," *RSC*, 4; quote from Erasmus Darwin Fenner, *History of the Epidemic Yellow Fever, at New Orleans, Louisiana, in 1853* (New York: Hall, Clayton and Co., 1854), 21.

3. "Testimony of Mr. Vandelinden, Clerk of the Charity Hospital," *RSC*, 3; "Testimony of Dr. L. B. Lindsay," *RSC*, 9.

4. *RSC*, ix.

5. "Examination of Dyson" and "Louisiana Items," *Daily Picayune*, June 23, 1853; Ari Kelman, "New Orleans's Phantom Slave Insurrection of 1853: Racial Anxiety, Urban Ecology, and Human Bodies as Public Spaces," in *The Nature of Cities: Culture, Landscape, and Urban Space*, ed. Andrew Isenberg (Rochester, NY: University of Rochester Press, 2006), 6.

6. Quoted from Carrigan, *Saffron Scourge*, 61, 371.

7. "New Orleans in Midsummer," *Daily Crescent*, June 22, 1853; "The Yellow Fever Alarm," *Daily Picayune*, June 23, 1853; "Splinters," *Gleason's Pictorial Drawing-Room Companion*, July 1853, 173.

8. Fenner, *History of the Epidemic*, 25.

9. "The Plague in the South-West," *DBR* 15, no. 6 (December 1853): 609–611, 620; George Washington Cable, "Flood and Plague in New Orleans," *Century Illustrated Magazine*, July 1883, 428.

10. *Report of the Howard Association of New Orleans: Epidemic of 1853, with Addenda* (New Orleans, 1854), 23–28, ms. RC211.L9 H6 1853, HNOC; "The Orphans," *Daily Picayune*, August 23, 1853.

11. See "Died," *The Tennessean*, September 21, 1853; "Touching," *Burlington Courier*, September 29, 1853; *Glasgow Herald*, September 5, 1853.

12. "Benefit to the Sufferers," *Daily Picayune*, September 19, 1853; "Relief for New Orleans," *Cooper's Clarksburg Register* (Virginia), August 24, 1853; "The Plague in the South-West," *DBR* 15, no. 6 (December 1853): 633; *San Francisco Daily Alta*, September 24, 25, and 26, 1853; "Donations," *Daily Picayune*, September 7, 1853.

13. William L. Robinson, *The Diary of a Samaritan: By a Member of the Howard Association of New Orleans* (New York: Harper and Brothers, 1860), 150–151; "The Yellow Fever in New Orleans," *Zion's Herald* (Boston), July 23, 1868; Bishop Leonidas Polk, "The Following Prayer," August 9, 1853, ms. BV283.Y4E6 1853, HNOC; Theodore Clapp, "Is God Capable of Being Angry?," *Daily Picayune*, September 2, 1853.

14. "The Pestilence in New Orleans," *Daily Journal* (Wilmington, NC), August 15, 1853; Mary Copes to Joseph Copes, September 9 and 18, 1853, Joseph S. Copes Papers, box 10, folder 9, ms. 733, LRC.

15. Quotes from Bennet Dowler, *Tableau of the Yellow Fever of 1853 with Topographical, Chronological, and Historical Sketches of the Epidemics of New Orleans since Their*

Origin in 1796 (New Orleans: Office of the Picayune, 1854), 60–61; E. D. Fenner, "Report on the Epidemics of Louisiana," *AMA* 7 (1854): 459; Carrigan, *Saffron Scourge*, 73. For lists of the dead, see Stanford Chaillé, "The Vital Statistics of New Orleans, from 1769 to 1874," *NOMSJ* (July 1874): 6–7; *The Epidemic Summer: List of Interments in All the Cemeteries of New Orleans* (New Orleans: Proprietor of the True Delta, 1853), 1–67.

16. Theodore Clapp, "A Discourse, Delivered in the First Congregational Church," *Daily Picayune*, September 4, 1853; *RSC*, 221.

17. *RSC*, 452–453; for funding sources, see 458–461.

18. Bennet Dowler, "Review—On the Sanitary Commission of New Orleans," *NOMSJ* 11, no. 4 (January 1855): 526–529; Karlem Reiss, "The Rebel Physiologist—Bennet Dowler," *Journal of the History of Medicine and Allied Sciences* 16, no. 1 (January 1961): 39.

19. McFarlane, "A Review of the Yellow Fever, Its Causes," in *The Epidemic Summer*, v–x.

20. Quoted from *The Cause and Prevention of Yellow Fever at New Orleans and Other Cities in America* (New York, 1857), 11; "Work for the Council," *Daily Picayune*, November 10, 1853.

21. Carrigan, *Saffron Scourge*, 74; Barton quoted in the *Bee* quoted in Edward H. Barton, *The Cause and Prevention of Yellow Fever, Contained in the Report of the Sanitary Commission of New Orleans* (Philadelphia: Lindsay and Blakiston, 1855), 262–264.

22. Ben Freedman, "The Louisiana State Board of Health, Established 1855," *American Journal of Public Health* 41, no. 10 (October 1951): 1279–1281; *Acts Passed by the Second Legislature of the State of Louisiana, Session of 1855* (New Orleans: Emile La Sere, 1855), Act 336, 471–477; John Duffy, ed., *The Rudolph Matas History of Medicine in Louisiana* (Baton Rouge: LSU Press, 1958), 2:186.

23. "Fruits of the New-Orleans Quarantine," *The Bee*, July 11, 1855; Board of Aldermen, *Report upon the Wealth, Internal Resources, and Commercial Prosperity of the City of New Orleans* (New Orleans: Bulletin Book and Job Office, 1855), 7, 13–14; Sven Beckert, *Empire of Cotton: A New History of Global Capitalism* (New York: Knopf, 2014), 98–135.

24. Cable, "Flood and Plague," 426.

25. "Sketches of Character. No. LXXV. The Anti-Panic Man," *Daily Delta*, August 13, 1853; Duffy, *Rudolph Matas*, 2:162.

26. This is a composite quote assembled by Kenneth Stampp from Southern journals during the late 1850s. Kenneth Stampp, *The Peculiar Institution: Slavery in the Ante-Bellum South* (New York: Vintage Books, 1956), 7. For proslavery thought, see Drew Gilpin Faust, *The Ideology of Slavery: Proslavery Thought in the Antebellum South, 1830–1860* (Baton Rouge: LSU Press, 1981); Larry Tise, *Proslavery: A History of the Defense of Slavery in America, 1701–1840* (Athens: University of Georgia Press, 2004); Walter Johnson, "The Pedestal and the Veil: Rethinking the Capitalism / Slavery

Question," *JER* 24 (Summer 2004): 299–308; Kenneth Kiple and Virginia King, "The African Connection: Slavery, Disease and Racism," *Phylon* 41, no. 3 (3rd Qtr. 1980): 211–222.

27. Richard Hofstadter, "The Paranoid Style in American Politics," *Harper's Magazine*, November 1964, 77–86. See also Eugene Genovese, *The World the Slaveholders Made: Two Essays in Interpretation* (New York: Pantheon Books, 1969), 119; James Breeden, "States-Rights Medicine in the Old South," *Bulletin of New York Academy of Medicine* 52, no. 3 (March–April 1976): 348–372. See also Kelman, *A River and Its City*, 107–109.

28. For cultural hegemony, Gramsci, and "dominant fundamental" ideologies, see T. J. Jackson Lears, "The Concept of Cultural Hegemony: Problems and Possibilities," *AHR* 90, no. 3 (June 1985): 567–593.

29. J. C. Simonds, *An Address on the Sanitary Condition of New Orleans* (New Orleans: D. Davies, Son, and Co., 1851), 7; Barton, *Cause and Prevention*, 262–263.

30. For the arguments forwarded in 1861 to convince non-slaveholding whites to rally to the Confederacy, see "The Non-Slaveholders of the South," *DBR* 30, no. 1 (January 1861): 67–77.

31. "Faithful and Bold New Orleans," *True American*, November 12, 1838; *Daily Picayune*, July 18, 1838.

32. "Editorial Correspondence," *Daily Picayune*, May 14, 1853.

33. Matthew Karp, *This Vast Southern Empire: Slaveholders at the Helm of American Foreign Policy* (Cambridge, MA: Harvard University Press, 2016), 183–187; Todd L. Savitt and James Harvey Young, eds., *Disease and Distinctiveness in the American South* (Knoxville: University of Tennessee Press, 1988), 1–28.

34. "An American," *National Intelligencer and Washington Advertiser*, November 19, 1806.

35. "An American."

36. Medicus, "For the Gazette," *Natchez Gazette*, April 15, 1826.

37. "Domestic Statistics," *DBR* 1, no. 4 (April 1846): 379–382.

38. E. H. Barton, *Introductory Lecture on the Climate and Salubrity of New-Orleans and Its Suitability for a Medical School* (New Orleans: E. Johns and Co., 1835), 8; Nott, "Life Insurance at the South *DBR* 3, no. 5 (May 1847): 362–364.

39. "New-Orleans and Its Unwholesomeness," *New York Tribune*, September 19, 1855; "New Orleans and the Tribune," *Daily Picayune*, September 29, 1855.

40. John C. McKowen, *Murder as a Money-Making Art* (Baton Rouge: Benton Print, 1901), 3–4.

41. Cable, "Flood and Plague," 425.

42. "The Acclimated Man," *Daily Delta*, August 1, 1853.

43. *Gibson's Guide and Directory of the State of Louisiana, and the Cities of New Orleans and Lafayette* (New Orleans: J. Gibson, 1838), iv, 288–289, 37.

44. James McMartin to Peter McMartin, February 9, 1849, Peter McMartin Papers, N-YHS.

45. Isaac H. Charles to John Edward Siddall, September 18 and November 18, 1847, Isaac H. Charles Letters, ms. 621, LSU.

46. Bartlett for Smith and Bro. to T. Smith & Co., August 12, 1847, T. Smith & Company Papers, mss. 930, 1116, 1232, etc., LSU. See also Jo Ann Carrigan, "Privilege, Prejudice, and the Strangers' Disease in Nineteenth-Century New Orleans," *JSH* 36, no. 4 (November 1970): 568–578, here 570–572.

47. E. H. Durell to sisters, July 5, 1853, August 26, 1855, E. H. Durell Papers, N-YHS.

48. George Washington Cable, *The Creoles of Louisiana* (New York: Charles Scribner's Sons, 1884), 292–293, 297.

49. Bennet Dowler, *Researches upon the Necropolis of New Orleans, with Brief Allusions to Its Vital Arithmetic* (New Orleans: Bills and Clark, 1850), 5; H., "Advice That Will Not Be Taken," *Daily Delta*, July 1, 1855.

50. James Wynne, *Report on the Vital Statistics of the United States, Made to the Mutual Life Insurance Company of New York* (New York: H. Bailiiere, 1857), 164.

51. Sharon Ann Murphy, *Investing in Life: Insurance in Antebellum America* (Baltimore: Johns Hopkins University Press, 2010), 246; Murphy, "Life Insurance in the United States through World War I," in *EH.Net Encyclopedia*, ed. Robert Whaples, August 14, 2002, https://eh.net/encyclopedia/life-insurance-in-the-united-states-through-world-war-i/.

52. Sharon Ann Murphy, "Securing Human Property: Slavery, Life Insurance, and Industrialization in the Upper South," *JER* 25, no. 4 (Winter 2005): 617–618; Jonathan Levy, *Freaks of Fortune: The Emerging World of Capitalism and Risk in America* (Cambridge, MA: Harvard University Press, 2009), 60–67, esp. 63, 95; *The Revised Statues of Louisiana* (New Orleans: J. Claiborne, 1856), 461.

53. Davis and Copes to Latting and Hitchcock, December 31, 1856, Joseph S. Copes Papers, box 11, folder 17, ms. 733, LRC.

54. A typical issue of the *Picayune* had a dedicated "Insurance" section advertising life companies from Boston to Edinburgh. See, for example, "Insurance," *Daily Picayune*, November 23, 1851; Nott, "Life Insurance," 358; Josiah Nott, "Statistics of Southern Slave Population with Especial Reference to Life Insurance," *DBR* 4, no. 3 (November 1847): 286–287, at 275.

55. Arthur H. Bailey, "On the Rates of Extra Premium for Foreign Travelling and Residence," *Journal of the Institute of Actuaries* 15, no. 2 (1869): 77–94.

56. Daniel Bouk, *How Our Days Became Numbered: Risk and the Rise of the Statistical Individual* (Chicago: University of Chicago Press, 2015); Bouk, "The Science of Difference: Developing Tools for Discrimination in the American Life Insurance Industry" (PhD diss., Princeton University, 2009), 125–126.

57. William Bard to Henry White, August 23, 1833, GA-3, and William Bard to William Atkinson, December 31, 1833, GA-4, New York Life and Trust Company Records, ms. 797 1830–1878 N567, HBS. For standard table rates, see Timothy Alborn and Sharon Ann Murphy, eds., *Anglo-American Life Insurance* (London: Pickering and Chatto, 2013), 1:44–47.

58. Charles Gill, "Actuary's Report to the Board of Trustees of the Mutual Life Insurance Company of New York," reprinted in Emory McClintock, "Charles Gill: The First Actuary in America, pt. 4," *Transactions of the Actuarial Society of America* 15, nos. 51–52 (1914), append. F, 258–264.

59. MONY, *HAR* (1865), 49–50.

60. William Bard to William Atkinson, December 31, 1833, New York Life and Trust Company Records, ms. 797 1830–1878 N567, GA-4, HBS; Murphy, *Investing in Life*, 34–36.

61. For the extra scrutiny given to Southern policy-seekers, see policies no. 1688, William A. Dawson, July 20, 1847, and no. 2006, H. W. Kuhtmann, March 9, 1848, New England Mutual Life Insurance Company Records, ms. 797 1844–1999 N532, HBS.

62. Gill, "Actuary's Report," 248–249, 260–263; Bouk, "The Science of Difference," 125.

63. John A. Stevenson, *A Century of Security Expressing the Spirit of William Penn, 1847–1947* (New York: Newcomen Society of England, 1946), 17; Allen Flitcraft, *Synopsis of Risks Assumed and Benefits Guaranteed by Forty-Four Life Insurance Companies* (Oak Park, IL: self-pub., 1894), 37, 55, 73; Flitcraft, *Contracts of the Most Important Life Insurance Companies of the United States of America* (Chicago: self-pub., 1888), 15, 26–27.

64. William Bard to George Atkinson, May 15, 1834, New York Life and Trust Company Records, GA-4, ms. 797 1830–1878 N567, HBS; Murphy, *Investing in Life*, 33–35.

65. Nott, "Life Insurance," 358–376; James Monroe Hudnut, *Semi-Centennial History of the New York Life Insurance Company, 1847–1895* (New York: New York Life Insurance Co., 1895), 35; MONY, *HAR* (1864), 46–47; "Life Insurance," *Boston Daily Advertiser*, May 6, 1857.

66. Quoted from Murphy, *Investing in Life*, 36.

67. Jonathan Adams Allen, *Medical Examinations for Life Insurance* (New York: J.H. and C.M. Goodsell, 1872), 25–26; Charles Benjamin Norton, *Life Insurance: Its Nature, Origin and Progress* (New York: self-pub., 1852), 54.

68. Nott, "Acclimation and Adaptation of Races to Climate," *American Journal of the Medical Sciences* 32, no. 64 (October 1856), 329.

69. Policy no. 568, Robert Purvis, January 15, 1845, New England Mutual Life Insurance Company Records, ms. 797 1844–1999 N532, HBS.

70. Policy no. 527, John M. Gould, January 15, 1845, New England Mutual Life Insurance Company Records, ms. 797 1844–1999 N532, HBS.

71. MONY, *HAR* (1858), 26.

72. "Life Insurance," *Bankers Magazine, and Statistical Register* 13, no. 10 (April 1859): 771.

73. Quoted from Murphy, *Investing in Life*, 37.

74. "Life Insurance," *Times Picayune*, August 11, 1841; Levy, *Freaks of Fortune*, 90.

75. MONY, *HAR* (1858), 80.

76. MONY, *HAR* (1866), 24.

77. New England Mutual Life Insurance Company, *HAR* (1859), 10–11; MONY, *HAR* (1866), 24.

78. Sayler quoted from Hudnut, *Semi-Centennial History*, 124.

79. MONY, *HAR* (1866), 23; "Life Assurance," *The Plantation* 1, no. 9 (March 1870): 154; *Proceedings and Debates of the Convention of Louisiana* (New Orleans: Besancon, Ferguson and Co., 1845), 20–32; "Song of the Yellow Fever Demons," *Daily Picayune*, September 27, 1842; Elisha Harris, "Hygienic Experience in New Orleans during the War," *Southern Medical and Surgical Journal* 21 (Augusta, GA: E. H. Pughe, 1867): 81.

80. Bryan Edwards, *The History, Civil and Commercial, of the British Colonies in the West Indies* (London: B. Crosby, 1801), 2:160; Tise, *Proslavery*, 77–81.

81. Philip Tidyman, "A Sketch of the Most Remarkable Diseases of the Negroes in the Southern States," *Philadelphia Journal of the Medical and Physical Sciences* 12 (1826): 325–327, at 306. See also Rana Hogarth, "The Myth of Innate Racial Differences between White and Black People's Bodies: Lessons from the 1793 Yellow Fever Epidemic in Philadelphia, Pennsylvania," *American Journal of Public Health* 109, no. 10 (2019): 1339–1341.

82. "William H. Holcombe, "Queer Things about Yellow Fever," *Southwestern Christian Advocate*, February 6, 1879; "Yellow Jack," *Daily Picayune*, October 18, 1844; "False Alarm about the Yellow Fever," *New York Times*, December 19, 1853; Margaret Humphreys, "No Safe Place: Disease and Panic in American History," *American Literary History* 14, no. 4 (Winter 2002): 845–857.

83. George Fitzhugh, *Sociology of the South, or the Failure of Free Society* (Richmond, VA: A. Morris, 1854), 225.

84. For polygenism, see Alfred Brophy, *University, Court, and Slave: Proslavery Academic Thought and Southern Jurisprudence, 1831–1861* (Oxford: Oxford University Press, 2016), 233.

85. Josiah Nott and George Gliddon, *Types of Mankind* (Philadelphia: J.B. Lippincott, Grambo and Co., 1854), 68.

86. Josiah Nott and George Gliddon, *Indigenous Races of the Earth; Or, New Chapters of Ethnological Inquiry* (Philadelphia: J. B. Lippincott & Co., 1857), 366–367; Josiah Nott, *Two Lectures on the Natural History of the Caucasian and Negro Races* (Mobile, AL: Dade and Thompson, 1844), 32. See also Eric Herschthal, *The Science of*

Abolition: How Slaveholders Became the Enemies of Progress (New Haven, CT: Yale University Press, 2021), 205–216.

87. Josiah Nott, "Facts upon Yellow Fever—Its Progress Northward," *DBR* 19, no. 4 (October 1855): 444; Nott, "Statistics of Southern Slave Population," 281; Nott and Gliddon, *Types of Mankind,* 68; Nott and Gliddon, *Indigenous Races,* 367, 380.

88. Samuel Cartwright, "Salutary Influences of the Jussieua Grandiflora," in Daniel Drake, *A Systematic Treatise, Historical, Etiological and Practical, on the Principal Diseases of the Interior Valley of North America* (Cincinnati: Winthrop B. Smith and Co., 1850), 82; Cartwright, "Prevention of Yellow Fever," *Ohio Medical and Surgical Journal* 6, no. 1 (1853): 217, 223; Cartwright, "Report on the Diseases and Physical Peculiarities of the Negro Race," *NOMSJ* 7 (May 1851): 691–715, here 700–701; Cartwright, "Ethnology of the Negro or Prognathous Race: A Lecture Delivered Nov. 30, 1857, before the N.O. Academy of Science" (New Orleans: n.p., 1857), 9.

89. Samuel Cartwright, "Negro Freedom an Impossibility under Nature's Laws," *DBR* 30 (May–June 1861): 651; Cartwright, "Ethnology of the Negro," 9, 11.

90. Cartwright, "Ethnology of the Negro," 2–3. See also Chris D. E. Willoughby, "Running Away from Drapetomania: Samuel A. Cartwright, Medicine, and Race in the Antebellum South," *JSH* 84, no. 3 (2018): 579–614.

91. Matthew Estes, *A Defence of Negro Slavery, as It Exists in the United States* (Montgomery: Press of the Alabama Journal, 1846), 49, 154–162, 49–50.

92. Tidyman, "Remarkable Diseases," 311–312.

93. Cartwright, "Ethnology of the Negro," 5, 2–3; "Editorial and Miscellaneous," *NOMNHG* 2, no. 1 (March 1855): 40.

94. John Van Evrie, *Negroes and Negro "Slavery": The First an Inferior Race; the Latter Its Normal Condition* (New York, 1861), 251; Van Evrie, *Anti-Abolition Tracts.—No.1. Abolition and Secession; or, Cause and Effect* (New York: Van Evrie, Horton and Co., 1864), 7; Van Evrie, *Free Negroism: Or, Results of Emancipation in the North and the West India Islands, Etc.* (New York: Van Evrie, Horton and Co., 1862), 6; George M. Fredrickson, *The Black Image in the White Mind: The Debate on Afro-American Character and Destiny, 1817–1914* (New York: Harper & Row, 1971), 92–94.

95. "Yellow Fever and Slavery," *Weekly Delta,* September 25, 1853.

96. Tuckahoe, "Practical Abolitionism and the Yellow Fever," *Weekly Delta,* August 11, 1853; *Weekly Delta,* October 2, 1853.

97. William Harper, "Harper's Memoir on Slavery," in *The Pro-Slavery Argument, as Maintained by the Most Distinguished Writers of the Southern States* (Philadelphia: Lippincott, Grambo, and Co., 1853), 67–77, here 73.

98. Edward Hall Barton, "Climate, Products, and Health, North and South," *DBR* 20, no. 6 (June 1856): 725–726.

99. Barton, "Climate, Products, and Health," 736–740.

100. Barton, "Climate, Products, and Health," 715–740.

6. Incumbent Arrogance

1. Sven Beckert, *Empire of Cotton: A New History of Global Capitalism* (New York: Knopf, 2014), 243; Scott Marler, "'An Abiding Faith in Cotton': The Merchant Capitalist Community of New Orleans, 1860–1862," *Civil War History* 54, no. 3 (September 2008): 248; *Appleton's American Annual Cyclopedia and Register of Important Events of the Year 1862* (New York: D. Appleton and Co., 1865), 113–114; James Henry Hammond, *Speech of Hon. James H. Hammond, of South Carolina, on the Admission of Kansas, under the Lecompton Constitution: Delivered in the Senate of the United States, March 4, 1858* (Washington, DC: L. Towers, 1858).

2. James McPherson, *War on the Waters: The Union and Confederate Navies, 1861–1865* (Chapel Hill: University of North Carolina Press, 2012), chap. 3.

3. Benjamin F. Butler, *Butler's Book: A Review of His Legal, Political, and Military Career* (Boston: A.M. Thayer and Co., 1892), 396–398; "Some Experiences with Yellow Fever and Its Prevention," *North American Review* 147, no. 384 (November 1888): 530; Urmi Engineer Willoughby, *Yellow Fever, Race, and Ecology in Nineteenth-Century New Orleans* (Baton Rouge: LSU Press, 2017), 96–99.

4. Robert F. Wilkinson to William and Mary Wilkinson, December 21, 1862, Robert F. Wilkinson Letters, 1860–1865, N-YHS; Benjamin Butler, "Some Experiences with Yellow Fever and its Prevention," *North American Review* 147, no. 384 (November 1888): 530.

5. William Howard Russell, *My Diary North and South* (Boston: T. O. H. P. Burnham, 1863), 231, entry for May 22, 1862; "Talk on the Flags," *New Orleans Crescent,* May 7, 1862.

6. Eliza Ripley, *Social Life in Old New Orleans: Being Recollections of My Girlhood* (New York; D. Appleton, 1912), 273; Butler, *Butler's Book,* 399; Percy Ashburn, *History of the Medical Department of the United States Army* (New York: Houghton Mifflin, 1929), 68.

7. Butler, *Butler's Book,* 398; Ashburn, *History of the Medical Department,* 68; Butler, "Some Experiences with Yellow Fever and Its Prevention," 529–530.

8. Butler, "Some Experiences with Yellow Fever," 531; "Can It Be Excluded?," *Daily True Delta,* May 11, 1862.

9. Chester G. Hearn, *When the Devil Came Down to Dixie: Ben Butler in New Orleans* (Baton Rouge: LSU Press, 1997), 97–100; "Address of Thomas Overton Moore, Governor of Louisiana, to the Loyal People and True of the City of New Orleans," in Benjamin Butler and Jessie Ames Marshall, *Private and Official Correspondence of Gen. Benjamin F. Butler, during the Period of the Civil War* (Norwood, MA: Plimpton Press, 1917), 1:459–461.

10. Jo Ann Carrigan, "Yankees versus Yellow Jack in New Orleans, 1862–1866," *Civil War History* 9, no. 3 (September 1963): 248–260.

11. Butler, *Butler's Book*, 408–410; James Parton, *General Butler in New Orleans: History of the Administration of the Department of the Gulf in the Year 1862* (New York: Houghton Mifflin, 1862), 605.

12. Thomas A. Anderson to Tinnie Anderson, April 20, 1863, Warren C. Ogden Collection of Civil War Letters, ms. 329, LRC; Ambert Remington to parents, September 7, 1862, Ambert O. Remington Papers, folder 10, ms. 89, LRC.

13. *The Statutes at Large, Treaties, and Proclamations of the United States of America / By Authority of Congress* (Boston: Little, Brown, 1863), 12:597–600; Barbara Brooks Tomblin, *Bluejackets and Contrabands: African Americans and the Union Navy* (Lexington: University Press of Kentucky, 2009), 63–98.

14. "Instructions from the Secretary of the Navy to Flag-Officers regarding Enlistment of Contrabands," April 30, 1862, *ORN*, 23:80–81.

15. The majority of these deaths were likely from malaria. General Order No. 76, July 26, 1863, *ORN*, 25:327–328; John McIlwaine Bell, *Mosquito Soldiers: Malaria, Yellow Fever, and the Course of the Civil War* (Baton Rouge: LSU Press, 2010), 71.

16. "A Negro Military Police for Southern Cities," *Natchez Daily Courier*, May 28, 1862.

17. "The Negro as a Unionist," *Hartford Courant*, May 5, 1862.

18. Butler to Edwin Stanton, May 25, 1862, 1:516–521, here 520, and Butler to J. W. Phelps, July 30, 1862, 2:126, August 2, 1862, 2:143–144 in *Private and Official Correspondence of Gen. Benjamin F. Butler*; General Orders, No. 40, Department of the Gulf, in Joseph T. Wilson, *The Black Phalanx: A History of the Negro Soldiers of the United States in the War of 1775–1812, 1861–65* (Hartford, CT: American Publishing Company, 1888), 119.

19. Henry Halleck to Ulysses S. Grant, March 30, 1863, in *The Papers of Ulysses S. Grant*, ed. John Y. Simon (Carbondale: Southern Illinois University Press, 1979), 8:93n2; "Speech of Judge Ewing," *Weekly News-Democrat* (Emporia, KS), September 6, 1862.

20. Ira Berlin, Joseph P. Reidy, and Leslie S. Rowland, eds., *Freedom's Soldiers: The Black Military Experience in the Civil War* (Cambridge: Cambridge University Press, 1998), 38; Ira Berlin et al., eds., *Freedom: A Documentary History of Emancipation, 1861–1867*, series II (Cambridge: Cambridge University Press, 2010), vol. 1, chap. 15 and doc. 205F; Richard White, *The Republic for Which It Stands: The United States during Reconstruction and the Gilded Age: 1865–1896* (Oxford: Oxford University Press, 2017), 31–35.

21. Interview with Olivier Blanchard, Texas, 16:91, Slave Narratives; Margaret Humphreys, *Intensely Human: The Health of the Black Soldier in the American Civil War* (Baltimore: Johns Hopkins University Press, 2008), 49–50.

22. J. David Hacker, "A Census-Based Count of the Civil War Dead," *Civil War History* 57, no. 4 (December 2011): 307–348, esp. table 8.

23. J. D. B. De Bow, "Desolation in Louisiana.—The Sugar Crop—Labor, &c," *Daily Union and American* (Nashville, TN), May 5, 1866. For economic / agricultural /

environmental consequences of the war, see Judkin Browning and Timothy Silver, *An Environmental History of the Civil War* (Chapel Hill: University of North Carolina Press, 2020), 187–196; James McPherson, *Battle Cry of Freedom: The Civil War Era* (Oxford: Oxford University Press, 2003), 818–819; Erin Stewart Mauldin, *Unredeemed Land: An Environmental History of Civil War and Emancipation in the Cotton South* (Oxford: Oxford University Press, 2019), chap. 2.

24. Gavin Wright, *Old South, New South: Revolutions in the Southern Economy since the Civil War* (New York: Basic Books, 1986), chap 2.

25. Gretchen Long, *Doctoring Freedom: The Politics of African American Medical Care in Slavery and Emancipation* (Chapel Hill: University of North Carolina Press, 2012), 102–103.

26. James N. Gregory, *The Southern Diaspora: How the Great Migrations of Black and White Southerners Transformed America* (Chapel Hill: University of North Carolina Press, 2005), 12–13; Morgan D. Peoples, "'Kansas Fever' in North Louisiana," *LH* 11, no. 2 (Spring 1970): 121–135.

27. E. H. Durell to C., December 25, 1854, Edward H. Durell Papers, N-YHS.

28. Melanie Kiechle, "'Health Is Wealth': Valuing Health in the Nineteenth Century," *Journal of Social History* 54, no. 3 (2021): 775–798.

29. Michael A. Ross, "Resisting the New South: Commercial Crisis and Decline in New Orleans, 1865–85," *American Nineteenth Century History* 4, no. 1 (2003): 61; Richard White, *Railroaded: The Transcontinentals and the Making of Modern America* (New York: W.W. Norton, 2011), chap. 1.

30. Ronald M. Labbé and Jonathan Lurie, *The Slaughterhouse Cases: Regulation, Reconstruction, and the Fourteenth Amendment* (Lawrence: University of Kansas Press, 2003), 53; Dennis Rousey, *Policing the Southern City: New Orleans, 1805–1889* (Baton Rouge: LSU Press, 1996), 114–119.

31. *Report of the Board of Health to the Legislature of the State of Louisiana, January 1867* (New Orleans: J.O. Nixon, 1867), 3–4; "Health of the City," *New Orleans Medical and Surgical Journal* (November 1866): 421; "Editorial: On the Health of the City," *Southern Journal of Medical Science* 1 (August 1866): 395.

32. Bowen quoted from Elisha Harris, "Hygienic Experiences in New Orleans during the War," *Southern Journal of Medical Sciences* 1 (1866): 30; E. D. Fenner, "Remarks on the Sanitary Conditions of the City of New Orleans, during the Period of Federal Military Occupation, from May 1862 to March 1866," *Southern Journal of Medical Sciences* (1866): 23–24.

33. "Longer Quarantine Is Folly," *Daily Picayune*, August 22, 1867; "Health of the City," *Daily Picayune*, August 27, 1867.

34. Jim Downs, *Sick from Freedom: African-American Illness and Suffering during the Civil War and Reconstruction* (Oxford: Oxford University Press, 2012), chaps. 3 and 4.

35. David MacKay to Captain A. B. Armstrong, October 7, 1867, Special Orders, Freedmen's Hospital, New Orleans, roll 1, M1483, 2, NARA; Eric Foner, *Reconstruction:*

America's Unfinished Revolution, 1863–1877 (New York: Harper and Row, 1988), 151–152; Surgeon-in-Chief, September 3, 1867, Records of the Field Offices for the State of Louisiana, Bureau of Refugees, Freedmen, and Abandoned Lands, 1865–1872, roll 11, M1905, 217, NARA.

36. Freedman's Bureau Records, Register of Patients, Medical Department, Freedmen's Bureau, vol. 86, roll 25, target 4, 116–132, NARA; Abstracts of Interments at Freedmen's Cemetery, New Orleans, RG 105, LA, 6–9, NARA.

37. "The Wolf Is In," *Daily Picayune*, August 29, 1867; Stanford Chaillé, "Vital Statistics of New Orleans, from 1769 to 1874," *NOMSJ*, n.s., 2 (July 1874): 13.

38. *New Orleans Bee*, September 22, 1867; *Commercial Reports Received at the Foreign Office from Her Majesty's Consuls in 1869* (London: Harrison and Sons, 1870), 390; "Affairs in the City," *Daily Picayune*, July 20, 1869.

39. Don H. Doykle, *New Men, New Cities, New South: Atlanta, Nashville, Charleston, Mobile, 1860–1910* (Chapel Hill: University of North Carolina Press, 1990), 22–39; Joe Gray Taylor, *Louisiana Reconstructed, 1863–1877* (Baton Rouge: LSU Press, 1974), 318–319; William Cronon, *Nature's Metropolis: Chicago and the Great West* (New York: W.W. Norton, 1991), 298.

40. R. Scott Huffard Jr., *Engines of Redemption: Railroads and the Reconstruction of Capitalism in the New South* (Chapel Hill: University of North Carolina Press, 2019), chap. 4; Ross, "Resisting the New South," 65.

41. David R. Goldfield, "The Urban South: A Regional Framework," *AHR* 86, no. 5 (December 1981): 1015–1016.

42. It took until 1883 for cotton receipts at New Orleans to attain their prewar levels. Wright, *Old South, New South,* 39–42; White, *Railroaded;* Harold D. Woodman, *King Cotton and His Retainers: Financing and Marketing the Cotton Crop of the South 1800–1925* (Washington D.C.: Beard Books, 2000), 271–280; Kenneth Weiher, "The Cotton Industry and Southern Urbanization," *Explorations in Economic History* 4 (1977): 120–140; Foner, *Reconstruction,* 395; "Must We Lose Texas?," *Daily Picayune,* May 18, 1869.

43. Scott Nelson, *Iron Confederacies: Southern Railways, Klan Violence, and Reconstruction* (Chapel Hill: University of North Carolina Press, 1999), 83.

44. *Acts Passed by the General Assembly,* 2 leg., 1 sess., 1866, 198–200; "The Southern El-Dorado," *DBR* 1, no. 3 (March 1866): 254; "Immigration from New England," *New Orleans Daily Crescent,* June 25, 1866.

45. "Emigration to Louisiana," *Harper's Weekly,* September 4, 1869, 563; E. Russ Williams, "Louisiana's Public and Private Immigration Endeavors: 1866–1893," *LH* 15, no. 2 (Spring 1974): 155–158.

46. "Our Vital Statistics," *New-Orleans Times,* June 4, 1874; "Immigration Movements," *New-Orleans Times,* December 17, 1873. For postbellum boosterism, see K. Stephen Prince, *Stories of the South: Race and the Reconstruction of Southern Identity, 1865–1915* (Chapel Hill: University of North Carolina Press, 2014), 110–115.

47. Edward King, *The Great South: A Record of Journeys* (Hartford, 1875), 99, here 314; C. Vann Woodward, *Origins of the New South, 1877–1913* (Baton Rouge: LSU Press, 1951), 114–115.

48. White, *Republic for Which It Stands*, 416. See also Wright, *Old South, New South*, 75–78; Richard Campanella, "An Ethnic Geography of New Orleans," *JAH* 94, no. 3 (December 2007): 707; Elizabeth Fussell, "Constructing New Orleans, Constructing Race: A Population History of New Orleans," *JAH* 94, no. 3 (December 2007): 847–848.

49. John Blassingame, *Black New Orleans, 1860–1880* (Chicago: University of Chicago Press, 1973), 223–225.

50. Interview with Lizzie Chandler in *Mother Wit: The Ex-Slave Narratives of the Louisiana Writers' Project,* ed. Ronnie Clayton (New York: P. Lang, 1990), 43.

51. Steven Hahn, *A Nation under Our Feet: Black Political Struggles in the Rural South, from Slavery to the Great Migration* (Cambridge, MA: Harvard University Press, 2003), 320–334, 341–345; Nell Irvin Painter, *Exodusters: Black Migration to Kansas after Reconstruction* (New York: Norton, 1976), 22–30, 184; James Campbell, *Middle Passages: African American Journeys to Africa, 1787–2005* (New York: Penguin Press, 2006), 107–113.

52. "Wanted Situation," *Daily Picayune,* April 2, 1898; "Wanted," *Daily Picayune,* March 5, 1879; "Help Wanted," *Times Democrat,* June 12, 1887; "Employment Wanted," *Daily Picayune,* July 18, 1872; "Notice to Cotton Factors," *New-Orleans Times,* May 26, 1873.

53. "Yellow Fever Made Contagious by Fear—The Moral Treatment," *Daily Picayune,* October 22, 1888.

54. William H. Holcombe, "Queer Things about Yellow Fever," *Southwestern Christian Advocate,* February 6, 1879; Holcombe, "Characteristics and Capabilities of the Negro Race," *Southern Literary Messenger* 33, no. 6 (December 1861): 402–403.

55. "Testimony by a Louisiana Planter before the Smith-Brady Commission," April 25, 1865, cited in Berlin et al., *Freedom: A Documentary History,* 3:610.

56. For an excellent discussion of the "extinction" hypothesis, see Downs, *Sick from Freedom,* 102–111. "Will the Freed Negro Race at the South Die Out?," *The Liberator,* September 22, 1865.

57. Harvey L. Byrd, "Yellow Fever," *Philadelphia Medical Times and Register* 3, no. 46. (August 1873): 727.

58. Joseph Holt, *History of the Yellow Fever Epidemic in the Fourth District* (New Orleans, 1879); "Our Vital Statistics," *New-Orleans Times,* June 4, 1874.

59. Interviews with Henry C. Pettus, 2: 341, pt. 5; Walter Jones, 2:171, pt. 4; Ellis Jefson, 2:44, pt. 4, Arkansas, Slave Narratives.

60. Moon-Ho Jung, *Coolies and Cane: Race, Labor, and Sugar in the Age of Emancipation* (Baltimore: Johns Hopkins University Press, 2006), 107–180; *The South-Western* (Shreveport, LA), November 15, 1854; Willoughby, *Yellow Fever,* 107. For decline in sugar, see King, *The Great South,* 79–82.

61. *Newberry Weekly Herald* (Newberry, SC), March 7, 1866; De Bow, "Desolation in Louisiana."

62. "How the Experiment Has Worked," *Charleston Daily News,* December 12, 1867; "The Coast Lands of Texas," *Daily Picayune,* December 16, 1866.

63. Warmoth cited in Ted Tunnell, *Crucible of Reconstruction: War, Radicalism, and Race in Louisiana, 1862–1877* (Baton Rouge: LSU Press, 1984). Foner, *Reconstruction,* 379–389; Mark W. Summers, *Railroads, Reconstruction, and the Gospel of Prosperity: Aid under the Radical Republicans* (Princeton, NJ: Princeton University Press, 1984), 14–15.

64. Quoted from Ross, "Resisting the New South," 64. See also Tuffly Ellis, "The New Orleans Cotton Exchange: The Formative Years, 1871–1880," *JSH* 39, no. 4 (November 1973): 545–564; Howard Rabinowitz, *The First New South, 1865–1920* (Charlottesville: University of Virginia Press, 1992), 55, 63.

65. LeeAnna Keith, *The Colfax Massacre: The Untold Story of Black Power, White Terror, and the Death of Reconstruction* (Oxford: Oxford University Press, 2008), 125–150; Leo Pfeffer, *This Honorable Court: A History of the United States Supreme Court* (Boston: Octagon Books, 1965), 200. See also Michael A. Ross, "Justice Miller's Reconstruction: The Slaughter-House Cases, Health Codes, and Civil Rights in New Orleans, 1861–1873," *JSH* 64, no. 4 (November 1998): 949–976; Taylor, *Louisiana Reconstructed,* 191.

66. Labbé and Lurie, *The Slaughterhouse Cases,* 1–11, 40–41, 32.

67. *Slaughter-House Cases,* 83 U.S., 498; White, *Republic for Which It Stands,* 282–284.

68. Richard L. Hume and Jerry B. Gough, *Blacks, Carpetbaggers, and Scalawags: The Constitutional Conventions of Radical Reconstruction* (Baton Rouge: LSU Press, 2008).

69. "Suggestive," *Pickens County Herald and West Alabamian* (Carrolton, AL), September 6, 1871.

70. Eric Foner, *Reconstruction,* 262–263; Lawrence N. Powell, "Reinventing Tradition: Liberty Place, Historical Memory, and Silk Stocking Vigilantism in New Orleans Politics," *Slavery and Abolition* 20 (1999): 127–149; James G. Dauphine, "The Knights of White Camelia and the Election of 1868," *LH* 30 (1989): 173–188; Melissa Meek Hennessey, "Race and Violence in Reconstruction New Orleans: The 1868 Riot," *LH* 20 (1979): 77–92.

71. Stanford Chaillé, *Intimidation and the Number of White and of Colored Voters in Louisiana in 1876* (New Orleans: Picayune Office, 1877), 34.

72. Testimony of J. D. McGill, January 8, 1879, report no. 855, Tensas Parish, in *Louisiana in 1878: Report of the United States Senate Committee to Inquire into Alleged Frauds and Violence in the Elections of 1878* (Washington, DC: US Government Printing Office, 1879), 212–225.

73. *Annual Report of the Board of Health to the General Assembly of Louisiana, December 31, 1869* (New Orleans: n.p., 1870), 7–8; "New Orleans and the Yellow Fever," *Louisiana Democrat* (Alexandria), October 11, 1871.

74. "New Orleans and the Yellow Fever," *Louisiana Democrat* (Alexandria), October 11, 1871. See also Humphreys, *Yellow Fever and the South,* chaps. 3–4; John Ellis, "Businessmen and Public Health in the Urban South during the Nineteenth Century: New Orleans, Memphis, and Atlanta," *BHM* 44, no. 3 (May–June 1970): 197–212, 346–71; David R. Goldfield, "The Business of Health Planning: Disease Prevention in the Old South," *JSH* 42, no. 4 (November 1976): 557–570.

75. "The Penalty of Deception," *New Orleans Republican,* October 18, 1876.

76. Ellen Shields to Michel Musson, August 9, 1878, Degas and Musson Families Papers, box 1, folder 15, ms. 266, LRC.

77. *Congressional Record: Containing the Proceedings and Debates of the Forty-Seventh Congress, First Session* 12 (Washington, DC: US Government Printing Office, 1882), 6897; Ernst von Hesse-Wartegg, *Travels on the Lower Mississippi, 1879–1880: A Memoir,* ed. and trans. Frederic Trautmann (1881; repr., Columbia: University of Missouri Press, 1990), 54, 63.

78. "New Orleans: A Sad State of Affairs," *Chicago Tribune,* August, 20, 1878.

79. "The Prospect," *Morning Star and Catholic Messenger,* October 13, 1878.

80. "Our City's Slanderers," *Daily Picayune,* August, 25, 1878.

81. *An Address from the Auxiliary Sanitary Association of New Orleans, to the Other Cities and Towns in the Mississippi Valley* (New Orleans: L. Graham, 1879), 2–3; Kiechle, "Health Is Wealth," 1–25; John Duffy, *Sanitarians: A History of American Public Health* (Champaign: University of Illinois Press, 1992).

Epilogue

1. Joseph Jones, "Comparative Pathology of Malarial and Yellow Fevers," *Proceedings of the Louisiana State Medical Society* (New Orleans: n.p., 1879), 135–136; Jo Ann Carrigan, *The Saffron Scourge: A History of Yellow Fever in Louisiana, 1796–1905* (Lafayette: University of Louisiana at Lafayette Press, 1994), 132–135; Gustavus B. Thornton, "Memphis Sanitation and Quarantine, 1879 and 1880," in American Public Health Association, *Public Health Papers and Reports,* vol. 6 (December 1880): 198; James O. Breeden, "Joseph Jones and Public Health in the New South," *Louisiana History* 32, no. 4 (Autumn 1991): 365.

2. "The Close of the Quarantine Season," *NOMSJ* 18 (December 1890): 483–484.

3. Michael A. Ross, "Resisting the New South: Commercial Crisis and Decline in New Orleans, 1865–85," *American Nineteenth Century History* 4, no. 1 (2003); Tuffly Ellis, "The New Orleans Cotton Exchange: The Formative Years, 1871–1880," *JSH* 39, no. 4 (November 1973): 561.

4. "The Mississippi versus Chicago," *Daily Picayune,* January 1, 1881; "Our Western Guests," *Daily Picayune,* January 11, 1878; Ernst von Hesse-Wartegg, *Travels on the Lower Mississippi, 1879–1880: A Memoir,* ed. and trans. Frederic Trautmann (Columbia:

University of Missouri Press,1990), 149 (orig. pub. 1881). See also Theophilus Bond and Daniel Arthur Rudd, *From Slavery to Wealth, the Life of Scott Bond: The Rewards of Honesty, Industry, Economy and Perseverance* (Madison, AK: Journal Printing Co., 1917), 361.

5. "Yellow Fever," *St. Joseph Gazette* (Missouri), July 22, 1883. See also Thomas Lathrop Stedman, *Twentieth Century Practice: Tuberculosis, Yellow Fever, and Miscellaneous* (New York: William Wood and Co., 1900), 20: 451; Edmond Souchon, *Educational Points concerning Yellow Fever, to Be Spread Broadcast by the Press, Pulpit, School Teachers and Others, and by All Men of Good Will* (New Orleans: n.p., 1898), 2; John C. McKowen, *Murder as a Money-Making Art: A Social Study* (Baton Rouge: Benton Print, 1901), 41.

6. McKowen, *Murder,* 52.

7. Samuel Freeman Miller to William Pitt Ballinger, June 29, 1879, Samuel Freeman Miller Correspondence, box 2, folder 4, MSS65919, Library of Congress.

8. William Gorgas, *Sanitation in Panama* (New York: D. Appleton, 1915), 25.

9. Algernon Badger to George Y. Badger, October 14, 1897, and November 11, 1897, Algernon Badger Family Papers, ms. 1080, LRC.

10. Carrigan, *Saffron Scourge,* 195–196.

11. For slow-building disasters, see Andy Horowitz, *Katrina: A History, 1915–2015* (Cambridge, MA: Harvard University Press, 2020), 1–18.

12. McKowen, *Murder,* 5.

Acknowledgments

When I started my PhD in 2013, I could not have predicted that my life would be consumed by yellow fever, nor that I would finish this book almost ten years later in a world consumed by another deadly virus. This pandemic has often been isolating. But it has also renewed my deep appreciation for the many wonderful colleagues and loved ones who helped me write this book, offering advice, pulling me back from the edge, making me laugh, and giving the most precious gift of all—time.

Numerous colleagues have read this manuscript in whole or in part or otherwise provided material support. I am grateful to Greg Ablavsky, Nora Barakat, Rabia Belt, Jennifer Burns, Joel Cabrita, Richard Carwadine, Gordon Chang, Nicholas Cole, David Como, Tom Cutterham, Brian DeLay, Jane Dinwoodie, Jeannette Estruth, Paula Findlen, Zephyr Frank, Estelle Freedman, Gary Gerstle, Jay Gitlin, Jeffrey Glover, Lawrence Goldman, Bob Gordon, Annette Gordon-Reed, Fiona Griffiths, Mark Harrison, Mandy Izadi, Sveinn Jóhannesson, Mara Keire, Ari Kelman, Amalia Kessler, Nonie Kubie, Josh Lappen, Ana Minian, Justine Modica, Sharon Ann Murphy, Sarah Pearsall, Bob Proctor, Jack Rakove, Jessica Riskin, Richard Roberts, Aron Rodrigue, Daniel Rowe, Carol Sanger, Priya Satia, Londa Schiebinger, Bruce Schulman, Parth Shil, Matthew Sommer, Amy Dru Stanley, Laura Stokes, Alan Taylor, Peter Thompson, Annie Twitty, Conevery Valenčius, Mikael Wolfe, Gavin Wright, and Ali Yaycioglu. My deepest thanks to you all.

Kären Wigen has offered great historical advice over long walks; walks; the marvelous Allyson Hobbs has the unparalleled ability to make me (and everyone) smile; Caroline Winterer never fails to get into the nuts and bolts of history over wine and cheese in her backyard. My fellow assistant-professor travelers and neighbors Rowan Dorin, Steven Press, and Jonathan Gienapp have earned special thanks. They have all read many (often embarrassingly rough) chapters. Their probing questions , pointed feedback, and excellent friendship were just what the doctor ordered. A few stalwarts read the entire manuscript. I am eternally grateful to James Campbell, Richard White, Seth Rockman, and J. R. Mc-Neill for taking part in my manuscript workshop and for their sharp comments at a crucial stage—this book is infinitely better because of you.

At Stanford, I have been fortunate to work with brilliant students. Erin Wenokur pored through volumes of city council records and offered her insights. Ravi Veriah Jacques read and commented on the entire manuscript, providing characteristically excellent feedback. Alastair Su taught me about capitalism, Paul Nauert deepened my appreciation for environmental history, and Magdalene Zier and Tanner Allread helped me stick (I hope) to the letter of the law.

I have been lucky to find a community of passionate scholars in the history of medicine, race, and disease. Urmi Engineer Willoughby—the doyenne of yellow fever in New Orleans—is a brilliant historian, as are Christopher Willoughby, Wangui Muigai, Eric Herschthal, Melanie Kiechle, Elaine LaFay, Maria Montalvo, Julia Mansfield, Carolyn Roberts, Jonathan Lande, and Mary Hicks. I thank each of them for their intellectual companionship and friendship.

I remain indebted to Pekka Hämäläinen, who continues to be a world-class advisor and cherished friend. Pekka has always pushed me to think bigger and better—and not to discount craft. I owe an unpayable intellectual debt to Katherine Mooney, who has kicked my butt since I was 19 years old, always takes my calls when I need to hammer out a thought, and read through this book multiple times. She is the definition of a good egg. I feel deep appreciation Emily Greenfield, who read, edited, and critiqued this book in full—and got me out of my house for invigorating and laughter-filled walks during the pandemic. Emily did not pull her punches in her criticism and for this I am exceedingly grateful—I will always return the favor.

It is an honor to publish with Kathleen McDermott as my editor. My appreciation extends to the rest of the team at Harvard University Press and to Wendy Nelson and Sherry Gerstein who saved me from numerous infelicities, as well as the anonymous referees who provided feedback on the entire manuscript. They, as well as editors and anonymous reviewers at the American Historical Review helped me to hone key ideas in this book. (Portions of Chapters 3 and 4 were first published as "Immunity, Capital, and Power in Antebellum New Orleans," *American Historical Review* 124, no. 2 [2019]: 424–455.)

Archivists from New Orleans to London to Boston have helped me locate materials and imparted their deep knowledge of collections and manuscripts. Many people in the History Department at Stanford, including Brenda Finkel, Burcak Keskin Kozat, and Maria van Buiten, provided logistical and administrative support without which I would have been lost. At the Stanford Humanities Center, Jenny Martinez arranged a wonderful manuscript workshop in 2020. Special thanks also to my agent, Kathleen Anderson, who saw the potential in this project long before there were words on the page.

Many friends provided me with a bed on research trips and lent an ear. I love and thank you: Bob Jeffrey and Trevor Adley, Tatiana Schlossberg, Parker Mitchell, Maggie Bower, Bright Dickson, Lily Colman Osborn, Alexandra Hughes Browne, Dave Chapin, Sarah Dean, Luke Studebaker and Anna Robinson-Sweet, Jefferson St. John, Thomas Fröhlich and Nikki Shure, Billy Cheringal and Aileen Fernandes, Charlie Warren and Anne Kauth Warren, and Katie Englehart. You have all made this book immeasurably better, and so much more fun to write. So have Sue and Jeff Epstein, who have truly made California feel like home.

My greatest thanks are reserved for my family. The Geylin-Tannis crew—Rosanne, Michael, Rachel, and Kevin—have been fabulous sounding boards. The McAllister-Olivarius clan has provided me with unparalleled support throughout the writing of this book (and indeed my whole life). I'm lucky to have fabulous siblings, the curious and creative Chase Olivarius-McAllister and our resident doctor Jack Olivarius-McAllister. I am also proud to have such a brilliant and courageous mother, Ann Olivarius, as well as an eagle-eyed and imminently patient father, Jef McAllister—a world-class writer and editor who inspired me to be a historian in the first place.

Finally, thank you to the person that makes everything better, Joe Geylin. Joe has read more drafts of this book than I can count and has endured a never-ending recital of gruesome yellow fever stories over dinner. He has done so with a smile on his face. Joe is the best historian I know and has always been there when I needed him most—I could not ask for a better friend and partner.

Index

Note: page numbers in *italics* refer to illustrations; those followed by "n" indicate endnotes